Mark E. Oppenlander
Editor

Neurosurgical Care of Athletes

Springer

Editor
Mark E. Oppenlander
Department of Neurological Surgery
University of Michigan
Ann Arbor, MI
USA

ISBN 978-3-030-88226-6 ISBN 978-3-030-88227-3 (eBook)
https://doi.org/10.1007/978-3-030-88227-3

This Springer imprint is published by the registered company Springer Nature Switzerland AG
The registered company address is: Gewerbestrasse 11, 6330 Cham, Switzerland

Introduction

The impact of sports-related neuro trauma is increasingly recognized, both in the medical literature and in the lay press. Athletes who participate in collision sports are subject to the inherent risks of neuro trauma, including concussion, structural brain injury, spinal cord injury, spinal column fracture, and peripheral nerve injury. While literature exists in each of these individual medical fields, a comprehensive overview of all sports-related neuro trauma is lacking.

This text aims to provide a modern and up-to-date overview of the evaluation and management of sports-related neuro trauma. The primary target audience is the "sports neurosurgeon," who can be found on the sidelines of collision sports at all levels of play from high school to professional, or who may care for these athletes in the acute setting in hospital or the outpatient clinics. The reach of this book, however, will also extend to professionals in other fields of medicine. Indeed, within this text are topics outside the typical neurosurgical specialty, ranging from chiropractic care in the evaluation and treatment of elite athletes to alternative medical therapies for concussion.

The importance of the emerging "sports neurosurgeon" subspecialty is exemplified by the adoption of a policy by the National Football League to require an Unaffiliated Neurotrauma Consultant on-field for player safety. This policy also speaks to the recent public awareness of the importance of recognizing and treating sports-related neuro trauma. This text aims to capitalize on this trend and become a multi-specialty reference to anyone interested in the field.

This text will serve as a comprehensive resource for physicians and researchers involved in sports-related neuro trauma. All chapters are prepared by experts in their fields and include the most up-to-date scientific and clinical information. It is my wish through introduction of this text to provide a summary of the current status of the field, thereby guiding patient management and stimulating investigative efforts.

Mark E. Oppenlander
Department of Neurological Surgery
University of Michigan
Ann Arbor, MI, USA

Contents

Contributors

Hussam Abou-Al-Shaar Department of Neurological Surgery, University of Pittsburgh Medical Center, Pittsburgh, PA, USA

Tim Adamson Carolina Neurosurgery & Spine Associates, Charlotte, NC, USA

Arjang Ahmadpour Department of Neurosurgery, University of Chicago Medical Center, Chicago, IL, USA

Andrea Almeida University of Michigan-Flint, Flint, MI, USA

Bara Alsalaheen University of Michigan-Flint, Flint, MI, USA

Julian E. Bailes Department of Neurosurgery, North Shore Hospital, Evanston, IL, USA

Daniel L. Barrow Emory University, Atlanta, GA, USA

Christopher M. Bonfield Vanderbilt Department of Neurosurgery, Vanderbilt University Medical Center, Nashville, TN, USA

Daipayan Guha Department of Neurological Surgery, University of Pittsburgh Medical Center, Pittsburgh, PA, USA

Nicholas F. Hug Department of Neurosurgery, Stanford University, Stanford, CA, USA

Megan M. Jack Neurological Surgery, Mayo Clinic, Rochester, MI, USA

Michael Jensen Department of Neurosurgery, Stanford University, Stanford, CA, USA

Soren Jonzzon Vanderbilt Department of Neurosurgery, Vanderbilt University Medical Center, Nashville, TN, USA

Jacob R. Joseph Department of Neurosurgery, University of Michigan, Ann Arbor, MI, USA

Allan D. Levi Department of Neurosurgery, University of Miami Miller School of Medicine, Miami, FL, USA

Matthew T. Lorincz University of Michigan, Michigan NeuroSport, Ann Arbor, MI, USA

Gordon Mao Department of Neurosurgery, Johns Hopkins University School of Medicine, Baltimore, MD, USA

Joseph C. Maroon Department of Neurological Surgery, University of Pittsburgh Medical Center, Pittsburgh, PA, USA

Mansour Mathkour Department of Neurosurgery, Tulane Medical Center, New Orleans, LA, USA

Vincent J. Miele Department of Neurological Surgery, University of Pittsburgh Medical Center, Pittsburgh, PA, USA

Michael A. Miller Palmer College of Chiropractic, Professional Football Chiropractic Society Hall of Fame, Norwood, MA, USA

Steve Monk Atrium Health Carolinas Medical Center, Department of Neurosurgery, Charlotte, NC, USA

Christian Mustroph Emory University, Atlanta, GA, USA

David O. Okonkwo UPMC/University of Pittsburgh, Department of Neurological Surgery, Pittsburgh, PA, USA

Vimal Patel Department of Neurosurgery, North Shore Hospital, Evanston, IL, USA

Aneek Patel Department of Neurosurgery, New York University School of Medicine, New York, NY, USA

David Peters Atrium Health Carolinas Medical Center, Department of Neurosurgery, Charlotte, NC, USA

David A. Purger Department of Neurosurgery, Stanford University, Stanford, CA, USA

Gerald Rodts Emory University, Atlanta, GA, USA

Katharine Seagly University of Michigan, Traumatic Brain Injury Rehabilitation Program, Ann Arbor, MI, USA

Allen K. Sills Vanderbilt Department of Neurosurgery, Vanderbilt University Medical Center, Nashville, TN, USA

Brandon W. Smith Neurological Surgery, Mayo Clinic, Rochester, MI, USA

Robert J. Spinner Neurological Surgery, Mayo Clinic, Rochester, MI, USA

William J. Steele III Department of Neurosurgery, University of Miami Miller School of Medicine, Miami, FL, USA

Frank A. De Stefano School of Medicine, Kansas City University, Kansas City, MO, USA

Alan R. Tang Vanderbilt Department of Neurosurgery, Vanderbilt University Medical Center, Nashville, TN, USA

Nicholas Theodore Department of Neurosurgery, Johns Hopkins University School of Medicine, Baltimore, MD, USA

Valentina Vasenina Department of Neurosurgery, University of Chicago Medical Center, Chicago, IL, USA

Ayobami L. Ward Department of Neurosurgery, University of Michigan, Ann Arbor, MI, USA

Thomas J. Wilson Department of Neurosurgery, Stanford University, Stanford, CA, USA

Aaron M. Yengo-Kahn Vanderbilt Department of Neurosurgery, Vanderbilt University Medical Center, Nashville, TN, USA

Khaled J. Zaza Department of Anesthesiology and Perioperative Medicine, University of Pittsburgh Medical Center, Pittsburgh, PA, USA

Scott L. Zuckerman Vanderbilt Department of Neurosurgery, Vanderbilt University Medical Center, Nashville, TN, USA

Chapter 1
Pre-Participation Screening for the Sports Neurosurgeon

Soren Jonzzon, Aaron M. Yengo-Kahn, Christopher M. Bonfield, Allen K. Sills, and Scott L. Zuckerman

Role of the Neurosurgeon in Sports

The number of neurosurgeons serving in roles as team-affiliated physicians is expanding. In recent decades, several prominent sports neurosurgeons have paved the way for future involvement (Table 1.1). While coaches, parents, and certified athletic trainers (AT) can manage many of the common injuries, having a neurosurgeon involved in athlete management can add additional expertise and perspective while also facilitating the care of more catastrophic injuries. Examples of catastrophic injuries include cranial or spinal fractures and brain or spinal cord injuries resulting in severe disability. While these types of sports injuries are rare, they often have life-changing implications. Amongst youth, collegiate and professional football between 1947 and 1999, there were 497 brain-injury related deaths, which is potentially an underestimation [1]. Additionally, 200 high school and collegiate football players suffered permanent cervical spinal cord injuries and 66 suffered permanent brain injuries during a 21 year window from 1977–1998 [2]. Neurosurgeons manage these catastrophic injuries routinely, and can seamlessly transfer their experience to provide care for the same injuries in athletes.

S. Jonzzon · A. M. Yengo-Kahn · C. M. Bonfield · A. K. Sills · S. L. Zuckerman (✉)
Vanderbilt Department of Neurosurgery, Vanderbilt University Medical Center, Nashville, TN, USA
e-mail: Soren.jonzzon@vumc.org; A.yengo@vumc.org; Chris.bonfield@vumc.org; Allen.sills@vumc.org

M. E. Oppenlander (ed.), *Neurosurgical Care of Athletes*,
https://doi.org/10.1007/978-3-030-88227-3_1

Table 1.1 Prominent neurosurgeons in sports

Dr. Richard C. Schneider	Dr. Richard C. Schneider, largely considered the father of sports neurosurgery, was a collegiate swimmer and lacrosse player who would go on to be chair of the University of Michigan Neurological Surgery Department. During his career, he provided major contributions to neurosurgery as well as athletics. He would go on to describe anterior cord syndrome, clarify central cord syndrome, as well as deepen our understanding of teardrop fractures and second-impact syndrome [56–62]. He started a laboratory to model head and neck injury and was intimately involved in the development of modern-day football helmets with his work guiding major rule changes to improve player safety [63–65]
Dr. Robert C. Cantu	Dr. Robert C. Cantu trained at mass general hospital and would later serve as the team physician for a local high school, which sparked his interest in minor head injuries. He served as the first chairman of American Association of Neurological Surgeons (AANS) section on sports medicine. His work includes one of the first attempts to standardize sport-related concussion (SRC) management through a grading system with return-to-play guidelines, and everlasting emphasis on the importance of recovery in avoiding complications of SRC, including second impact syndrome [62, 66]. He remains the head of several sports injury registries and serves as a consultant to the National Football League (NFL) [63]
Dr. Joseph C. Maroon	Dr. Joseph C. Maroon was a collegiate American football player and trained at the University of Indiana. He served as a local advisor for sports teams and ultimately as the Pittsburgh Steelers' team neurosurgeon. He was the second chair of the AANS section on sports medicine. He helped to develop the immediate post-concussion assessment and cognitive test (ImPACT), one of the first, and most frequently utilized, computerized neurocognitive testing system [67, 68]. This information provided insight into the timeline of recovery. Computerized neurocognitive testing is now often considered an essential component of the return-to-play process at all levels of sports [63]. Additionally, he has published on post-concussion syndrome and possible non-pharmacological treatments [69]
Dr. Julian E. Bailes	Dr. Julian E. Bailes was an All-State high school American football player in Louisiana before playing in college at Northwestern State. He trained at Louisiana State University and would go on to be the fourth AANS Section on Sports Medicine Chair. He coedited a book *Neurological Sports Medicine: A guide for Physicians and Trainers* [70]. He also made significant contributions to rule changes made in football to improve player safety including return-to-play guidelines in spinal cord injury and delineated the risks of heatstroke in athletes [63, 71–73]. Dr. Bailes is on the forefront of chronic traumatic encephalopathy (CTE) research and was involved in the highly publicized early case reports of CTE [74, 75]. His work in this domain led to his portrayal as a leading character in the movie *Concussion*, which outlined his work and contributions to the field. His impact has extended beyond just football to other sports such as boxing where he has contributed to ringside evaluation, analyzing when to halt a match for safety concerns, and delineated the role of the neurosurgeon for the sport [76–78]
Dr. Allen K. Sills	In 2020, the Chief Medical Officer (CMO) of the NFL is also a neurosurgeon, Dr. Allen K. Sills. Dr. Sills began his career working with the Memphis Grizzlies, Mississippi State Athletics, Vanderbilt University Athletics, Southeastern Conference Sports, and the Nashville Predators. Dr. Sills has focused his leadership on sport-related concussion (SRC) and the ongoing Coronavirus pandemic

The multi-disciplinary care of athletes is an evolving area of medicine, and many healthcare practitioners provide high-level care to athletes. Orthopedic surgeons represent the classic team physician, provide an invaluable service with regards to managing musculoskeletal injuries, and often lead the medical care of athletes; however, brain injuries may be outside the scope of their training. Additional members of the sports medicine team include internists, emergency medicine doctors, oral surgeons, ophthalmologists, plastic surgeons, chiropractors, and sometimes neurologists. Furthermore, experienced nurse practitioners and physician's assistants that specialize in sports medicine can be vital members of the team [3]. Importantly, certified ATs are some of the most vital members of the sports medicine team, especially at lower levels of play, where physicians are less present. ATs have invaluable knowledge of the team and their players and are often with the team daily. A prerequisite to success for any team physician is a close relationship with the team's AT.

Though the focus of this chapter is on pre-participation screening, it should be briefly noted that neurosurgeons can participate in sports through a variety of mechanisms. Additional areas of involvement include: event coverage to assess and manage acute brain and spine injuries, development and implementation of a concussion plan including return to play protocols, education within the community for other physicians, coaches, athletes, schools and/or parents, as well as participation in regulatory agencies to support these stakeholders.

Epidemiology of Sport-Related Concussion and Catastrophic Neurologic Injuries

Given the breadth of sports that require pre-participation screening, a brief discussion of the epidemiology surrounding sport-related concussion (SRC) and catastrophic injuries is helpful in contextualizing the landscape of neurologic injuries in sports. Though professional athletes receive significant attention, the majority of the burden of injury falls amongst youth and high school athletes. Moreover, resources for medical care at these lower levels are often sparse compared to the professional level.

SRC and mild traumatic brain injury (mTBI) are significant contributors to rates of injury, particularly in contact sports. It is estimated that there are between 1.6 and 3.8 million SRCs annually in the United States, which represents 5–9% of all sports injuries [4]. Additionally, this number is widely considered underreported as concussions may either go undiagnosed or an athlete may downplay symptoms, so they may continue to participate. Catastrophic neurologic injuries, defined as a severe injury to the brain or spine, are not common occurrences yet require typically emergency care and attention. Examples of these injuries include: subarachnoid hemorrhage (SAH), epidural hemorrhage (EDH), subdural hemorrhage (SDH), intraparenchymal hemorrhage (IPH), diffuse cerebral edema (DCE), and diffuse axonal injury (DAI). In a 26 year window amongst middle school and high school athletes of various sports, 980 individuals or 0.6 per 100,000 participants suffered a catastrophic injury [5]. Of note, 635 of those individuals were football players with a rate of 1.78 per 100,000 participants [5]. In high school sports, the average rate of catastrophic injury is 0.6 per 100,000 participants per year, which correlates with 37.7 catastrophic injuries per year in the U.S. Though rare, the presence of catastrophic injuries in sports of all levels allows neurosurgeons to play an important role in acutely managing these injuries, as well as to participate in the return to play process.

Pre-Participation Screening

Pre-participation screening includes a focused neurologic history with an in-depth concussion history and consideration of baseline cognitive, balance, and symptom assessments. Most scholastic-based sports require some type of preparticipation screening process, where neurosurgeons can play an important role. Much of this process is done by the athlete's pediatrician or primary care physician, yet neurosurgeons' expertise can help with complex patients with those with prior neurological conditions.

What Sports Require Screening?

Sports are often categorized into contact and non-contact sports, and contact level has major implications for subsequent brain and spine injury risk. The American Academy of Pediatrics has released analyses of medical conditions affecting sports conditions. Historically, the academy has defined sports into 3 categories of contact: contact, limited-contact, and noncontact. We have slightly modified these categorizations to differentiate collision sports that confer a higher risk of catastrophic injury (Table 1.2) [6, 7]. Based on this modified classification, collision sports includes sports with frequent and potentially high velocity player-player contact such as football and hockey, while contact sports include soccer and basketball. Limited contact sports include baseball, volleyball, and horseback riding while noncontact sports include golf, swimming, tennis, amongst others.

All sports require screening. Typically, SRC screening focuses on collision sports that are often most popular, such as football, soccer, hockey, and basketball; however, the impact of SRC extends far beyond these common sports. Amongst collegiate athletes, rates of concussion were highest among wrestlers, occurring

Table 1.2 Classification of sport

Collision	Contact and Collision	Limited Contact	Noncontact
Boxing Football (tackle) Ice hockey Lacrosse (men's) Martial arts Rodeo Rugby Wrestling	Basketball Diving Field hockey Lacrosse (women's) Ski jumping Soccer Team handball Water polo	Baseball/softball Bicycling Cheerleading Canoeing/kayaking (white water) Fencing Field events Floor hockey Football (flag) Gymnastics Handball Horseback riding Racquetball Skating Skiing[a] Skateboarding[a] Snowboarding[a] Squash Surfing (water/wind) Ultimate Frisbee Volleyball	Archery Badminton Body building Bowling Canoeing/kayaking (flat water) Crew or rowing Curling Dancing Track and Field Golf Weightlifting Race walking Riflery Rope jumping Running Sailing Scuba diving Swimming Table tennis Tennis Track Weightlifting

[a]It should be noted that these "extreme sports" require helmets and have a higher risk for severe injuries, though they are limited contact
Adapted from two sources: [6, 79]

almost 11 times per 10,000 athletic events [8]. Though American football bears the highest SRC rate across all high school sports, it ranks 13th amongst National Collegiate Athletic Association (NCAA) sports in recurrent concussions, which are often the source of long-term symptoms and delayed return to school and play [8, 9]. Other NCAA sports such as men's ice hockey, women's field hockey, men's basketball, and women's soccer all had higher rates of repeat concussions in a study from 2009–2014 [8].

With respect to SRC, mechanisms of injury vary significantly between sports. In contact and collision sports, the most common injury is player-player contact, but many injuries seen in limited contact and noncontact sports such as baseball, swimming, gymnastics, and tennis are a product of player-surface or contact with equipment during competition [8]. Additionally, SRC are not limited to team sports. For example, many head injuries suffered during equestrian sports are severe and represent a significant health burden that should not be overlooked [10].

Neurological History

Knowing a patient's neurological history can assist medical decision-making, clearance, and return to play [11]. Often times, the historical information used in the decision-making process is based on subtle differences and clarifications that may not be elicited by individuals who are not aware of those subtleties. Important aspects of the neurological history for an athlete include:

- *Any major brain or spine injuries*: Any type of severe cranial trauma or spine trauma related to sports or any other accidents such as motor vehicle collisions must be identified.
- *Concussion history:* Quantification and qualification of this history is essential. The athlete's number of prior concussions, approximate time missed for the concussion, and severity of symptoms must be delineated. It is important to be holistic and not focus solely on the athletic impact. Concussions can affect school, relationships, and psychologic status. These can also serve as adjuncts to assess for severity of concussion in patients unable to recall specific symptoms [11].
- *Seizure history*: Athlete's seizure history is important to document as patients who have TBI are at an increased risk of having seizures. Having a baseline seizure disorder including febrile seizures are important as they may suggest an increased likelihood of seizure in the setting of concussion or TBI [12].
- *Headache history*: Knowing an athlete's headache status is important for symptomatic management. Understanding the specifics of headache type, frequency and quality are critical for evaluation of post-injury headaches. A poor understanding of baseline headache history can lead to an athlete returning to play too soon or being held out of competition longer than is necessary. Additionally, athletes who have conditions such as headache are more likely to develop post-concussion syndrome [11].
- *Psychiatry conditions/medications*: Athletes who have a psychiatric condition or are on any type of mood-altering drug should be thoroughly assessed. This gives a baseline symptom and medication requirement that can be used for comparison in post injury management. Additionally, athletes with a family or personal history of psychiatric conditions are more than 5 times as likely to develop post-concussion symptoms [13].
- *History of learning disability*: Athletes with learning disabilities including attention deficit hyperactivity disorder (ADHD), as well as those who need special education, and/or require repetition of grades may demonstrate higher rates of concussion, lower baseline neurocognitive test scores, more baseline and post-concussion symptoms and/or prolonged recovery [13–18].
- *Hydrocephalus or shunt device*: Athletes having a history of these conditions are more complex medically in the setting of injury and symptomatic presentation from their baseline condition may overlap with concussion symptoms [12, 19].
- *Family history of medical conditions*: First degree family histories of headache, epilepsy, and psychiatric conditions are of critical importance as athletes in

youth sports may have a predisposition or undiagnosed condition given varying age of onset of different conditions. The family history may provide a way to screen for development of these baseline conditions that can affect post-concussion assessment [13].

It is incredibly important to be specific in assessing all these aspects of the athlete's history. Often, asking a blanket question regarding an athlete's neurological history may lead to missed or incorrect information, most often due to simple misunderstanding of what is important to mention. Athletes tend to focus more on their history of musculoskeletal injury and may minimize their prior neurologic issues due to the perception of lack of severity or minimal missed time from sport. Young, high performing athletes may simply deny any past medical history when asked broadly, but detailed inquiry about missed games or practices may reveal a variety of injuries that were not mentioned in the first response. For example, asking if they have ever missed any games for any reason will be higher yield than simply asking if they have ever had any injuries. Additionally, direct questioning such as, *"Have you ever had or been diagnosed with a concussion?"* will provide better information than asking if they have any general medical problems. It is important to assess patient understanding of medications that they may take. For example, if a patient takes an antiseizure medication, it is important to ask if they understand why they take that medication.

Baseline Testing

In addition to a complete history and exam, athletes often require baseline cognitive assessment, balance assessment, visual assessment, and baseline symptom inventory. With respect to SRC, many school systems obtain annual or biannual baseline neurologic screening – a battery of neurologic and/or neurocognitive tests – prior to initiation of competition, in order for athletes who suffer a SRC to be compared to their own performance, rather than normative values. The most commonly used cognitive assessment is the computerized ImPACT battery, which provides objective measures of memory, attention, visual, and verbal problem solving [20]. Balance is typically tested using the modified Balance Error Scoring System (mBESS), which measures balance loss during 3 different poses [21]. The Sport Concussion Assessment Tool (SCAT) combines a neurologic screening, cognitive assessment, balance evaluation and the Post-Concussion Symptom Scale (PCSS) into a single efficient and comprehensive evaluation either on the field or in the clinic [22]. Baseline measures are often obtained by a neuropsychologist or AT, and though the neurosurgeon is not the one performing these tests, every sports neurosurgeon should be familiar with all baseline tests given their relevance in the post-concussion testing. These tests may be administered in an office individually or in a team/group setting at the beginning of the season.

Screening for Specific Cranial and Spinal Conditions

While there are many factors that determine the safety of an athlete's participation in sport, studies looking at various cranial or spinal conditions and their safety profile for participation have been published in an attempt to guide providers. Unfortunately, much of the prior literature consists of summative reviews rather than primary data. Some of the most relevant studies on cranial and spinal conditions are summarized for in Tables 1.3 and 1.4, respectively. Though neurosurgeons involved in these complex decisions would appreciate all-encompassing guidelines, most studies suggest that each athlete must be considered on a case-to-case basis given the complexity of a neurological patient, the athlete's desired long-term goals, level of competition, and type of sport (contact, limited-contact, non-contact). Below, we aim to provide guidance for individual conditions based on the available literature. While each one of these conditions could be the subject of a single chapter, we briefly summarize some of the relevant studies and present the most up-to-date recommendations regarding commonly encountered neurologic conditions.

Table 1.3 Cranial conditions

Condition	Author, year	Synopsis
Arachnoid cyst	Zaben et al. 2020 [19]	Survey of pediatric neurosurgeons in the UK All respondents allow participation in soccer 91.2%, 55.9%, and 53% allow participation in skiing, rugby, and taekwondo respectively
	Strahle et al. 2016 [23]	112 patients who played a variety of sports No patients with permanent neurological injury or injury requiring treatment by surgical intervention Two patients with subdural hygroma Safe to participate
	Miele et al. 2006 [12]	Expert commentary Possible increased risk of bleeding but not proven Recommend risk-benefit discussions with patient/family Not an absolute contraindication to play
Brain tumor	Stanuszek et al. 2020 [26]	42 patients 6–18 years with brain tumors 71.4% safely returned to contact sports, but not collision sports Predictors of not returning to play included worse WHO grade, tumor location, neurological deficit, hydrocephalus, and additional oncological treatment
	Davis et al. 2009 [25]	Expert commentary on an athlete with a tectal glioma and an athlete with a frontal meningioma Cleared to compete in contact sports if no neurological deficit and complete bony fusion after craniotomy One expert felt presence of a cyst should restrict athlete

Table 1.3 (continued)

Condition	Author, year	Synopsis
Cavum septum pellucidum	Gardner et al. 2016 [80]	Case matched study of 17 retired professional football players Increased prevalence and severity of cavum septum pellucidum No known clinical significance
	Miele et al. 2006 [12]	Expert summary Often result of trauma and not clinically relevant Isolated disease should not preclude participation
Chiari malformation	Zaben et al. 2020 [19]	Survey of pediatric neurosurgeons in the UK Paucity of evidence regarding Chiari and CSF obstruction Most decisions made based on personal experience of the physician
	Strahle et al. 2016 [28]	328 patients with a mean age of 10.7 with Chiari I malformation (CM-I) playing a variety of sports No increase catastrophic injuries Safe to participate in sports
	Meehan et al. 2015 [27]	147 patients ages 11–19 with diagnosed Chiari malformation playing a variety of sports No increase catastrophic injuries Case-by-case decision
	Harrell et al. 2010 [81]	Case report CM-I safe to participate in sport unless there is: Syringomyelia, obliteration of subarachnoid space, indention of anterior medulla, symptoms thought to be related to CSF flow
	Miele et al. 2006 [12]	Expert summary Syringomyelia, obliteration of the subarachnoid space, indentation of the anterior medulla, or symptomatic disease are contraindications for participation in sport Against participation if CM-I is diagnosed during concussion diagnosis/evaluation
	Callaway et al. 1996 [82]	Case report and expert consensus on CM-I causing functional spinal stenosis Syringomyelia, obliteration of the arachnoid space, or indentation of the anterior medulla are contraindications for contact sports
Previous craniotomy	Laker, 2011 [29]	Expert summary Precludes sport participation for 1 year Later participation should be evaluated by a multi-specialty team
	Miele et al. 2006 [12]	Expert summary Three concerns of previous craniotomy are bone flap weakness, fragility of underlying tissue, and possible CSF flow abnormalities None of these permanently preclude participation

(continued)

Table 1.3 (continued)

Condition	Author, year	Synopsis
Seizures	Capovilla et al. 2016 [32]	ILAE task force statement Benefit of seizure control in physical activity and sports participation exceeds the risk of participation Sports tiered by risk factors Consider seizure type, frequency, triggers, timing, and patient/family attitude towards possible risk
	Stanuszek et al. 2015 [83]	407 children hospitalized for seizure 3.4% associated with physical exertion or sport
	Pinikahana et al. 2009 [31]	225 patients with epilepsy 16.4% cited physical exercise as a provoking factor
	Miele et al. 2006 [12]	Expert summary Potential risks associated with participation are outweighed by the benefit of participation in other aspects of health No restriction to participation Caution should be taken with sports involving risk of fall especially from height
	Nakken et al. 2005 [30]	1677 pediatric patients in multiple cohorts 0.3–6.0& cite physical activity as a provoking factor
	Sahoo et al. 2004 [84]	Expert summary Risks of sports are outweighed by the seizure control benefits of exercise Case-by-case evaluation of athletes
	Frucht et al. 2000 [85]	400 epilepsy patients 0.5% cite physical activity as a provoking factor
Shunt	Zaben et al. 2020 [19]	Survey of pediatric neurosurgeons in the UK Paucity of evidence regarding CSF flow and sport participation Most decisions made based on personal experience
	Miele et al. 2006 [12]	Expert summary Low complication rate Most common are shunt dysfunction or fracture Most neurosurgeons do not prohibit noncontact sports, but most restrict contact sports
	Blount et al. 2004 [33]	Survey of 92 pediatric neurosurgeons >75% of physicians had not seen sport-related complication of shunt Shunt dysfunction or fracture were most common No evidence to suggest that restriction from sport is necessary
Vascular lesions	Sousa Nanji et al. 2015 [86]	738 cases of SAH 57.5% of cases were associated with physical activity 1.2% of cases were associated with sports, 1 sport related trauma Sport induced SAH is uncommon and has milder presentation
	Davis et al. 2009 [35]	Expert commentary on cavernoma No strong evidence for or against participation An incidental, asymptomatic cavernoma clear for participation

Table 1.4 Clearance and RTP in athletes with cervical spine pathology

Author, year	Synopsis
Richards et al. 2020 [87]	73 golf/tennis/swimming athletes with cervical spine surgery Median (range) age 69 (33–90); older athlete population ACDF 63%; 19% cervical laminectomy; 18% cervical laminectomy/fusion 81% returned to preoperative sport practice; 68% returned to golf; 31% returned to tennis; 82% returned to swimming
Schroeder et al. 2020 [44]	Modified Delphi consensus among cervical spine surgeons 1–2 level ACDF appropriate for RTP; not for 3-level ACDF Asymptomatic athletes with cervical stenosis OK for play (canal >10 mm 90.5%; resolved MRI findings >13 mm 81.3%)
Kang et al. 2016 [43]	Review concluding that 1-level ACDF can safely return to play No consensus regarding 2–3 level ACDF; most studies say contraindication to RTP Poor consensus on other cervical procedures
Molinari et al. 2016 [88]	Review of 9 studies, 175 patients 1-level ACDF appropriate for RTP; controversy over all else 6 months is appropriate time for RTP after fusion-procedure
Tempel et al. 2015 [89]	5 professional athletes with T2 hyperintensity on MRI after spinal cord contusion 4/5 underwent ACDF; 1 nonoperative Signal change was NOT a contraindication if no symptoms The 2 athletes that have RTP have had no sequelae
Maroon et al. 2013 [42]	15 pro athletes underwent 1-level ACDF (7 football; 8 wrestlers) Transient neuropraxia most common presentation 13/15 athletes RTP between 2–12 months

Cranial Conditions

Arachnoid Cyst

In a study of 112 athletes with arachnoid cyst, there were no subjects who suffered permanent neurological injury, and complication rates related to sports were very low [23]. In an expert commentary by Miele et al. the authors consider the theoretical increased risk of subdural or intra-cyst hemorrhage, but there is no clinical evidence to support these concerns presently as reasons to limit sport participation [12]. However, a survey of UK neurosurgeons showed that there are inconsistencies between providers and the sport in question [19]. The authors of this chapter feel that at this point in time, there are no absolute contraindications for patient with arachnoid cysts to participate in sport, unless there is history of a prior cyst-related hemorrhage. However, parents and athletes should be counseled appropriately [24].

Brain Tumor

While brain tumors encompass a wide variety of pathologies and symptomatic features, Davis et al. showed that some experts believe athletes should be allowed to play if they do not have any neurological deficit or high-risk feature for sudden decompensation as a result of their tumor [25]. Additionally, it has been shown that athletes with tumors have safely returned to play, but predictors of their ability to participate include WHO grade, tumor location, neurological deficit, adjuvant oncological treatment and the presence of hydrocephalus [26]. Other considerations such as clearance for participation after undergoing craniotomy for resection are discussed in subsequent sections.

Chiari Malformation

Studies by Meehan et al. and Strahle et al. have shown that the risk of catastrophic injury in athletes with Chiari malformation is quite low, and report 0 cases in their studies [27, 28]. Additionally, an expert consensus by Miele et al. and a survey amongst pediatric surgeons by Zaben et al. show that it is typically safe for these athletes to participate, as long as they don't have high risk features including syringomyelia, obliteration of subarachnoid space, indentation of the anterior medulla, or symptoms thought to be related to changes in CSF flow [12, 19]. The presence of a syrinx or brainstem/spinal cord compression are contraindications to participation in sports, as these patients likely require surgery. Anecdotally, many providers would allow return to sports participation after successful Chiari malformation decompression, after full recovery and resolution of pre-operative symptoms, syrinx, and brainstem compression. Our practice throughout the last decade reflects this management approach.

Previous Craniotomy

Experts have suggested that athletes who have had a craniotomy for any type of pathology should wait at least 1 year prior to returning to competition, to allow fusion of the bone flap, especially those participating in contact sports [12, 29]. Previous concerns included the possibility of flap weakness, fragility of underlying tissue, or changes in CSF flow after operation [12, 29]. While a craniotomy itself does not prohibit participation, it is important to assess the athlete in the setting of their underlying pathology as well. Previously treated and resolved pathology should not impede sport participation (benign brain tumor, resolved aneurysm with no rupture); however, unresolved conditions requiring further treatment should be considered cautiously (subtotal resection, etc.).

Seizure

While the rates of epileptic seizures being provoked by physical activity vary greatly, ranging from 0.3–16% of all seizures, the consensus is that the benefit of sport participation from a seizure control standpoint and other comorbidities strongly outweigh the risk of seizure provocation [30, 31]. In a task force statement by the International League Against Epilepsy (ILAE) on Sports and Epilepsy, the authors recommend that individuals should not be restricted from athletic competition due to seizures [32]. However, careful consideration should be given to seizure type, specifically drop-attacks and those involving loss of consciousness, especially for sports involving heights. A neurologist's input for these patients can also be very helpful.

Shunt

In three studies surveying pediatric neurosurgeons on their experience treating sport-related shunt complications, the overwhelming majority have seen very low rates of sport-related shunt complications [12, 19, 33]. In a survey of 92 pediatric neurosurgery providers, 77% had never observed a sport-related shunt complication, and the remaining 23% treated a total of 25–30 complications. The most common complications were broken shunt catheters or shunt dysfunction, with only one acute intracranial hematoma observed. The authors concluded that the incidence of sport-related shunt complications in children was significantly less than 1%. Moreover, 90% of pediatric neurosurgeons did not restrict their patients' participation in non-contact sports, and for contact sports, 33% recommend no participation, 33% decided on a case-by-case and sport basis, and 33% allowed contact sport play. Given the low frequency and severity of complications, we believe that patients with VP shunts should be allowed to participate in athletic competition, though counseling should be offered about high-contact and collision sports that may create hardware disruption [12, 19, 33].

Vascular Lesions

Vascular lesions include a variety of conditions such as aneurysms, arteriovenous malformations (AVMs), and cavernomas. Routine screening for vascular lesions in athletes is not done. Incidental aneurysms should be evaluated and treated accordingly. Our anecdotal approach to incidentally found aneurysms is that if the aneurysm does not need to be treated based on the surgeon's assessment or rupture risk (though this is rare in a young person), the athlete can play with the understanding that the athlete may be at an increased risk compared to an athlete without an aneurysm. If the aneurysm does require treatment, and is successfully treated, the athlete can play after full recovery. For large AVMs, we would likely recommend against intense physical activity, but for other, smaller lesions, we recommend treatment on a case-by-case method, depending no sport, location, and size of the AVM. Like aneurysms, if fully treated, RTP after a full recovery is allowed. An 18-year-old football player suffered an AVM rupture during exercise, received radiosurgery, and successfully returned to play [34]. For cavernomas, Davis et al. provided an expert commentary stating that if a patient has an asymptomatic, incidentally found cavernoma, they should be able to participate in athletic competition [35].

Spinal Conditions

Spine pathology requiring screening includes congenital conditions, previous trauma, and postoperative clearance. Below we have broken down spine clearance by specific pathology, yet many reports focus on postoperative RTP. According to patient experiences from 98 neurosurgeons who operated on athletes, Saigal et al. [36] reported that 72% of patients with spinal instrumentation returned to sport, whereas 28% did not, and nearly all (97%) of patients that underwent uninstrumented spine procedures returned to sport. Football was the primary sport in 55% of cases. Similar percentages of pediatric (82%) and adult (92%) patients were allowed to RTP. The most controversial area regarding clearance of spinal conditions deals with the cervical spine, and relevant studies have been succinctly summarized in Table 1.4. Below we elaborate on specific preexisting and postoperative conditions.

Cervical Stenosis

Cervical stenosis, with or without an episode of neuropraxia, is perhaps the biggest controversy regarding spine clearance in athletes. The major decision point is stenosis with or without a symptomatic episode (most often transient quadriparesis), as symptoms usually unmask the previously unknown stenosis. Davis et al. [37] highlighted both these scenarios with expert commentary. For asymptomatic athletes, the experts acknowledged a lack of literature to guide the ultimate decision. Cantu and colleagues stated that effacement of CSF in an asymptomatic athlete represented functional stenosis, and players should not be allowed to participate in sport [38, 39]. However, others have argued for a more lenient approach, that after appropriate counseling with a neurosurgeon, athletes should be allowed to participate as long as they understand the inherent risk [37]. Moreover, the experts also agreed that previous Torg-Pavlov ratios may not be useful in athletes, as the ratio had a positive predictive value of 0.2% [37]. The experts also agreed that a transient episode of quadriparesis in an athlete, without radiographic stenosis, does not preclude RTP [37, 40]. Drawing from a systematic review of cervical contusions, Nagoshi et al. [41] describe two cases of spinal cord contusion without radiographic stenosis; one pediatric patient had no recurrent symptoms, and an adult experienced a recurrence after RTP. In the setting of stenosis, some returned successfully while others suffered permanent neurologic deficit, highlighting the heterogeneity of practices. Despite expert commentaries from spine surgeons involved in the care of professional athletes, no all-encompassing guidelines exist, and an individualized approach specific to athlete is recommended.

Cervical Surgery

The most literature exists surrounding clearance for play after anterior cervical discectomy and fusion (ACDF). Maroon et al. [42] reported 15 professional athletes after 1-level ACDF, and 13/15 athletes returned between 2–12 months. Overall, the consensus is that athletes who undergo 1 and 2-level ACDFs may return to play after fusion has been confirmed, whereas 3–4 level ACDF is likely a contraindication to participation in sport. Two reviews have provided similar conclusions regarding 1 and 2-level ACDF [43, 44]. However, there is no current consensus on sport participation after cervical disc replacement, posterior cervical decompression and/or fusion, and posterior cervical laminoplasty.

Down's Syndrome and Atlantoaxial Instability

Individuals with Down's Syndrome have high rates of atlantooccipital (AO) and atlantoaxial (AA) instability, affecting approximately 7% to 27% of patients with Down's syndrome [45]. One study of 80 patients with Down's syndrome reported 17.5% with atlantooccipital instability, and 11.2% had atlantoaxial instability [46]. Yet, only 3.8% of patients had symptoms referable to the documented instability. The authors defined AO instability as the basion-dens interval (BDI) or the basion-axial interval (BAI) >12 mm, and AA instability as ADI of >3 mm. The authors widely concluded that follow-up was appropriate, rather than any immediate surgical action. With regard to sport, special Olympics and other activities can be a major source of enjoyment, pride, and confidence for this population. Myslieiec and colleagues summarized the literature and concurred with the Special Olympics Rules, [45, 47] flexion-extension x-rays should be obtained for any Down's Syndrome patient participating in most organized sports, including: butterfly stroke, diving, pentathlon, high jump, equestrian sports, artistic gymnastics, soccer, alpine skiing and any warm-up exercise placing undue stress on the head and neck [45]. Tassone and colleagues [48] summarized the pathophysiology of AO/AA instability and treatment recommendations. For asymptomatic athletes with AO/AA instability, no reports exist of neurologic injuries incurred from sport in athletes with Down's Syndrome, yet follow-up is crucial. Any concern over canal narrowing on x-ray warrants an MRI scan. If symptomatic, surgery may be appropriate, though operative treatment still has challenges. Younger age and other spinal anomalies may contribute to non-union rates, [49] and fusion to the occiput may be required, though it adds additional morbidity.

Os Odontoideum

Os ondotoideum is a congenital or acquired condition where the dens is separated from the body of C2. The tip of the dens, instead of connected to the inferior C2 body, is a separate, smooth ossicle, variable in shape and size, with an obvious gap from the shortened odontoid process. Little guidance exists regarding os odontoideum and sport participation. Similar to Down's syndrome patients, any evidence of cervical instability requires further workup, and surgery may be indicated if symptomatic, most often a C1/2 fusion. Any sign of instability, such as a pathologic increase in the atlanto-dens interval (ADI) requires further workup, and the athlete should not play until the workup is resolved. Also, evidence of stenosis should be evaluated and treated accordingly.

Stingers

Stingers, also known as "burners", are characterized by an intense, electric-like pain occurring unilaterally down one arm, associated with numbness and/or weakness in the arm and hand. Stingers typically last for 10 seconds or less, but can last for hours or even days, and are caused by transient compression or irritation of proximal nerve roots or more distal peripheral nerves, most often in the brachial plexus. Stingers are very common, especially in American football players due to the tackling technique of hitting between the neck and shoulder area. In a study of 57 NCAA football programs from 2009–2015, 229 stingers were reported with a rate of 2.04 per 10,000 athletic events [50]. One in five stingers (19%) were recurrent, and most injuries occurred during player contact (93%) during tackling (37%) and blocking (26%). First time stingers, once symptoms are resolved, can return to competition the same day after pain resolves and full range of motion and strength resume [51]. In many cases, the athlete may be out of the game for only minutes. Athletes with second-time stingers are withheld from the remainder of play that day, but can return once the pain resolves, assuming they remain with full strength. Third- and fourth-time stingers require cervical imaging, including flexion-extension x-rays and an MRI, as these recurrent injuries may be a sign of existing foraminal or central stenosis.

Lumbar Spine

For lumbar spine conditions, if the spinal cord is not involved, disc herniations and stenosis can be treated nonoperatively, and the athlete may return to play as long as they can tolerate the pain and no neurologic compromise is identified, such as a foot drop. Fractures and traumatic injuries require a workup for stability, and the athlete should not be cleared until this is completed. Several reports exist on clearance and return to play in athletes after lumbar spine surgery. Importantly, the risk is significantly less than cervical lesions, yet still worthy of discussion. Clearance for return to sport after lumbar decompressive surgery is fairly straightforward, most often occurring in the 6–12 week time period, yet more controversy exists over fusion. Hsu et al. [52] evaluated 342 North American professional athletes with lumbar disc herniations, and 226 (66.1%) required surgery. Professional baseball players had a higher return to play rate than other sports, whereas American football players had a lower rate than other sports; however, no specific return to play times were reported. In 87 NHL players with lumbar disc herniations, 31 treated nonoperatively, 48 undergoing discectomy, and 8 undergoing a single-level fusion, return to play was high for all athletes at 85% [53]. The lumbar fusion group did not show a decrease in games played per season or performance after surgery [53]. Moreover, return to play after lumbar fusion in golfers, a low contact sport, is high, with 50% returning to on-course play within 1 year of lumbar fusion surgery [54]. Larger fusions for spondylolisthesis or scoliosis correction should be counseled on an individual patient basis, and likely require a longer recovery period before return to play [55].

Conclusions

In an athlete with an existing neurologic condition or prior neurologic injury, clearance for participation is rarely straightforward, with many academic, sport, and personal factors to consider. Neurosurgeons are often asked to provide informed counseling for parents and athletes in these situations. Given the absence of accepted, all-encompassing guidelines, obtaining a full neurologic history and exam in each individual athlete is crucial, as each athlete is truly unique. Though neurosurgeons are charged with leading these complex decisions, in most cases, parents and athletes ultimately make the final decision to return or not after understanding the potential associated risks. Sports neurosurgeons should understand the factors important in pre-participation screening, lead the multi-disciplinary discussions involved in sport participation, and continue to improve the process of pre-participation screening.

Conflicts of Interest/Financial Disclosures None.

References

1. Cantu RC, Mueller FO. Brain injury-related fatalities in American football, 1945-1999. Neurosurgery. 2003;52(4):846–52; discussion 52-3.
2. Cantu RC, Mueller FO. Catastrophic football injuries: 1977-1998. Neurosurgery. 2000;47(3):673–5; discussion 5-7.
3. Zuckerman SL, Vance EH, Brett BL. Commentary: the Florida youth concussion law: a survey-based observational study of physician practices and their legislative awareness. Neurosurgery. 2019;85(5):E959–E61.
4. Harmon KG, Drezner JA, Gammons M, Guskiewicz KM, Halstead M, Herring SA, et al. American medical Society for Sports Medicine position statement: concussion in sport. Br J Sports Med. 2013;47(1):15–26.
5. Zemper ED. Catastrophic injuries among young athletes. Br J Sports Med. 2010;44(1):13–20.
6. Committee on Sports M, Fitness. American Academy of Pediatrics: medical conditions affecting sports participation. Pediatrics. 2001;107(5):1205–9.
7. Rice SG. American Academy of Pediatrics Council on sports M, fitness. Medical conditions affecting sports participation. Pediatrics. 2008;121(4):841–8.
8. Zuckerman SL, Kerr ZY, Yengo-Kahn A, Wasserman E, Covassin T, Solomon GS. Epidemiology of sports-related concussion in NCAA athletes from 2009-2010 to 2013-2014: incidence, recurrence, and mechanisms. Am J Sports Med. 2015;43(11):2654–62.
9. Kerr ZY, Chandran A, Nedimyer AK, Arakkal A, Pierpoint LA, Zuckerman SL. Concussion incidence and trends in 20 high school sports. Pediatrics. 2019;144(5).
10. Zuckerman SL, Morgan CD, Burks S, Forbes JA, Chambless LB, Solomon GS, et al. Functional and structural traumatic brain injury in equestrian sports: a review of the literature. World Neurosurg. 2015;83(6):1098–113.
11. Morgan CD, Zuckerman SL, Lee YM, King L, Beaird S, Sills AK, et al. Predictors of postconcussion syndrome after sports-related concussion in young athletes: a matched case-control study. J Neurosurg Pediatr. 2015;15(6):589–98.
12. Miele VJ, Bailes JE, Martin NA. Participation in contact or collision sports in athletes with epilepsy, genetic risk factors, structural brain lesions, or history of craniotomy. Neurosurg Focus. 2006;21(4):E9.

13. Legarreta AD, Brett BL, Solomon GS, Zuckerman SL. The role of family and personal psychiatric history in postconcussion syndrome following sport-related concussion: a story of compounding risk. J Neurosurg Pediatr. 2018;22(3):238–43.
14. Miller JH, Gill C, Kuhn EN, Rocque BG, Menendez JY, O'Neill JA, et al. Predictors of delayed recovery following pediatric sports-related concussion: a case-control study. J Neurosurg Pediatr. 2016;17(4):491–6.
15. Aggarwal SS, Ott SD, Padhye NS, Schulz PE. Sex, race, ADHD, and prior concussions as predictors of concussion recovery in adolescents. Brain Inj. 2020;34(6):809–17.
16. Brett BL, Kuhn AW, Yengo-Kahn AM, Solomon GS, Zuckerman SL. Risk factors associated with sustaining a sport-related concussion: an initial synthesis study of 12,320 student-athletes. Arch Clin Neuropsychol. 2018;33(8):984–92.
17. Cook NE, Iaccarino MA, Karr JE, Iverson GL. Attention-deficit/hyperactivity disorder and outcome after concussion: a systematic review. J Dev Behav Pediatr. 2020;41(7):571–82.
18. Houck ZM, Asken BM, Bauer RM, Kontos AP, McCrea MA, McAllister TW, et al. Multivariate Base rates of low scores and reliable decline on ImPACT in healthy collegiate athletes using CARE consortium norms. J Int Neuropsychol Soc. 2019;25(9):961–71.
19. Zaben M, Manivannan S, Petralia C, Bhatti I, Patel C, Leach P. Patient advice regarding participation in sport in children with disorders of cerebrospinal fluid (CSF) circulation: a national survey of British paediatric neurosurgeons. Childs Nerv Syst. 2020;36(11):2783–7.
20. Manderino LM, Gunstad J. Performance of the immediate post-concussion assessment and cognitive testing protocol validity indices. Arch Clin Neuropsychol. 2018;33(5):596–605.
21. Buckley TA, Munkasy BA, Clouse BP. Sensitivity and specificity of the modified balance error scoring system in concussed collegiate student athletes. Clin J Sport Med. 2018;28(2):174–6.
22. Echemendia RJ, Meeuwisse W, McCrory P, Davis GA, Putukian M, Leddy J, et al. The sport concussion assessment tool 5th edition (SCAT5): background and rationale. Br J Sports Med. 2017;51(11):848–50.
23. Strahle J, Selzer BJ, Geh N, Srinivasan D, Strahle M, Martinez-Sosa M, et al. Sports participation with arachnoid cysts. J Neurosurg Pediatr. 2016;17(4):410–7.
24. Zuckerman SL, Prather CT, Yengo-Kahn AM, Solomon GS, Sills AK, Bonfield CM. Sport-related structural brain injury associated with arachnoid cysts: a systematic review and quantitative analysis. Neurosurg Focus. 2016;40(4):E9.
25. Davis G, Marion DW, George B, Le Roux P, Laws ER, McCrory P. Clinics in neurology and neurosurgery of sport: mass lesions. Benign brain tumours. Br J Sports Med. 2009;43(8):619–22.
26. Stanuszek A, Milczarek O, Rubinkiewicz M, Rymarowicz J, Kwiatkowski S. Return to play after brain tumor surgery in children. Childs Nerv Syst. 2020.
27. Meehan WP 3rd, Jordaan M, Prabhu SP, Carew L, Mannix RC, Proctor MR. Risk of athletes with Chiari malformations suffering catastrophic injuries during sports participation is low. Clin J Sport Med. 2015;25(2):133–7.
28. Strahle J, Geh N, Selzer BJ, Bower R, Himedan M, Strahle M, et al. Sports participation with Chiari I malformation. J Neurosurg Pediatr. 2016;17(4):403–9.
29. Laker SR. Return-to-play decisions. Phys Med Rehabil Clin N Am. 2011;22(4):619–34, viii.
30. Nakken KO, Solaas MH, Kjeldsen MJ, Friis ML, Pellock JM, Corey LA. Which seizure-precipitating factors do patients with epilepsy most frequently report? Epilepsy Behav. 2005;6(1):85–9.
31. Pinikahana J, Dono J. Age and gender differences in initial symptoms and precipitant factors of epileptic seizures: an Australian study. Epilepsy Behav. 2009;16(2):231–9.
32. Capovilla G, Kaufman KR, Perucca E, Moshe SL, Arida RM. Epilepsy, seizures, physical exercise, and sports: a report from the ILAE task force on sports and epilepsy. Epilepsia. 2016;57(1):6–12.
33. Blount JP, Severson M, Atkins V, Tubbs RS, Smyth MD, Wellons JC, et al. Sports and pediatric cerebrospinal fluid shunts: who can play? Neurosurgery. 2004;54(5):1190–6; discussion 6-8.

34. Smith MS, Friedman WA, Smith KB, Pass AN Sr, Clugston JR. Intracranial arteriovenous malformation in a college football player and return-to-play considerations. Clin J Sport Med. 2014;24(6):e62–4.
35. Davis G, Fabinyi G, Le Roux P, McCrory P. Clinics in neurology and neurosurgery of sport. Mass lesions: cavernoma. Br J Sports Med. 2009;43(11):866–8.
36. Saigal R, Batjer HH, Ellenbogen RG, Berger MS. Return to play for neurosurgical patients. World Neurosurg. 2014;82(3–4):485–91.
37. Davis G, Ugokwe K, Roger EP, Benzel EC, Cantu RC, Rogers M, et al. Clinics in neurology and neurosurgery of sport: asymptomatic cervical canal stenosis and transient quadriparesis. Br J Sports Med. 2009;43(14):1154–8.
38. Cantu RC, Li YM, Abdulhamid M, Chin LS. Return to play after cervical spine injury in sports. Curr Sports Med Rep. 2013;12(1):14–7.
39. Rosenthal BD, Boody BS, Hsu WK. Return to play for athletes. Neurosurg Clin N Am. 2017;28(1):163–71.
40. Dailey A, Harrop JS, France JC. High-energy contact sports and cervical spine neuropraxia injuries: what are the criteria for return to participation? Spine (Phila Pa 1976). 2010;35(21 Suppl):S193–201.
41. Nagoshi N, Tetreault L, Nakashima H, Nouri A, Fehlings MG. Return to play in athletes with spinal cord concussion: a systematic literature review. Spine J. 2017;17(2):291–302.
42. Maroon JC, Bost JW, Petraglia AL, Lepere DB, Norwig J, Amann C, et al. Outcomes after anterior cervical discectomy and fusion in professional athletes. Neurosurgery. 2013;73(1):103–12; discussion 12.
43. Kang DG, Anderson JC, Lehman RA Jr. Return to play after cervical disc surgery. Clin Sports Med. 2016;35(4):529–43.
44. Schroeder GD, Canseco JA, Patel PD, Hilibrand AS, Kepler CK, Mirkovic SM, et al. Updated return-to-play recommendations for collision athletes after cervical spine injury: a modified Delphi consensus study with the Cervical Spine Research Society. Neurosurgery. 2020;87(4):647–54.
45. Mysliwiec A, Posluszny A, Saulicz E, Doroniewicz I, Linek P, Wolny T, et al. Atlanto-axial instability in people with Down's syndrome and its impact on the ability to perform sports activities - a review. J Hum Kinet. 2015;48:17–24.
46. El-Khouri M, Mourao MA, Tobo A, Battistella LR, Herrero CF, Riberto M. Prevalence of atlanto-occipital and atlantoaxial instability in adults with down syndrome. World Neurosurg. 2014;82(1–2):215–8.
47. Special Olympics. Participation by individuals with Down Syndrome who have Atlantoaxial Instability 2020. Available from: ab https://www.specialolympics.ca/sites/default/files/athleteEligibility.pdf.
48. Tassone JC, Duey-Holtz A. Spine concerns in the special Olympian with down syndrome. Sports Med Arthrosc Rev. 2008;16(1):55–60.
49. Nader-Sepahi A, Casey AT, Hayward R, Crockard HA, Thompson D. Symptomatic atlanto-axial instability in down syndrome. J Neurosurg. 2005;103(3 Suppl):231–7.
50. Green J, Zuckerman SL, Dalton SL, Djoko A, Folger D, Kerr ZY. A 6-year surveillance study of "stingers" in NCAA American football. Res Sports Med. 2017;25(1):26–36.
51. Paulus S, Kennedy DJ. Return to play considerations for cervical spine injuries in athletes. Phys Med Rehabil Clin N Am. 2014;25(4):723–33.
52. Hsu WK, Jenkins TJ. Management of Lumbar Conditions in the elite athlete. J Am Acad Orthop Surg. 2017;25(7):489–98.
53. Schroeder GD, McCarthy KJ, Micev AJ, Terry MA, Hsu WK. Performance-based outcomes after nonoperative treatment, discectomy, and/or fusion for a lumbar disc herniation in National Hockey League athletes. Am J Sports Med. 2013;41(11):2604–8.
54. Shifflett GD, Hellman MD, Louie PK, Mikhail C, Park KU, Phillips FM. Return to golf after lumbar fusion. Sports Health. 2017;9(3):280–4.

55. Sellyn GE, Hale AT, Tang AR, Waters A, Shannon CN, Bonfield CM. Pediatric thoracolumbar spine surgery and return to athletics: a systematic review. J Neurosurg Pediatr. 2019:1–11.
56. Kahn EA, Schneider RC. Chronic neurological sequelae of acute trauma to the spine and spinal cord. I. the significance of the acute-flexion or tear-drop fracture-dislocation of the cervical spine. J Bone Joint Surg Am. 1956;38-A(5):985–97.
57. Schneider RC. A syndrome in acute cervical spine injuries for which early operation is indicated. J Neurosurg. 1951;8(4):360–7.
58. Schneider RC. Chronic neurological sequelae of acute trauma to the spine and spinal cord. Part V. the syndrome of acute central cervical spinal-cord injury followed by chronic anterior cervical-cord injury (or compression) syndrome. J Bone Joint Surg Am. 1960;42-A:253–60.
59. Schneider RC. Cervical spine and spinal cord injuries. Mich Med. 1964;63:773–86.
60. Schneider RC, Cherry G, Pantek H. The syndrome of acute central cervical spinal cord injury; with special reference to the mechanisms involved in hyperextension injuries of cervical spine. J Neurosurg. 1954;11(6):546–77.
61. Schneider RC, Thompson JM, Bebin J. The syndrome of acute central cervical spinal cord injury. J Neurol Neurosurg Psychiatry. 1958;21(3):216–27.
62. Cantu RC, Voy R. Second impact syndrome. Phys Sportsmed. 1995;23(6):27–34.
63. Dunn IF, Dunn G, Day AL. Neurosurgeons and their contributions to modern-day athletics: Richard C. Schneider Memorial Lecture Neurosurg Focus. 2006;21(4):E1.
64. Kindt GW, Schneider RC, Robinson JL. A method of comparing the impact absorption characteristics of football helmets. Med Sci Sports. 1971;3(4):203–9.
65. Levy ML, Ozgur BM, Berry C, Aryan HE, Apuzzo ML. Birth and evolution of the football helmet. Neurosurgery. 2004;55(3):656–61; discussion 61-2.
66. Cantu RC. Guidelines for return to contact sports after a cerebral concussion. Phys Sportsmed. 1986;14(10):75–83.
67. Collins MW, Field M, Lovell MR, Iverson G, Johnston KM, Maroon J, et al. Relationship between postconcussion headache and neuropsychological test performance in high school athletes. Am J Sports Med. 2003;31(2):168–73.
68. Maroon JC, Lovell MR, Norwig J, Podell K, Powell JW, Hartl R. Cerebral concussion in athletes: evaluation and neuropsychological testing. Neurosurgery. 2000;47(3):659–69; discussion 69-72.
69. Maroon JC, Lepere DB, Blaylock RL, Bost JW. Postconcussion syndrome: a review of pathophysiology and potential nonpharmacological approaches to treatment. Phys Sportsmed. 2012;40(4):73–87.
70. Bailes JE, Day AL. Neurological sports medicine : a guide for physicians and athletic trainers. Rolling Meadows, Ill.: American Association of Neurological Surgeons; 2001.
71. Bailes JE, Cantu RC, Day AL. The neurosurgeon in sport: awareness of the risks of heatstroke and dietary supplements. Neurosurgery. 2002;51(2):283–6; discussion 6-8.
72. Hobbs JG, Young JS, Bailes JE. Sports-related concussions: diagnosis, complications, and current management strategies. Neurosurg Focus. 2016;40(4):E5.
73. Manley G, Gardner AJ, Schneider KJ, Guskiewicz KM, Bailes J, Cantu RC, et al. A systematic review of potential long-term effects of sport-related concussion. Br J Sports Med. 2017;51(12):969–77.
74. Omalu BI, DeKosky ST, Minster RL, Kamboh MI, Hamilton RL, Wecht CH. Chronic traumatic encephalopathy in a National Football League player. Neurosurgery. 2005;57(1):128–34; discussion –34.
75. Omalu BI, Hamilton RL, Kamboh MI, DeKosky ST, Bailes J. Chronic traumatic encephalopathy (CTE) in a National Football League Player: case report and emerging medicolegal practice questions. J Forensic Nurs. 2010;6(1):40–6.
76. Miele VJ, Bailes JE. Objectifying when to halt a boxing match: a video analysis of fatalities. Neurosurgery. 2007;60(2):307–15; discussion 15-6.
77. Miele VJ, Bailes JE, Voelker JL. Boxing and the neurosurgeon. Clin Neurosurg. 2002;49:396–406.

78. Miele VJ, Norwig JA, Bailes JE. Sideline and ringside evaluation for brain and spinal injuries. Neurosurg Focus. 2006;21(4):E8.
79. Zuckerman SL, Totten DJ, Rubel KE, Kuhn AW, Yengo-Kahn AM, Solomon GS. Mechanisms of injury as a diagnostic predictor of sport-related concussion severity in football, basketball, and soccer: results from a regional concussion registry. Neurosurgery. 2016;63(Suppl 1):102–12.
80. Gardner RC, Hess CP, Brus-Ramer M, Possin KL, Cohn-Sheehy BI, Kramer JH, et al. Cavum septum Pellucidum in retired American pro-football players. J Neurotrauma. 2016;33(1):157–61.
81. Harrell BR, Barootes BG. The type I Chiari malformation in a previously asymptomatic college athlete: addressing the issue of return to athletic participation. Clin J Sport Med. 2010;20(3):215–7.
82. Callaway GH, O'Brien SJ, Tehrany AM. Chiari I malformation and spinal cord injury: cause for concern in contact athletes? Med Sci Sports Exerc. 1996;28(10):1218–20.
83. Stanuszek A, Wnekowicz E, Kuzniar E, Krakowska K, Gergont A, Kacinski M. Seizure-precipitating factors in relation to medical recommendations: especially those limiting physical activity. J Child Neurol. 2015;30(12):1569–73.
84. Sahoo SK, Fountain NB. Epilepsy in football players and other land-based contact or collision sport athletes: when can they participate, and is there an increased risk? Curr Sports Med Rep. 2004;3(5):284–8.
85. Frucht MM, Quigg M, Schwaner C, Fountain NB. Distribution of seizure precipitants among epilepsy syndromes. Epilepsia. 2000;41(12):1534–9.
86. Sousa Nanji L, Melo TP, Canhao P, Fonseca AC, Ferro JM. Subarachnoid Haemorrhage and sports. Cerebrovasc Dis Extra. 2015;5(3):146–51.
87. Richards A, Pines A, Rubel NC, Mauler D, Farnsworth J, Zhang N, et al. Return to golf, tennis, and swimming after elective cervical spine surgery. Cureus. 2020;12(8):e9993.
88. Molinari RW, Pagarigan K, Dettori JR, Molinari R Jr, Dehaven KE. Return to play in athletes receiving cervical surgery: a systematic review. Global Spine J. 2016;6(1):89–96.
89. Tempel ZJ, Bost JW, Norwig JA, Maroon JC. Significance of T2 hyperintensity on magnetic resonance imaging after cervical cord injury and return to play in professional athletes. Neurosurgery. 2015;77(1):23–30; discussion –1.

Chapter 2
On Field Assessment of the Athlete

Christian Mustroph, Gerald Rodts, and Daniel L. Barrow

Introduction

Providing proficient on field neurosurgical care of athletes requires a team-based approach encompassing health professionals from various specialties in order to address diverse pathologies. Settings range from middle school soccer fields to professional stadiums, and healthcare professionals face unique challenges including external social pressures, unique mechanisms of injury, and physical barriers to the patient from protective equipment. By following injury protocols, planning and practicing ahead, and getting input and engagement from athletes, coaches, and trainers we can strive to identify, treat, and mitigate the negative impact of neurologic injuries on athletes.

The best practices for managing on-the-field athletes begin with pre-competition planning, with communication and meetings among game officials, medical and athletic staff. Game-day meetings help to review injury protocol, refresh personnel on the location of necessary medical equipment, and set the groundwork for communication during the game. Staff should familiarize themselves with the location of required equipment including first aid-supplies, location of ambulance and paramedic personnel, automatic emergency defibrillator, and equipment needed to remove protective sports equipment such as facemasks. Action plans have been shown to prevent death from sudden cardiac arrest in athletes but require communication among coaches, medical staff, and emergency medical technicians. These action plans also apply to the neurosurgical care of athletes [1, 2].

C. Mustroph · G. Rodts · D. L. Barrow (✉)
Emory University, Atlanta, GA, USA
e-mail: daniel.barrow@emory.org

M. E. Oppenlander (ed.), *Neurosurgical Care of Athletes*,
https://doi.org/10.1007/978-3-030-88227-3_2

Neurosurgeons have been at the forefront of prevention and management of neurotrauma including concussions, brachial plexus injuries, cervical spine "stingers," and spinal cord injury. Early recognition of brain injury or concussion may prevent long term effects of neurotrauma such as chronic traumatic encephalopathy (CTE). Neurosurgery training programs ensure competency in evaluating, examining, and managing patients with traumatic brain and spinal cord injury. Thus, neurosurgeons are well-prepared for assessment of neurotrauma in athletes. The Center for Disease Control (CDC) estimates 1.6–3.8 million annual sports related concussions (SRC) in the US [3]. Additionally, 12% of spinal cord injuries in the US are sports related [4]. The advent of return to play laws addressing concussions and head injuries beginning in 2009 have further increased demand for neurosurgical care of athletes and rapid assessment of athletes during play [5]. This high volume of neurotrauma in athletes precludes the demand being met by neurosurgeons alone and, therefore, other professionals are playing more prominent roles in assessing and managing neurological issues in athletes, especially outside of a hospital setting.

Orthopedists receive training on managing spinal cord injury while also treating athletes for a wide array of musculoskeletal injuries. Neurologists and physiatrists help to recognize, treat and rehabilitate patients who have experienced neurotrauma. The majority of concussions are diagnosed and treated by emergency room or primary care physicians [4]. It is prudent for all healthcare providers to have the basics in assessing for neurotrauma to facilitate appropriate management and care of athletes.

Identification of Injured Athletes

The rapid identification of an injured athlete results in timely and appropriate neurosurgical care. It can be difficult to identify a potential injury in the midst of competitive play with players, coaches, and families more focused on the outcome of competition than potential injuries. Due to its diverse symptomatology, neurotrauma can be difficult to identify in an athlete and it is estimated that 19% of sports related traumatic brain injuries are overlooked [6]. No biomarkers, imaging techniques, or monitoring devices have been shown to be effective in the midst of competition to diagnose a neurologic injury [7]. Diagnosis of neurotrauma and concussion relies on evaluation of neurological, vestibular, oculomotor, visual and neurocognitive function [8, 9]. While some possible perturbations may be monitored while an athlete remains in play, many require stoppage of play. This poses the first initial challenge of identifying a potential neurologic injury in order to evaluate the player on the field or on the sideline.

Physician-witnessed trauma to the head or spine with concerns for possible neurologic injury should result in stoppage of play to allow for evaluation, or for the athlete to be transported to the sideline for examination. Symptoms including (but not limited to) temporary loss of consciousness, focal weakness, disorientation, confusion, fencing posturing, amnesia, nausea, vomiting, and slurred speech should prompt rapid evaluation. Ancillary support staff play a critical role in identifying injured athletes. Athletic trainers, coaches, referees, and other players may observe injuries or trauma which a sideline physician may have missed. Referees and teammates may have vantage points that allow them to better view trauma and detect neurologic deficits in players at their side more rapidly than physicians positioned on the sideline. Though most concussions will occur in the immediate vicinity of the primary action of play, it is important to be aware that some concussions will occur "out of direct sight" in the periphery of the play.

Renewed media focus on concussions and CTE has led to increased education on concussion symptomatology. Unfortunately, although increased concussion knowledge has been linked to increased self-reporting, increased concussion education has not resulted in a significant increase in self-identification. Self-identification rates for concussion are about 50% in high-school athletes and, therefore, self-reporting alone is not an adequate means of screening for concussion [10]. There are a number of barriers to self-identification as well as self-reporting. Self-identification requires the athlete to be aware of the signs and symptoms of a neurological injury. For many athletes in contact sports, the subtler signs of concussion or other neurological injury may be unknown to the athlete from lack of education or tendency to assume minor symptoms are just part of the game. Common phrases such as "he got his bell rung" have been used so ubiquitously that many uninitiated athletes and coaches may believe a transient alteration in level of consciousness or other subtle neurological symptoms can be ignored. Self-reporting requires both recognition and the desire to protect one's health and well-being. Many athletes will purposefully ignore symptoms and signs to enable them to continue to participate in a sport they love, and in some instances must play for their financial well-being and living.

Collegiate and professional sports have adopted review systems to identify and tag potential traumatic injury with concern for brain or spine injury. The National Football League (NFL) began making use of certified athletic trainers ("ATC spotters") beginning in 2011 which has since expanded to other professional sports including hockey. The ATC spotters are typically located higher above the field, rink or court of play so that they have a broader vantage point. The primary goal of the ATC spotter is to alert sideline personnel to potential injuries. In addition to an ATC spotter which monitors the game, an additional ATC spotter or physician reviews video footage and live TV/Cable broadcast of the game, tagging potential injuries. During the 2017 NFL regular season, 456 incidents were reported using the spotter system with only 7 stoppages of play total [11]. The low number of interruptions demonstrates how a video review system can improve the sensitivity of a monitoring system without significantly influencing the flow of play.

Assessment on the Field of Play

When an injury requiring medical attention is identified, the medical team should follow a predetermined algorithm to stabilize, evaluate, and treat the patient. The principles of basic life support should be followed with the healthcare workers or support staff evaluating airway, breathing, and circulation prior to proceeding with evaluation for further injury. While the regimented approach helps to ensure that no critical aspects of patient stabilization are missed, many aspects of basic life support can be assessed simultaneously. A patent airway can be identified through verbal responses. Breathing can be observed by watching for chest rise, while circulation can be assessed by measuring a peripheral pulse. With the basics of airway, breathing, and circulation secured, the patient can be evaluated for neurologic deficits. Disability and mental status can be rapidly assessed using the alert, verbal pain, unresponsive (AVPU) scale or the Glasgow coma scale (GCS). During the disability evaluation, concerns for neurologic deficits from spinal cord injury may become apparent. The evaluation for spinal cord injury should include a motor and sensory examination and determination of the presence of paresthesia or numbness. The athlete should be questioned about cervical, thoracic, or lumbar spinal pain or tenderness to palpation, and focal weakness. If any concern for spinal injury arises, spinal precautions should be strictly maintained.

In cases of suspected spinal cord injury athletes should be secured to a rigid spine board for stabilization and transportation to a level 1 or 2 trauma center [12]. Multiple techniques have been described for transferring a patient including the 6-plus-person (6+) lift, the lift-and-slide, the logroll spine board transfer, and the use of a scoop stretchers. The 6-plus-person lift and lift-and-slide transfer techniques have been demonstrated to reduce lateral flexion, axial rotation, and lateral translation of the spine compared to the logroll [13]. Similarly, the logroll has been shown to increase overall head movement when compared to the lift-and-slide [14]. The Inter-Association Task Force for Appropriate Care of the Spine-Injured Athlete has advocated the use of the 6+ lift in combination with a scoop stretcher [15].

The removal of helmet and protective equipment remains controversial. Removal of helmets and shoulder pads may cause increased spinal movement, while removal of the facemask in American football can be done with minimal motion of the cervical spine [16, 17]. Furthermore, removal of either the helmet or shoulder pads alone in hockey and football has been shown to disrupt atlanto-occipital alignment [18, 19]. The removal of protective equipment is left to the discretion of the healthcare provider and depends on the injury, personnel available to assist, and need for exposure. If removal is not needed for resuscitation, it is reasonable to keep protective equipment in place until removal in a hospital.

The unconscious athlete provides a set of unique challenges. Following the principles of basic life support, the athlete must first be assessed for a patent airway. In order to gain better access to the patient's airway, protective equipment such as helmets or facemasks may need to be removed. Depending on the sport and helmet, various tools are available for removing facemasks and helmets and it is imperative that medical staff be familiar with this equipment prior to the start of competition.

Breathing is evaluated by listening for breath sounds, observing chest movement, or auscultating if a stethoscope is readily available. If insufficient ventilation is determined, assisted ventilations may be given and the athlete may require intubation. Circulation is assessed by feeling for peripheral or central pulses, blood pressure measurement, cardiac auscultation or for monitoring for signs of decreased perfusion. If abnormalities are noted, emergency services or EMTs, if present on scene, should be notified immediately.

Sideline Assessment of Ambulatory Patient

After an athlete has been evaluated on the field and is medically stable, they can be taken to the sideline where a more detailed neurological examination can occur. The evaluator should be attentive to any red flag signs or symptoms, including headache, blurred or double vision, confusion, altered mental status, paresthesia, numbness, and weakness. A standardized assessment should be used on the sideline with which the examiner is familiar. Multiple assessment tools have been developed to assess for sports related concussion and TBI and these continue to evolve over time.

The Standardized Assessment of Concussion (SAC), developed in 1997, aims to test for reduced orientation, immediate memory, concentration, and delayed recall following concussion [20]. Questions assess orientation to time by asking the month, date, day of week, year, and time within 1 hour. Five words are listed and tested for immediate recall and again at the conclusion of the exam. Lastly, concentration is tested by reordering digits and listing the months of the year in reverse giving a cumulative score out of 30. A decline in score after injury reflects a 95% sensitivity and 76% specificity in differentiating between a concussed and uninjured patient [18].

The Maddocks questions were developed in 1995 from Australian rules football [21]. Questions inquire about location, the time period of the game, who scored last, the opponent and outcome of a previous game. Similar questions have been validated in children under the age of 13 and include questions about location, current time in respect to lunch, last class subject, and the child's teacher's name [22]. The Maddocks questions provide a sensitive tool for identifying concussion but due to their high false positive rate, they are often combined with other diagnostic tools.

A detailed exam is also able to uncover signs of concussion [23]. The neurologic examination includes testing of all cranial nerves. New cranial nerve palsies in the setting of recent trauma should prompt immediate neuroimaging. Individual muscle group testing and reflexes can help reveal signs of significant neurologic injury, whether central or peripheral. In addition to potentially revealing a hemiparesis, individual muscle testing can also identify radicular deficits in patients with stinger complaints (e.g., paresthesias, radicular pain, neck pain, peri-scapular pain, weakness).

After the initial sideline diagnosis, the medical staff must decide whether the player can safely remain in the game. The decision of whether to remove a player from play is based on initial diagnosis, the risk of further injury, need for further testing and imaging. When available, sideline review of video replay can be helpful in analyzing the mode of impact and the player's immediate behavior and movements following injury. There are certain symptoms and signs that are clear and unequivocal indicators for disqualification from further play, or what is referred to as a "No Go". This includes loss of consciousness or unresponsiveness, confusion, anterograde amnesia, new and/or persistent symptoms, seizure activity, diplopia, repeated vomiting, or focal neurological deficits. A player removed from competition should undergo continued monitoring and potentially further assessment in the locker room.

Locker Room Assessment of Injured Player

The sport concussion assessment tool (SCAT) created in 2004 brought together multiple methods of assessing neurologic function including the Maddocks questions, SAC, and neurologic exam. The SCAT has undergone multiple updates, most recently in 2016 to the SCAT5 which is to be used by healthcare professionals in patients age 13 and older. The Child SCAT5 is used in children ages 5–12, while the CRT5 is meant for use by non-physicians. The SCAT5 is made up of an on-the-field and off -the-field assessment which should be administered in no less than 10 minutes. The immediate assessment includes red-flag symptoms encompassing neck pain or tenderness, double vision, weakness or tingling/burning, severe or increasing headache, seizure or convulsion, loss of consciousness, deteriorating conscious state, vomiting, and increasingly restless, agitated or combative state. Observable signs whether witnessed by members on the sideline or video include lying motionless, balance and gait difficulty, blank or vacant look, and facial injury after head trauma. The Maddocks questions and GCS are incorporated into the SCAT5 followed by assessing the cervical spine for pain, range of motion, and limbs for normal strength and sensation. The second portion of the examination is intended to be conducted in a quiet environment at near resting heart rate. The patient is screened for presence of one of 22 symptoms and given a symptoms severity score. Cognitive screening is performed using the SAC and balance examined using the modified balance error scoring system (mBESS). The mBESS aims to measure postural stability [24]. Athletes are asked to balance in double leg, single leg, and tandem gaits with their eyes closed. Scores are tabulated and compared to pre-injury baseline or normative values [25].

Post-Competition and Game End Repeat Examination

Athletes removed from a game should be re-examined for resolution, persistence, or worsening of symptoms. Most athletes with mild head injury can be observed for 2 hours before being released to a monitor [26, 27]. When allowed to leave the

Table 2.1 Clinical Decision Rules for Imaging in Concussion

New Orleans criteria
Computed tomography is required for patients with minor head injury with any one of the following findings. The criteria apply to patients who also have a Glasgow coma scale score of 15
Headache
Vomiting
Older than 60 years
Drug or alcohol intoxication
Persistent anterograde amnesia (deficits in short-term memory)
Visible trauma above the clavicle
Seizure
Canadian CT head rule[a]
Computed tomography is only required for patients with minor head injury with any one of the following findings:
Patients with minor head injury who present with a Glasgow coma scale score of 13 to 15 after witnessed loss of consciousness, amnesia or confusion
High risk of neurosurgical intervention
1. Glasgow coma scale lower than 15 at 2 hours after injury
2. Suspected open or depressed skull fracture
3. Any sign of basal skull fracture[b]
4. Two or more episodes of vomiting
5. 65 years or older
Medium risk for brain injury detection by computed tomographic imaging
1. Amnesia before impact of 30 or more minutes
2. Dangerous mechanism[c]

[a]the rule is not applicable if the patient did not experience trauma, has a Glasgow coma scale score lower than 13, is younger than 16 years, is taking warfarin or has a bleeding disorder, or has an obvious open skull fracture

[b]signs of basal skull fracture include hemotympanum, racoon eyes, cerebrospinal fluid, otorrhea or rhinorrhea, Battle's sign

[c]dangerous mechanism is a pedestrian struck by motor vehicle, an occupant ejected from a motor vehicle, or a fall from an elevation of 3 or more feet or 5 stairs

locker room, athletes and their families or monitors must be vigilant for progressive symptoms including worsening headache, weakness, nausea, vomiting, and increased somnolence. The appearance of such symptoms should prompt further medical evaluation.

The majority of mild TBI has no imaging findings on CT with only 10% demonstrating hemorrhage [28]. The Canadian CT head rule, Nexus Criteria, and New Orleans Criteria can help to identify athletes requiring neuroimaging (Table 2.1) [29–31]. Patients with a GCS less than 15, two hours after injury, open or depressed skull fractures, signs of basal skull fracture (hemotympanum, racoon eyes, CSF otorrhea or rhinorrhea, Battle's sign), more than two vomiting episodes and age greater than 65 years have a high risk of needing neurosurgical intervention and require head imaging. Patients with amnesia for more than 30 minutes prior to injury or undergoing a dangerous mechanism (fall from elevation of more than 3 feet) have a medium risk of having evidence of brain injury on CT and should obtain a head CT.

Following the diagnosis of concussion, athletes will require monitoring for resolution of symptoms and for retesting. Return to play is recommended when all symptoms have resolved, and baseline SCAT-5 or other testing has returned to baseline. This topic will be covered in another chapter of this book.

In conclusion, neurosurgical care of the athlete in the competitive setting requires a multitude of important steps. Education of athletes, trainers and coaches in recognizing the signs of brain or spine trauma is essential. Pre-game communication with game officials, coaches, athletic trainers, and emergency personnel can establish location of resources (x-ray, closest appropriate hospital, ambulance, crash cart, etc.) and help ensure efficient flow of medical activity in the event of injury. Physicians and allied professionals are encouraged to remove athletes from the arena of play to allow for proper evaluation if there is any question of a brain or spine injury.

Conclusion: Neurosurgical assessment and treatment of athletes requires a structured approach to identify, stabilize, evaluate, and monitor injured participants. Rapid triage and appropriate treatment of patients is aided by pre-competition planning, education, and a team-based approach. Through early identification of neurologic injuries, removing athletes from play for screening or monitoring, and promptly transferring those with more severe injuries to medical facilities, the sports neurosurgeon can help mitigate the adverse effects neurologic injuries have on athletes.

References

1. Weisfeldt ML, Sitlani CM, Ornato JP, Rea T, Aufderheide TP, Davis D, et al. Survival after application of automatic external defibrillators before arrival of the emergency medical system: evaluation in the resuscitation outcomes consortium population of 21 million. J Am Coll Cardiol. 2010;55(16):1713–20.
2. Drezner JA, Courson RW, Roberts WO, Mosesso VN, Link MS, Maron BJ. Inter-association task force recommendations on emergency preparedness and Management of Sudden Cardiac Arrest in high school and college athletic programs: a consensus statement. Heart Rhythm. 2007;4(4):549–65.
3. Langlois JA, Rutland-Brown W, Wald MM. The epidemiology and impact of traumatic brain injury: a brief overview. J Head Trauma Rehabil. 2006;21(5):375–8.
4. Chan CW, Eng JJ, Tator CH, Krassioukov A. Epidemiology of sport-related spinal cord injuries: a systematic review. J Spinal Cord Med. 2016;39(3):255–64.
5. Tomei KL, Doe C, Prestigiacomo CJ, Gandhi CD. Comparative analysis of state-level concussion legislation and review of current practices in concussion. Neurosurgical Focus FOC. 2012;33(6):E11.
6. Theadom A, Starkey NJ, Dowell T, Hume PA, Kahan M, McPherson K, et al. Sports-related brain injury in the general population: an epidemiological study. J Sci Med Sport. 2014;17(6):591–6.
7. McCrea M, Meier T, Huber D, Ptito A, Bigler E, Debert CT, et al. Role of advanced neuroimaging, fluid biomarkers and genetic testing in the assessment of sport-related concussion: a systematic review. Br J Sports Med. 2017;51(12):919–29.

8. Sussman ES, Ho AL, Pendharkar AV, Ghajar J. Clinical evaluation of concussion: the evolving role of oculomotor assessments. Neurosurgical Focus FOC. 2016;40(4):E7.
9. Feddermann-Demont N, Echemendia RJ, Schneider KJ, Solomon GS, Hayden KA, Turner M, et al. What domains of clinical function should be assessed after sport-related concussion? A systematic review. Br J Sports Med. 2017;51(11):903–18.
10. Register-Mihalik JK, Guskiewicz KM, McLeod TC, Linnan LA, Mueller FO, Marshall SW. Knowledge, attitude, and concussion-reporting behaviors among high school athletes: a preliminary study. J Athl Train. 2013;48(5):645–53.
11. Mack C, Myers E, Barnes R, Solomon G, Sills A. Engaging athletic trainers in concussion detection: overview of the National Football League ATC spotter program, 2011-2017. J Athl Train. 2019;54(8):852–7.
12. Macias CA, Rosengart MR, Puyana JC, Linde-Zwirble WT, Smith W, Peitzman AB, et al. The effects of trauma center care, admission volume, and surgical volume on paralysis after traumatic spinal cord injury. Ann Surg. 2009;249(1):10–7.
13. Del Rossi G, Horodyski MH, Conrad BP, Di Paola CP, Di Paola MJ, Rechtine GR. The 6-plus-person lift transfer technique compared with other methods of spine boarding. J Athl Train. 2008;43(1):6–13.
14. Del Rossi G, Horodyski M, Powers ME. A comparison of spine-board transfer techniques and the effect of training on performance. J Athl Train. 2003;38(3):204–8.
15. Mills BM, Conrick KM, Anderson S, Bailes J, Boden BP, Conway D, et al. Consensus recommendations on the prehospital Care of the Injured Athlete with a suspected catastrophic cervical spine injury. Clin J Sport Med. 2020;30(4):296–304.
16. Kleiner D, Almquist JL, Bailes J, Burruss P, Feuer H, Griffin LY, et al. Prehospital care of the spine-injured athlete: a document from the inter-association task force for appropriate care of the spine-injured athlete. J Athl Train. 2001;36:4–29.
17. Swartz EE, Mihalik JP, Beltz NM, Day MA, Decoster LC. Face mask removal is safer than helmet removal for emergent airway access in American football. Spine J. 2014;14(6):996–1004.
18. Metz CM, Kuhn JE, Greenfield ML. Cervical spine alignment in immobilized hockey players: radiographic analysis with and without helmets and shoulder pads. Clin J Sport Med. 1998;8(2):92–5.
19. Tierney RT, Mattacola CG, Sitler MR, Maldjian C. Head position and football equipment influence cervical spinal-cord space during immobilization. J Athl Train. 2002;37(2):185–9.
20. McCrea M, Kelly JP, Kluge J, Ackley B, Randolph C. Standardized assessment of concussion in football players. Neurology. 1997;48(3):586–8.
21. Maddocks DL, Dicker GD, Saling MM. The assessment of orientation following concussion in athletes. Clin J Sport Med. 1995;5(1):32–5.
22. Brooks MA, Snedden TR, Mixis B, Hetzel S, McGuine TA. Establishing baseline normative values for the child sport concussion assessment tool. JAMA Pediatr. 2017;171(7):670–7.
23. Matuszak JM, McVige J, McPherson J, Willer B, Leddy J. A practical concussion physical examination toolbox. Sports Health. 2016;8(3):260–9.
24. Guskiewicz KM, Ross SE, Marshall SW. Postural stability and neuropsychological deficits after concussion in collegiate athletes. J Athl Train. 2001;36(3):263–73.
25. Petit KM, Savage JL, Bretzin AC, Anderson M, Covassin T. The sport concussion assessment Tool-5 (SCAT5): baseline assessments in NCAA division I collegiate student-athletes. Int J Exerc Sci. 2020;13(3):1143–55.
26. Servadei F, Teasdale G, Merry G. Defining acute mild head injury in adults: a proposal based on prognostic factors, diagnosis, and management. J Neurotrauma. 2001;18(7):657–64.
27. Blostein P, Jones SJ. Identification and evaluation of patients with mild traumatic brain injury: results of a national survey of level I trauma centers. J Trauma. 2003;55(3):450–3.
28. Jeret JS, Mandell M, Anziska B, Lipitz M, Vilceus AP, Ware JA, et al. Clinical predictors of abnormality disclosed by computed tomography after mild head trauma. Neurosurgery. 1993;32(1):9–15; discussion −6.
29. Stiell IG, Wells GA, Vandemheen K, Clement C, Lesiuk H, Laupacis A, et al. The Canadian CT head rule for patients with minor head injury. Lancet. 2001;357(9266):1391–6.

30. Mower WR, Gupta M, Rodriguez R, Hendey GW. Validation of the sensitivity of the National Emergency X-radiography utilization study (NEXUS) head computed tomographic (CT) decision instrument for selective imaging of blunt head injury patients: an observational study. PLoS Med. 2017;14(7):e1002313.
31. Bouida W, Marghli S, Souissi S, Ksibi H, Methammem M, Haguiga H, et al. Prediction value of the Canadian CT head rule and the New Orleans criteria for positive head CT scan and acute neurosurgical procedures in minor head trauma: a multicenter external validation study. Ann Emerg Med. 2013;61(5):521–7.

Chapter 3
Spinal Injury in Athletes: Prevalence and Classification

Gordon Mao and Nicholas Theodore

Abbreviations

AIS	ASIA Impairment Scale
ASIA	American Spinal Injury Association
CCN	Cervical cord neuropraxia
CSI	Cervical spine injury
MVA	Motor vehicle accident
NSCISC	National Spinal Cord Injury Statistical Center
SCI	Spinal cord injury
SLIC	Subaxial Injury Classification
TAL	Transverse atlantal ligament
TLICS	Thoracolumbar Injury Classification and Severity

Introduction

Athletic competition is a common cause of traumatic spinal cord injury (SCI). In fact, sports-related injuries contribute to 8.7% of SCI cases in the United States and are a leading cause of SCI only behind motor vehicle accidents, falls and violence [54]. Spinal injuries are common across all age groups, from high school athletics to collegiate- and professional-level sports. These injuries can be devastating and have long-lasting effects on athletes and their families.

G. Mao · N. Theodore (✉)
Department of Neurosurgery, Johns Hopkins University School of Medicine, Baltimore, MD, USA
e-mail: theodore@jhmi.edu

M. E. Oppenlander (ed.), *Neurosurgical Care of Athletes*,
https://doi.org/10.1007/978-3-030-88227-3_3

Sports-related spinal injuries are separated into cervical and thoracolumbar spine injuries. Cervical injuries include insults to the C1 vertebra as well as the craniocervical junction downward to the C7–T1 disc space and facet joints. Common causes of cervical spine injuries include both direct-contact sports such as American football, wrestling, ice hockey, and baseball; and non-contact sports such as diving, skiing, snowboarding, and cheerleading. Thoracolumbar injuries include those that occur from the T1 vertebra downward, through the lumbar and sacral spine to the coccyx. Thoracolumbar sports injuries are even more prevalent than cervical sports injuries, and frequently occur during both direct-contact sports such as football and hockey, as well as sports with frequent jumping and landing, such as basketball and downhill skiing or snowboarding.

The term "spinal injury" is broad and may be used to describe direct damage to the spinal column, the neural elements that make up the spinal cord, the 31 pairs of exiting spinal nerve roots, and the surrounding paraspinous muscles that allow for movement and maintenance of erect posture. The spinal column itself includes the boney vertebral elements, the intervertebral discs, and the surrounding stabilizing ligamentous structures that support the vertebral column against gravity and preserve normal, anatomic alignment during movement. Minor injuries to the spinal column generally affect the paraspinous musculature and fascia, which absorb the brunt of the trauma and spare the underlying spinal column and neural elements from severe injuries. Major spinal injuries from high-energy sports trauma can cause significant damage to the spinal column, leading to acute mechanical instability, or neurologic injury that causes different patterns of weakness and numbness in the torso and extremities. High-impact injuries can also result in epidural hematoma, angulated or comminuted vertebral fractures, or catastrophic fracture–dislocations—all of which can result in the violation of the spinal canal with resulting SCI and pronounced neurologic deficit. Of the 11,000 cases of SCI in the US per annum, the second leading cause of SCI in the young adults (ie, patients under the age of 30) is sports participation [66].

Cervical Spine Injuries

Incidence

The cervical spine supports the weight of the head and provides flexibility that allows extensive range of motion of the head. Cervical spine injuries can manifest in a wide spectrum of physiologic and neurologic symptoms, both transient and permanent. Mild injuries can present primarily with pain and spasm from soft tissue injury without structural instability or neurologic impairment. In other instances, non-catastrophic cervical injuries can include transient neurologic phenomena from radicular or plexus injuries, such as stingers or burners, and mild cord insult causing cord neuropraxia. Cervical cord neuropraxia (CCN) generally comprises transient sensory disturbance of the upper or lower extremities with resolution in 10 to

15 minutes [9], secondary to hyperflexion or hyperextension neck movements in individuals with existing spinal stenosis. Stingers, or transient unilateral or bilateral dysesthesia of the upper extremities, can also occur in patients with milder injuries secondary to brachial plexus traction. Less commonly, catastrophic cervical injuries can cause acute mechanical instability from disruption of osteoligamentous structures, as well as neurologic deficit from nerve root injury or acute SCI.

Because of the high range of motion in the cervical spine, injuries can occur in a variety of positions. Catastrophic injuries involving SCI or traumatic malalignment typically occur with axial impact to the top of the head with the neck in flexion. In the neutral (ie, lordotic) position, the impact energy is dissipated by both the paravertebral musculature and the intervertebral discs. However, at 30 degrees of flexion, the energy is transferred directly through the spinal column up to the failure point when a flexion injury (eg, flexion tear drop fracture, facet dislocation) or pure compression (eg, burst fracture, acute disc herniation) injury occurs [9].

A severe, sudden twist to the neck or a severe blow to the head or neck can cause a neck fracture. Sports involving violent physical contact (eg, football, ice hockey, rugby, and wrestling) carry a greater risk of neck fracture. Spearing an opponent in football or rugby can cause a neck injury, as can non-contact activities like gymnastics—for example, if the gymnast misses the high bar during a release and falls. Cervical spine injuries can range from subluxations and dislocations with or without neurologic symptoms to fractures with or without neurologic symptoms.

The US Consumer Product Safety Commission tracks product-related injuries through its National Electronic Injury Surveillance System. According to the Consumer Product Safety Commission, an estimated 23,720 neck fractures were treated at US hospital emergency departments in 2018. Of these, an estimated 3194 fractures (13.47%) were related to sports. Cervical injuries can occur both in contact sports, such as soccer and rugby, and in non-contact sports, such as gymnastics and cycling. Between 2000 and 2015, the number of sporting-related cervical fractures increased by 30%, driven primarily by a 300% increase in cycling-related injuries [75]. Gender-related differences also exist in SCI patients, due to the underlying differences in the popularity of various sports between men and women (Fig. 3.1). Cycling was the most common cause of cervical fractures in men, whereas horseback riding was the most common cause in women [18]. Nearly one-quarter of cervical spine injuries (CSIs) in young persons under 15 years of age are sport related, and 85% of sport-related CSIs result in tetraplegia [54]. More than 250 new sport-related CSIs occur each year [54].

The risk of injury varies among sports. Ice hockey players are among those at highest risk of CSIs [83]. American tackle football has the highest number of catastrophic cervical spine injuries among all sports played in the United States, due to the high level of participation, with more than 1.5 million active players ranging from middle school to professional levels [83]. American football does, however, maintain an overall low rate of cervical spine injuries [52]. Less than 1% of cervical spine injuries result in a serious fracture or SCI [48]. Just as the development of safer helmets reduced the incidence of traumatic brain injury in football in the 1970s, cervical spine injury rates likewise declined after the recognition and ban of

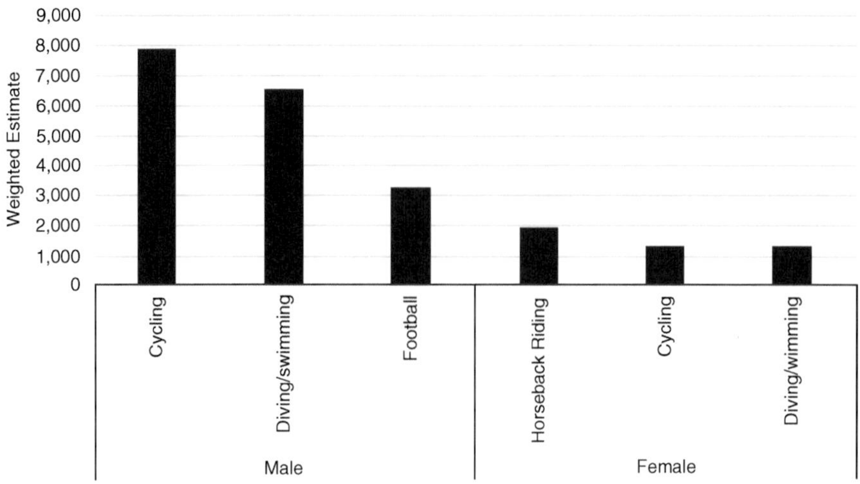

Fig. 3.1 Most frequent causes of cervical spine fractures in men versus women (Depasse [18])

dangerous maneuvers such as spear tackling in 1976, dropping the rate of quadriplegia by 80% over the subsequent decade [73]. CCN is estimated to occur in approximately 7 per 10,000 participants [72], and CSIs are estimated to occur in 10% to 15% of all football players—most commonly in linemen and defensive players. Similarly, rugby also has a high rate of cervical injury, particularly due to the lack of protective gear worn by the players and the aggressive style of play. During engagement, a rugby hooker player can sustain almost 0.75 tons of force. Overall, 10% of serious rugby injuries occur in the cervical spine, with SCI occurring in 25% of those cases [62].

Injuries are an inevitable consequence of horseback riding, as the rider's head may be up to 4 m (13 feet) from the ground and horses can travel at speeds up to 65 km/h (40 mph) [64]. In the US, as many as 30 million people will ride a horse each year [59], and a 1991 report of horseback riding injuries described 217 deaths in 10 states [14]. Horseback riding carries an injury rate of 1 per 350 hours of riding, which is 20-fold higher than the injury rate of motorcycling [29]. Unlike other sports in which the head often leads during movement, falls from horseback riding predominantly cause thoracolumbar injuries. Horseback riding accidents can be divided based on 2 methods of riding—the jockey style with the head forward, which presents a higher risk for cervical injury after a fall; and the classical style, where the head is held high and the rider lands on her buttocks [7].

Cervical spine sports-related injuries increased by 35% between 2000 and 2015, mainly due to an increase in cycling-related injuries. A 14-year Canadian study of severe cycling injuries identified spine injury as accounting for 45.7% of the 11,772 cases [60]. Studies in the US, Ireland, Australia, France, and Israel have all found evidence of increased cycling related-cervical spine injuries. During a 1-year period in Ireland, 70% of cycling-related spine trauma occurred in the cervical spine [13].

The authors of these studies attributed the increased popularity of cycling to its health benefits and the agreeable climate [18]. In a study specifically looking at off-road cycling, a similar 73% spine injury rate was seen, but off-road cycling was associated with higher relative rates of severe SCI (40% ASIA A) [21] compared with road cycling (12.5% overall) [13].

Cheerleading has evolved into a highly competitive sport that requires complex gymnastic maneuvers. At the high school and college levels, cheerleading is the leading cause of up to 50% of severe sports injuries, with the United States Consumer Product Safety Commission recognizing 1814 neck injuries occurring in collegiate cheerleaders in 2000 [10]. Collegiate cheerleading athletes sustain more injury proportionally than those at the high school level due to the increasing technical difficulty of the performances. The pyramid stunt and the basket toss are the most common scenarios for injury, mostly due to the high vertical distance reached by the participants, and the hard indoor gym surface [12]. In response to these risk factors, safety guidelines have been implemented to limit the maximum height of pyramids to 2 people at high school level and 2.5 body lengths at collegiate level, and to limit stunts such as the basket toss during wet conditions.

Although spinal injuries are infrequent in baseball, the relative rate of catastrophic cervical spine injuries remains high, as in cheerleading. A common scenario involves a base runner diving head-first toward the catcher and sustaining a compressive injury. Rules advise the runner to avoid the fielder, who has the right to base path [9], but this rule is not always followed. Little leagues have outright banned head-first sliding in favor of feet-first sliding.

Diving injuries in shallow water are another well-recognized cause of catastrophic cervical SCI. Although many recreational cervical spine diving injuries remain unreported, a European trauma center reported 7.7% of all cervical SCI to be from diving [63]. Both college and high school athletic associations now prohibit race diving in waters less than 4 feet in depth, and many community recreational pools are choosing to remove high-dive boards in favor of water slides to mitigate the risk of SCI.

Spine injuries in wrestling overwhelmingly occur in the cervical spine, notably when a wrestler lands directly on top of his head with his arms locked in a position unable to support his body weight, or when a wrestler attempts to roll but is landed on with the full weight of his competitor [9]. More injuries occur in the light- and middle-weight divisions frequently during a defensive posture during a takedown, followed by a kneeling or lying position. Vulnerable wrestlers in the defensive position often have their arms restrained, preventing protection of the neck [11]. Thus, the main safety mechanisms rely on both the referee and the coach maintaining vigilance, and a low threshold for stopping the match in dangerous circumstances.

Downhill skiing is another common cause of both cervical and thoracolumbar spine injuries. Although the rate of SCI is low—just 0.01 per 1000 ski days [51]—spinal injuries in downhill skiing actually appear to be increasing in the past 2 decades. Injuries tend to occur in younger male skiers, with risk factors including poorly groomed slopes, equipment failure, inclement weather, collision, high speeds, and overcrowded conditions. Injuries tend to occur at the end of the day, suggesting that fatigue is a major factor, and fatalities are typically from traumatic brain injury secondary to collision with stationary object.

Ice hockey is also a common source of cervical spine injury due to its high participation rate. Most injuries occur in the lower cervical spine, between C5–7, and do not result in SCI. Common mechanisms include axial loading to the top of the head from direct head contact with the boards after being checked from behind. A Canadian survey from 1966 to 1993 reported 241 cervical spine fractures from ice hockey [68].

Classification

Cervical spine injuries are generally classified based on a morphologic description of the fracture level and pattern, and traditionally divided into subaxial (C3–T1) and upper cervical (occipital condyle–C2) injuries. Traditionally, various common fracture patterns of the cervical spine have been described individually and attributed to eponymous physicians with specific grading systems attached in order to categorize fractures on a spectrum of severity, thereby guiding treatment practices. Since the 1980s, efforts have been made to create subaxial cervical injury classification schemes, but none of these early systems were widely adopted by spine surgeons due to their over-complexity in real-world application and lack of validation studies. More recently, in 2011, the Academy of Orthopedics has developed a more structured nomenclature system to describe upper cervical (Fig. 3.2) and subaxial spine injury (Fig. 3.3).

In a clinical context, cervical injuries resulting from participation in sports can be divided into the following syndromes:

- Acute cervical sprains/strains, including whiplash injury.
- Cervical spinal stenosis.
- Intervertebral disc lesions.
- Nerve root or brachial plexus injuries.
- Cervical fractures and dislocations.
- Transient or permanent quadriplegia from SCI.

Historically, upper cervical spine injuries have been considered a distinct entity due to the inherent anatomic differences in the morphology of the C1 and C2 vertebrae as well as the unique and high degrees of motion concentrated at the craniocervical junction and the C1–2 segment [20]. A significant degree of flexion–extension motion is contributed by the atlantooccipital joint between C1 and the cranium. The atlantoaxial joint between C1 and C2 is responsible for approximately 50% of cervical rotation. In particular, ligamentous structures are recognized for their high contribution to the stability of motion segments of the upper cervical spine. Upper cervical injuries are rare in sports and are more commonly seen in either a high-impact settings (eg, MVA, fall from height); however, they can occur with direct cervical trauma in sports such as diving and American football. We will describe

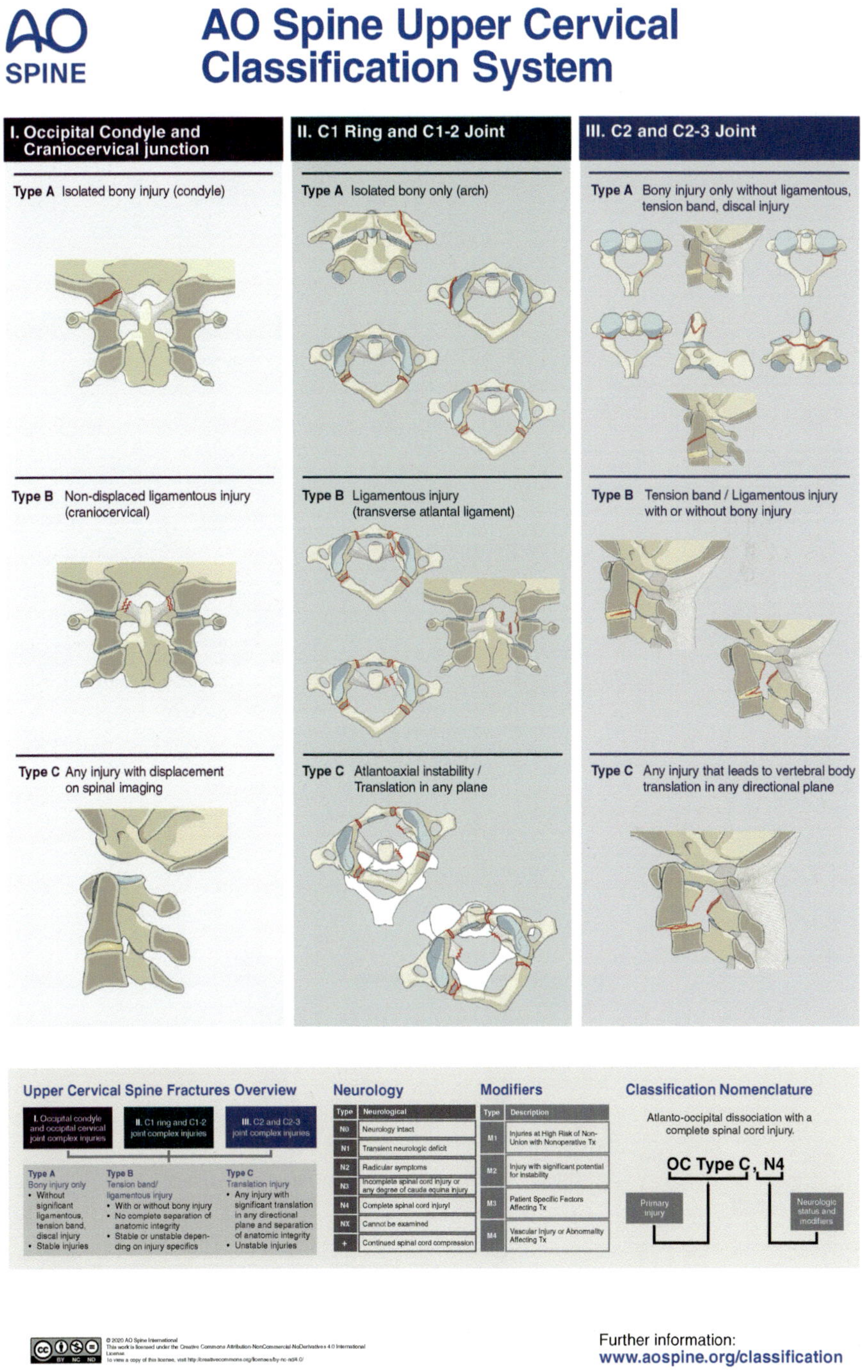

Fig. 3.2 Upper cervical spine classification. (Reprinted with permission from AOSpine International. © AOSpine International, Switzerland)

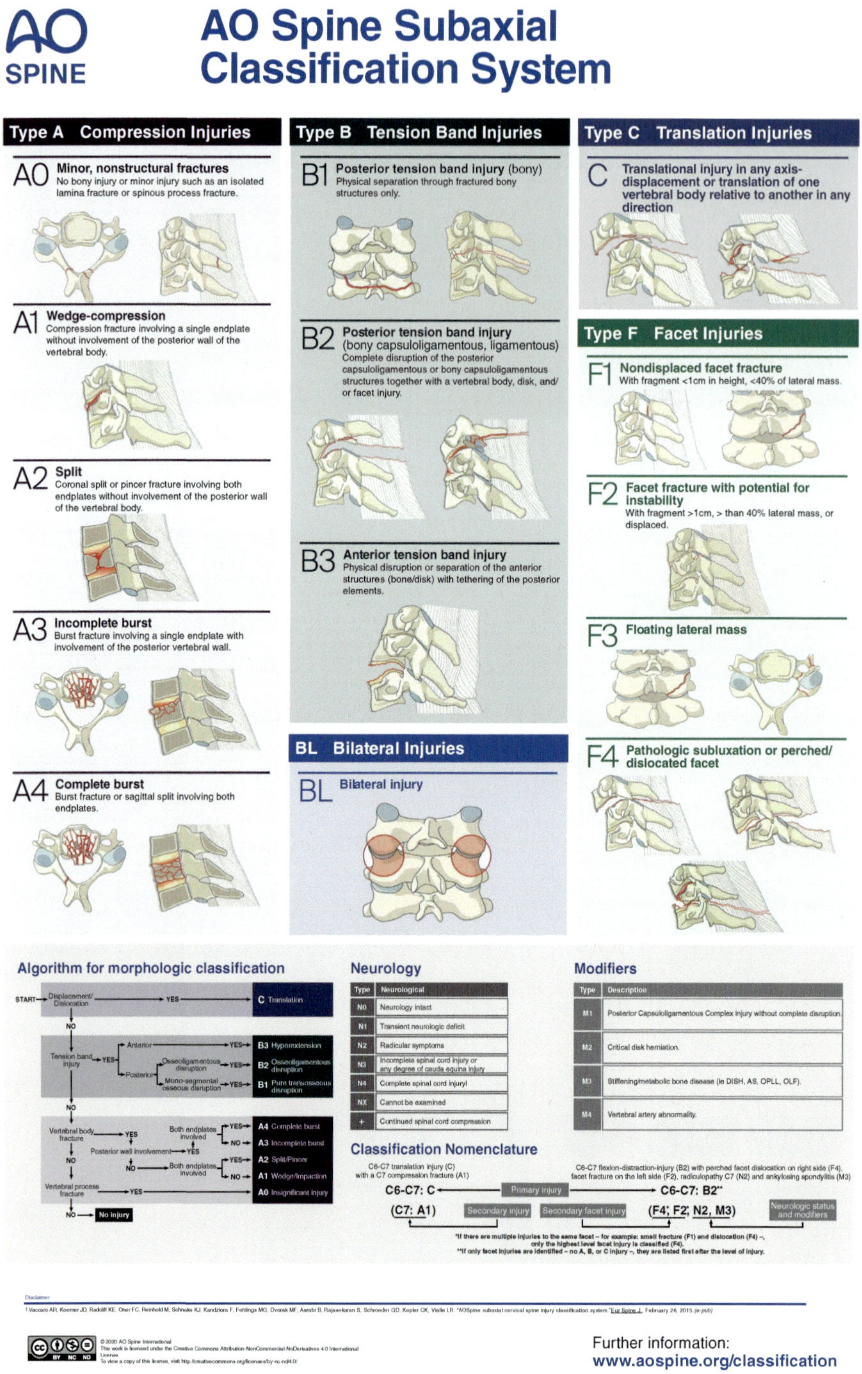

Fig. 3.3 Subaxial cervical spine classification. (Reprinted with permission from AOSpine International. © AOSpine International, Switzerland)

some of the older classification schemes as well as a new system developed by AOSpine.

Older classification systems of upper cervical spine injury are based on the specific level of injury as well as the morphology or potential for instability. Occipital condyle fractures are commonly described by the Anderson and Montesano system [4], which is based on the mechanism of injury and extent of fracture. Traumatic atlantooccipital dislocations are classified by the Traynelis system [74], which is based on direction of displacement, while the later Harborview system [8] graded the degree of displacement to predict stability.

Fracture of the C1 vertebra is classically referred to as a Jefferson fracture when it affects both the anterior and posterior rings. Jefferson fractures are described generally based on suspicion for transverse atlantal ligament (TAL) injury, which affects the stability of the C1–2 complex. Odontoid fractures are described morphologically by the Anderson and d'Alonzo system [3] based on involvement of the C2 body and location of the fracture line with respect to TAL. C2 pars fractures, known as Hangman fractures when occurring bilaterally, were described by 2 similar systems known the Francis and Effendi (modified by Levine-Edwards) systems. The Francis classification [30] separated fractures based on degree of fracture displacement (3.5 mm), C2–3 angulation (11 degrees), and C2–3 disc space involvement. The Effendi system [26, 45] divided fractures based on progressive degrees of ligamentous involvement, initially with posterior longitudinal ligament or disc disruption, and culminating in C2–3 facet capsule disruption.

The AOSpine upper cervical classification system was created in 2013 to unify and simplify existing classification systems. It divides injuries into 3 broad categories based on the spinal level affected—the occipital condyle and craniovertebral junction, the C1 vertebral body and C1–2 joint injuries, and C2 vertebral body and C2–3 joint issues. Each injury type is then subcategorized into 3 categories of increasing instability, beginning with isolated boney fracture, then additional ligamentous injuries, and finally, translational injuries. Additional case-specific "M" modifiers are available. M1 describes any ligamentous injuries with high potential for instability (eg, radiographic evidence of TAL disruption). M2 describes risk factors for nonunion, such as odontoid fracture with significant displacement (>5 mm) or angulation (>11 degrees). The M3 modifier describes patient comorbidities such as smoking, renal failure, or osteoporosis that would affect treatment. Finally, M4 describes any anatomic or vascular abnormality or injury that would affect treatment, such as the presence of vertebral artery injury.

The subaxial cervical spine is a region commonly affected by trauma. Various methods have also been proposed to classify these injuries. In isolation, these systems have been based on assumed mechanism of injury inferred from plain radiographs, ignoring the contribution of ligaments to stability and failing to account for underlying neurologic injury [76]. Allen and Ferguson [2] provided the first comprehensive description of such injuries based primarily on mechanism of trauma. This include the categories CF (compressive flexion), VC (vertical compression), DF (distractive flexion), CE (compressive extension), DE (distractive extension), and LF (lateral flexion). Each category was further subdivided into 2–5 severity stages to correlate with degree of neurologic risk. Although this was comprehensive, it has been difficult to apply clinically and lacks interobserver reliability [65]. Another classification system was later introduced by Harris [36]. Based on biomechanical, cadaveric, and pathological evidence that vector forces along the "central coordinating system" are fundamental determinants of cervical spine injuries, Harris and colleagues introduced yet another mechanistic classification based on the literature and clinical data [1]. Major vector forces in this system were flexion, extension, rotation, vertical compression, and lateral bending. Like the Allen method, this scheme was overly detailed and was never adopted into widespread use.

AOSpine developed a user-friendly unified subaxial classification system in 2016 [77]. By avoiding overly descriptive terminology often used in historical systems, injury morphology was used as the basis for recent algorithm-based systems instead of mechanism of injury. This comprehensive but simple classification system was developed with high intraobserver and interobserver reliability. It separates injuries broadly into compression injuries (type A), distraction injuries (type B), and translation injuries (type C), in a fashion similar to the AOSpine thoracolumbar injury classification (described below). Like thoracolumbar injuries, type A subaxial injuries are categorized on a continuum ranging from minor, nonstructural fractures to complete burst fractures, whereas type B injuries are split between anterior versus posterior tension band injuries. Unique to the subaxial classification is a fourth category (type F) specifically created to distinguish facet injury patterns from small, nondisplaced fractures affecting less than 40% of the lateral mass to true facet dislocations. Also similar to other AOSpine schemas, additional neurologic (N) and patient-specific modifiers (M) can optionally be added to capture the complete clinical picture of the spinal injury, ultimately assisting surgeons to select a treatment plan.

Management

Cervical spine injuries can be managed operatively or nonoperatively, depending on the biomechanical stability of the injury and the neurologic status of the patient. Different factors, such as the fracture pattern, suspected mechanism of injury, spinal alignment, and expected long-term stability will also help determine the treatment plan. Panjabi and White introduced the most widely accepted definition of clinical spinal stability: namely, the ability of the spine under physiology loads to limit displacement in order to prevent injury or irritation of the spinal cord and nerve roots, and to prevent major deformity or incapacitating pain due to structural changes [82]. In their seminal cadaveric biomechanical study, Panjabi and White systematically destroyed the facets and incrementally sectioned ligamentous structures in 8 cervical cadaveric specimens, and then examined behavior of the spine under physiologic bending moments. They demonstrated that overt instability occurred whenever displacement or listhesis progressed to 3.5 mm at rest or with any physiologic bending or 11 degrees of segmental angulation in the subaxial spine.

Milder cervical spine injuries without significant neurologic deficit or concerns for acute instability may be treated conservatively with symptomatic pain control, and sometimes serial imaging and follow-up, with or without a rigid orthosis. Cervical sprains isolated to paraspinous muscle and soft tissue injuries often require only physical therapy and pain control without imaging or rigid orthosis. Traumatic injury patterns typically involve either isolated ligamentous injuries without acute malalignment or deformity, or focal boney fractures of the vertebral body or posterior elements without significant fracture displacement, malalignment, or concomitant ligamentous injuries. These injuries will require a rigid collar for at least 4 to 6 weeks, followed by dynamic cervical spine radiographs to assess stability before the collar can be discontinued and the patient returned to certain activities.

Acutely or overtly unstable cervical injuries typically require surgical intervention. These are usually classified as AOSpine type B or C subaxial injuries, which involve both boney and ligamentous injuries, or more severe type F (facet) injuries with high risk for instability. Unstable injuries typically have greater involvement of ligamentous structures and higher risk of development of acute malalignment. Rigid bracing or application of a Halo vest can be alternatives to surgery in patients with unacceptably high medical risk from comorbidities or advanced age. However, many surgeons try to avoid prolonged bracing for unstable fracture patterns due to the long-term risk factors of braces, such as pressure ulcers or aspiration risks, as well as development of severe spinal deformity.

In general, acute cervical injuries that cause pronounced or progressive neurologic impairment require surgical intervention at the very least to relieve neural compression. Often times, neurologic injury is related to higher impact and severity mechanisms that are also associated with boney or ligamentous injuries that are chronically or acutely unstable. These circumstances often necessitate open surgery involving decompression of the neural elements with instrumentation and fusion of multiple segments.

These anatomic and neurologic considerations have been synthesized into a validated severity scoring system for subaxial cervical injuries. The Subaxial Injury Classification (SLIC) scoring system was developed by Vaccaro and the Spine Trauma Study Group in 2007. According to the SLIC system, patients with scores between 6 and 10 represent surgical candidates; those with scores between 1 and 3 are likely better candidates for immobilization by rigid orthosis (Table 3.1). Unlike older frameworks built on inferred injury mechanisms, the SLIC system is utilitarian in that it abandons these anatomic considerations for the 3 expert-consensus–determined major components of the injury. This scheme was validated by 20 spine surgeons across 11 cervical trauma cases, showing raters' agreement with treatment recommendations of the algorithm in 93.3% of cases [76].

Table 3.1 The Subaxial Injury Classification (SLICS) scale

Classification	
Injury morphology	No abnormality: 0 points
	Simple compression fracture: 1 point
	Burst fracture: 2 points
	Distraction (eg, perched facet joint, hyperextension cervical injuries): 3 points
	Rotation/translation (eg, facet dislocation, unstable teardrop or advanced flexion compression injury): 4 points
Discoligamentous complex	Intact: 0 points
	Indeterminate (eg, isolated interspinous widening, MRI signal change only): 1 point
	Disrupted (eg, disc space widening, facet perch or dislocation): 2 points
Neurologic status	Intact: 0 points
	Root injury: 1 point
	Complete cord injury: 2 points
	Incomplete cord injury: 3 points
	Incomplete with ongoing cord compression: 4 points

Thoracolumbar Spinal Injuries

Incidence

Between 75% and 90% of spinal injuries occur in the thoracolumbar spine, most commonly between T10 and L3 [37]. Low back pain is common in the general population, but almost 30% of athletes experience lumbar pain directly related to their sports participation [24]. Unlike cervical spine injuries, thoracolumbar injuries in athletes tend to separate into 2 distinct populations. The first is the acute, high-energy traumatic injury that typically occurs at the thoracolumbar junction with boney, and (often concordant) ligamentous injuries that can also be associated with SCI or root injuries. The second population comprises more chronic, degenerative stress injuries that occur in the lower lumbar spine secondary to the strenuous and repetitive flexion, extension, and loading activities involved in athletic training and competition [5]. In a study of collegiate athletes, just over 50% of lumbar injuries were found to be acute [40].

Age and anatomic considerations also influence the type of lumbar injury. Adolescent athletes experience more posterior-element injury secondary to skeletally immature spines [50], whereas adults tend to suffer from muscle strain and discogenic disease [25]. In general, sports involving repetitive hyperextension, axial loading (jumping), twisting, or direct contact carry higher risks of low-back injuries. In a study of 4790 collegiate athletes, the highest rates of lumbar injuries were seen in football players, gymnasts, and rowers, with an overall incidence of 7% among collegiate athletes [38]. Another study identified the setting of injury as predominantly during practice in 80% of cases, versus 14% during preseason, and 6% during competition [40].

American football is a common cause of thoracolumbar injuries, with 30.9% of all football injuries involving the lumbar spine [48] and 28% of lumbar injuries due to disc herniations at L4–5 and L5–S1 [33]. Axial loading is a common mechanism during heavy blocking and tackling maneuvers; therefore, defensive and offensive linemen are the players most commonly affected. Shear stress from sudden directional changes in non-contact scenarios can also lead to injuries. Pars fractures (spondylolysis) are also common affecting up to 50% of players [70], in part due to the inadequate locking of the lumbosacral spine that normally protects the spine since there are multiple concurrent forces on the athlete as they compete for possession of the ball [15].

Ice hockey players have a high prevalence for chronic low back pain—one study reported that 95% of players experienced chronic low back pain [39]. One long-term study over 15 years in players with a median age of 24 found that most athletes who developed back pain already had existing degenerative abnormalities on magnetic resonance imaging, and these abnormalities continued to progress throughout their careers. This study concluded that most back pain was the result of injuries sustained during adolescence that persisted through adulthood [6]. A study of Canadian hockey league players identified 18% of spinal injuries in the thoracolumbar spine, with the most common mechanism of injury as being checked from behind [69]. Furthermore, up to 44% of low back pain in youth hockey may be linked to spondylolysis [22].

The incidence of spinal injuries in snowboarding is almost 4 times higher than skiing. Most injuries are in the thoracolumbar spine [46] and secondary to overcrowded slopes and high-risk jumps. Jumping is estimated to be responsible for 80% of these injuries [67].

Basketball injuries are heavily concentrated in the lower extremities and lumbar spine due to the large amount of jumping and short sprints involved in the game. Lumbar injuries account for 10.2% of all National Basketball Association player injuries [23] based on a 17 year study. The majority of lumbar injuries were related to musculoskeletal strain and sprain, which accounted for 7.9% of injuries while disc disease accounted for another 0.9% [23].

Degenerative lumbar disease is also prevalent in baseball. One Major League Baseball study found a 11.7% injury rate between 2002 and 2008 [57], whereas a Japanese study showed a 60% prevalence of degenerative disc disease at the L4–5 and L5–S1 levels among professional players [34]. Indeed, 89.5% of baseball players report experiencing lower back pain during their lives [34].

Injury Classification

An understanding of the typical injury patterns in the thoracolumbar spine requires an understanding of the anatomic and biomechanical consideration of the thoracolumbar spine. The natural lumbar lordosis disperses axial loads both perpendicularly and horizontally through the disc space [25]. Flexion movements place the instantaneous axis of rotation at the center of the disc space, placing tension on the lumbodorsal fascia, erector spinae muscle groups, and gluteus maximus, whereas extension movements shift the instantaneous axis of rotation posteriorly within the disc space. The spinal column bears significant tensile and shear stress, as well as compressive loads, whereas the posterior soft tissues bears more resistive stress.

Minor and degenerative thoracolumbar injuries in athletes can be broadly classified into several patterns. Soft tissue injuries are the most common and divide into "sprains," which are ligamentous injuries, and "strains," which are injuries to the muscle, tendon, and musculotendinous junction [25]. These injuries typically present with localized paraspinous tenderness with superficial bruising and back pain exacerbated by bending or twisting at the waist. Pseudoradicular symptoms of radiation to the hip may be present, representing spasms extending to the fascia latae.

Disc herniations are also common. They can occur acutely during weight-lifting or strength training, or from a sudden twisting or pivoting movement. Athletes who are exposed to repetitive twisting, bending/flexion, or heavy lifting movements are vulnerable to lumbar disc herniations [25]. Bowling and collision sports both have higher risks of herniation [53]. Radicular symptoms typically occur in older athletes, while younger, adolescent, or collegiate athletes more often present with back pain and spasm likely due to the more viscous disc composition and lower chances of a large, sequestered disc free-fragment [32].

Minor fractures without any risk to spinal stability or neural elements also often occur. These injuries include thoracic and lumbar spinous process and transverse process fractures, as well as vertebral body endplate and wedge compression fractures. These fractures can occur after forceful rotation, flexion, compression, and direct blows. Athletes with these injuries typically report acute-onset localized pain, generally without any neurologic signs or symptoms.

More severe thoracolumbar injuries typically pose significant risk to mechanical stability and neurologic elements. Historically, various classification systems have been based on individual experience or retrospective series predicated on anatomic structures of the injury involvement as well as mechanisms of injury. Many systems were difficult to apply clinically, as they involved an impractical number of variables and were difficult to interpret. Serious efforts at creating a comprehensive morphology-based classification systems such as the Magerl system [47] were overly complex for clinical use and ultimately were never validated, revised, or updated. For many decades, there was a lack of a widely accepted universal classification system.

Kelley and Whiteside proposed the first biomechanical model of thoracolumbar stability in 1968, introducing the concept of the 2-column model—the anterior column (vertebral body) and the posterior column (neural arches) [41]. By the 1980s, McAfee et al. analyzed a series of 100 patients with unstable fracture complexes using modern computed tomography technology that offered insight into some of the important theoretical principles behind our current understanding of thoracolumbar stability, such as the integrity of the middle column osteoligamentous complex and the effects of translational injuries [49]. Another influential mechanical model, proposed by Francis Denis in 1983, is known as the 3-column thoracolumbar stability model. Denis became the first person to introduce a graduated system of instability rather than trying to clearly define each injury in a binary (ie, stable or unstable) fashion. The anterior column was composed of the anterior two-thirds of the vertebral body, while the middle column—often crucial in defining stability—was composed of the posterior longitudinal ligament and posterior one-third of the body. The posterior column was composed of the pedicles and other neural elements and dorsal ligamentous structures. Isolated violation of the anterior or posterior was therefore considered a more stable injury, while the addition each additional column increased the instability of the injury.

An international group of spine surgeons was assembled the American Academy of Orthopedics, known as the AOSpine Knowledge Forum, to formulate the current AOSpine thoracolumbar classification system (Fig. 3.4). This system takes into account morphological factors and other important clinical factors, such as neurologic status, with the goal of creating a simple but comprehensive classification scheme that could guide surgeons with treatment planning. This system was validated in a subsequent clinical study that found a moderate interobserver reliability coefficient (k = 0.56) and good intraobserver reliability coefficient (k = 0.68).

The AOSpine system separates injuries into 4 broad groups representing different injury mechanisms. Within each group, different subtypes are further delineated to distinguish severity or anatomic structures (eg, osseous vs ligamentous). Type A injuries involve various degrees of compression/axial-loading–related fractures. Type B injuries represent tension band injuries to key ligamentous structures anterior or posterior to the vertebral column. Type C injuries represent high-energy translational injuries in any plane or direction, and are considered uniformly structurally unstable. Additional modifier categories include neurologic status, which defines the degree of neurologic injury and presence of ongoing spinal cord compression, and patient-specific comorbidities that would affect surgical decision making or planning, such as presence of osteoporosis or ankylosing spondylitis.

Management Guidelines

Similar to the management of cervical spine injuries, traumatic thoracolumbar spine injury management is guided by the severity and stability of the injury complex, as well as the degree of neurologic impingement. Bracing, physical therapy, rest, and symptomatic pain relief are indicated with purely soft tissue paraspinous injuries that present with focal pain and back spasms that cause limitation of activity. Soft braces (ie, corsets) or no bracing can be used for injuries in which there is no concern for long-term chronic instability, whereas rigid (ie, clamshell) lumbar sacral orthosis or thoracic lumbar sacral orthosis braces can be used for more severe boney injuries, such as burst fractures, which have higher long-term risks for development of a focal kyphotic deformity.

Nonsurgical conservative management is reserved for injury complexes without pronounced or progressive neurologic injury or acute instability. Like cervical injuries, major neurologic compromise is typically an indication for urgent surgery for decompression and possible instrumented stabilization of the injury. Otherwise,

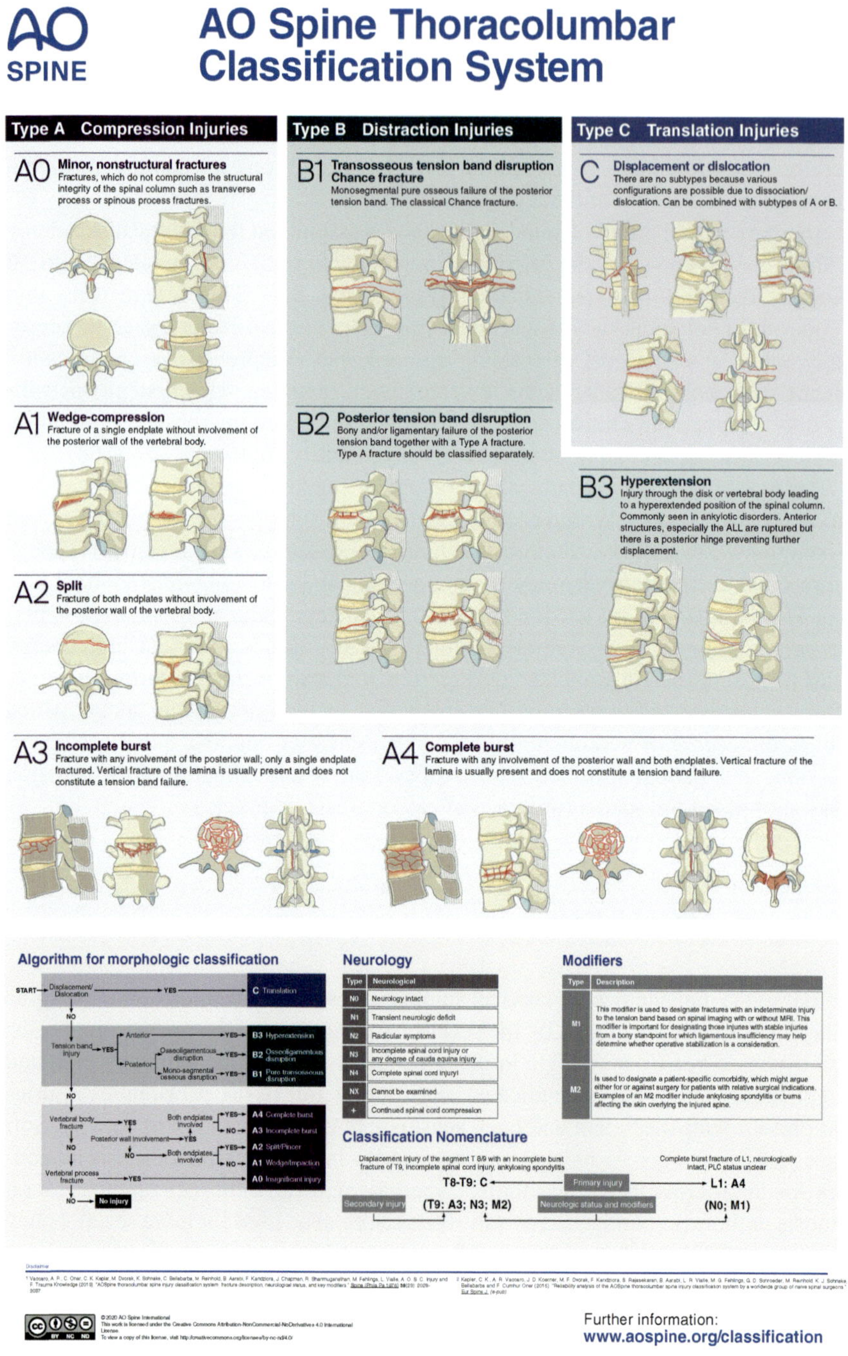

Fig. 3.4 Thoracolumbar classification. (Reprinted with permission from AOSpine International. © AOSpine International, Switzerland)

acutely unstable injuries without neurologic compromise will often also be surgical candidates for instrumented fixation or fusion procedures. Overtly unstable injuries typically involve at least 2 of the 3 columns [17] and represent AOSpine types B and C, especially with any translation or distraction noted on imaging.

Anatomic and neurologic considerations are similarly synthesized into a reproducible, valid, and easily performed scoring system known as the Thoracolumbar Injury Classification and Severity score (TLICS) score developed by Lee and the Spine Injury Trauma Group in 2005 [44]. TLICS was created based on an extensive review of the literature as well as consensus opinion from a diverse group of 40 spinal trauma surgeons from 15 trauma centers in the United States. This scoring system has been validated both retrospectively [78] and prospectively [79], with greater than 95% to 96% agreement with actual administered treatment.

This system combines point-based severity classification across 3 categories that serve as independent surgical indications for thoracolumbar injury. First, the immediate stability of the injury can be described by the morphology. Compression fractures with minimal instability are rated with 1 point, whereas high-energy distraction injuries are tallied at 4 points. Immediate and long-term stability also depend on the soft tissue ligamentous support around the spine that, in the thoracolumbar spine, is highly reliant on the integrity of the posterior ligamentous complex. Here a definite injury is given 3 points. Finally, neurologic compromise forms a distinct surgical decision-making branch point, so both the severity of the injury (ie, cord vs root injury) and responsiveness to intervention (ie, incomplete vs complete SCI) are given extra points. The total points from the 3 subcategories are summated for the final TLICS score (Table 3.2). Similar to the SLIC score, a score higher than or equal to 5 represents stronger surgical indication, whereas scores 0 to 3 represent evidence for conservative management. Often, magnetic resonance imaging is required to determine the posterior ligamentous complex score when the findings from computed tomography are indeterminate.

Table 3.2 Thoracolumbar Injury Classification and Severity Scale (TLICS)

Classification	
Morphology	Wedge compression fracture: 1 point
	Burst fracture: 2 points
	Translation/rotation: 3 points
	Distraction: 4 points
Posterior ligamentous complex	Intact: 0 points
	Suspected injury or indeterminate: 2 points
	Injured: 3 points
Neurologic involvement	Intact: 0 points
	Nerve root: 2 points
	Cord/conus medullaris (complete): 2 points
	Cord/conus medullaris (incomplete): 3 points
	Cauda equina: 3 points

Table 3.3 Top US Sports Contributing to SCI in 2019 (National Spinal Cord Injury Statistical Center 2019)

Sport	Male	Female	Total
Diving	1772	160	1932
Cycling	496	68	564
All-terrain vehicle/all-terrain cycle	218	37	255
Football	153	0	153
Skiing	170	19	189
Horseback riding	76	77	153
Surfing (including body surfing)	140	6	146

-Spinal Cord Injury

Incidence

Based on epidemiologic data from 2011, the global incidence of traumatic SCI is estimated at 23 million, or almost 180,000 new cases year each [43]. In the US, sports injuries account for 8.4% of all causes of SCI, ranking fourth behind MVAs, falls, and violence as contributors of traumatic SCI (Table 3.3) [55].

Rates of sports-related SCIs vary by country. A 2016 systematic review/meta-analysis of 54 studies identified wide variation in rates of traumatic SCI caused by athletics [16]. The 6 countries with the highest proportions of sports-related SCI were Russia (33%), Fiji (32%), New Zealand (20%), Iceland (19%), France (16%), and Canada (13%). Countries with the lowest proportion of SCIs caused by sports were Turkey (3%), Jordan (3%), Nepal (2%), Malaysia (2%), China (2%), and Nigeria (2%) [16]. Similarly, the popularity of different sports across the world affected their contributions to SCI, with skiing and winter sports causing 48% of sports related SCI in Scandinavian countries but only 1% of SCI in Ireland. The popularity of rugby in New Zealand contributes to its causing 74% of all sports-related SCI in that country, while it only contributes to 0.7% of sports-related SCI in Germany. The popularity of diving in China causes it to contribute to 65% of sports-related SCI in China, but just 8% in Germany. Similarly, horseback riding accounts for 42% of sports-related SCI in Ireland but only 1% in Japan.

Outcomes and location of SCI also vary based on pattern of activity and trauma from each sport. The cervical spine is the level most commonly affected across all sports—it is the cause of greater than 96% of SCI in diving and American football, but only 41% in snowboarding. Thoracic SCI is relatively more common in noncontact sports such as snowboarding and horseback riding, where it accounts for 25% to 30% of SCI cases with mechanism of injury more likely from falls rather than direct impact against another person or object [16].

Unfortunately, prognosis remains poor after sports-related SCI. NSCISC 40-year data from 1973 to 2013 show that only 1% of individuals who sustain sports-related SCI recover to neurologic baseline by discharge. The most common discharge neurologic examinations showed incomplete tetraplegia from incomplete cervical SCI (47%), followed by complete tetraplegia (37%), and incomplete and complete paraplegia (both 6%) [56].

Injury Classification

Traumatic SCI represents a wide range of pathology that can affect both presentation and prognosis. Classification systems have been developed to standardize the description of neurologic injury by qualifying the degree of residual neurological function and neurologic compromise based on sensory and motor functions below a specific spinal or neurologic level. They have been useful not only for reproducibility, but also for prognostication. Prior to the formation of the American Spinal Injury Association (ASIA) in 1973, the Frankel scale was the most commonly recognized SCI classification system. This scale (Table 3.4), developed in 1961, included 5 grades, from A to E, in decreasing severity. This legacy system posed several inherent limitations related to the lack of specificity in the grade descriptions. Specifically, the failure to define a distinct level of spine injury, and the ill-defined terms "motor-useful" and "motor-useless" in distinguishing grades C and D [61].

By 1982, ASIA created the ASIA Impairment Scale (AIS), which currently serves as the gold standard for evaluation of SCI both in clinical and academic setting (Fig. 3.5). This standardized exam is composed of a myotome-based motor examination, dermatome-based sensory examination, and an anorectal examination, the results of which are combined into a single neurologic injury level and an overall injury severity grade. The neurologic level is defined as the most caudal spinal level at which the sensory exam is normal, and the motor exam is at least 3/5 (ie, anti-gravity) on testing.

A notable and important distinction in the AIS is the delineation between complete and incomplete SCI. Many large retrospective registries have shown a

Table 3.4 Frankel Grading System

Grade	Injury
A	Complete neurological injury. No motor or sensory function detected below level of lesion
B	Preserved sensation only. No motor function detected below level of lesion, some sensory function below level of lesion preserved
C	Preserved motor, nonfunctional. Some voluntary motor function preserved below level of lesion, but too weak to serve any useful purpose. Sensation may or may not be preserved
D	Preserved motor, functional. Functionally useful voluntary motor function below level of injury is preserved
E	Normal motor function. Normal motor and sensory function below level of lesion, abnormal reflexes may persist

ASIA — American Spinal Injury Association

INTERNATIONAL STANDARDS FOR NEUROLOGICAL CLASSIFICATION OF SPINAL CORD INJURY (ISNCSCI)

ISCOS

Patient Name_______________ Date/Time of Exam_______________

Examiner Name_______________ Signature_______________

RIGHT — MOTOR KEY MUSCLES — SENSORY KEY SENSORY POINTS — Light Touch (LTR) Pin Prick (PPR)

LEFT — SENSORY KEY SENSORY POINTS — Light Touch (LTL) Pin Prick (PPL) — MOTOR KEY MUSCLES

C2, C3, C4

UER (Upper Extremity Right) / UEL (Upper Extremity Left):
- Elbow flexors C5
- Wrist extensors C6
- Elbow extensors C7
- Finger flexors C8
- Finger abductors (little finger) T1

T2, T3, T4, T5, T6, T7, T8, T9, T10, T11, T12, L1

Comments (Non-key Muscle? Reason for NT? Pain? Non-SCI condition?):

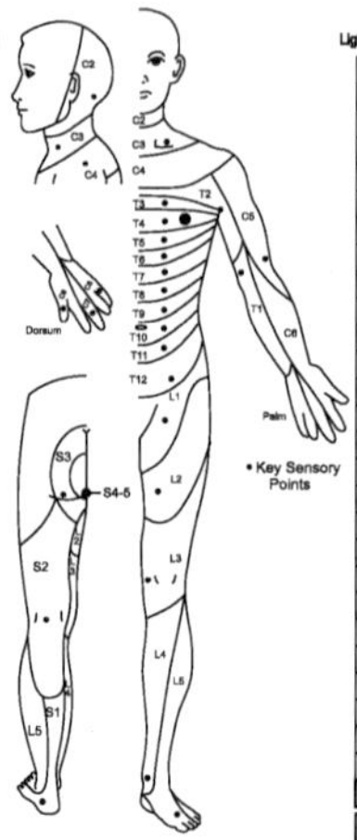

MOTOR (SCORING ON REVERSE SIDE)
0 = Total paralysis
1 = Palpable or visible contraction
2 = Active movement, gravity eliminated
3 = Active movement, against gravity
4 = Active movement, against some resistance
5 = Active movement, against full resistance
NT = Not testable
0*, 1*, 2*, 3*, 4*, NT* = Non-SCI condition present

SENSORY (SCORING ON REVERSE SIDE)
0 = Absent NT = Not testable
1 = Altered 0*, 1*, NT* = Non-SCI condition present
2 = Normal

LER (Lower Extremity Right) / LEL (Lower Extremity Left):
- Hip flexors L2
- Knee extensors L3
- Ankle dorsiflexors L4
- Long toe extensors L5
- Ankle plantar flexors S1

S2, S3, S4-5

(VAC) Voluntary Anal Contraction (Yes/No)

(DAP) Deep Anal Pressure (Yes/No)

RIGHT TOTALS (MAXIMUM) (50) (56) (56)

LEFT TOTALS (MAXIMUM) (56) (56) (50)

MOTOR SUBSCORES

UER ☐ + UEL ☐ = UEMS TOTAL ☐ — MAX (25) (25) (50)

LER ☐ + LEL ☐ = LEMS TOTAL ☐ — MAX (25) (25) (50)

SENSORY SUBSCORES

LTR ☐ + LTL ☐ = LT TOTAL ☐ — MAX (56) (56) (112)

PPR ☐ + PPL ☐ = PP TOTAL ☐ — MAX (56) (56) (112)

NEUROLOGICAL LEVELS (Steps 1-6 for classification as on reverse) — R L — 1. SENSORY 2. MOTOR

3. NEUROLOGICAL LEVEL OF INJURY (NLI)

4. COMPLETE OR INCOMPLETE? Incomplete = Any sensory or motor function in S4-5

5. ASIA IMPAIRMENT SCALE (AIS)

6. ZONE OF PARTIAL PRESERVATION (In injuries with absent motor OR sensory function in S4-5 only) — Most caudal levels with any innervation — R L — SENSORY MOTOR

Page 1/2

This form may be copied freely but should not be altered without permission from the American Spinal Injury Association.

REV 04/19

Muscle Function Grading

0 = Total paralysis

1 = Palpable or visible contraction

2 = Active movement, full range of motion (ROM) with gravity eliminated

3 = Active movement, full ROM against gravity

4 = Active movement, full ROM against gravity and moderate resistance in a muscle specific position

5 = (Normal) active movement, full ROM against gravity and full resistance in a functional muscle position expected from an otherwise unimpaired person

NT = Not testable (i.e. due to immobilization, severe pain such that the patient cannot be graded, amputation of limb, or contracture of > 50% of the normal ROM)

0*, 1*, 2*, 3*, 4*, NT* = Non-SCI condition present *

Sensory Grading

0 = Absent **1** = Altered, either decreased/impaired sensation or hypersensitivity

2 = Normal **NT** = Not testable

0*, 1*, NT* = Non-SCI condition present *

Note: Abnormal motor and sensory scores should be tagged with a '' to indicate an impairment due to a non-SCI condition. The non-SCI condition should be explained in the comments box together with information about how the score is rated for classification purposes (at least normal / not normal for classification).

When to Test Non-Key Muscles:

In a patient with an apparent AIS B classification, non-key muscle functions more than 3 levels below the motor level on each side should be tested to most accurately classify the injury (differentiate between AIS B and C).

Movement	Root level
Shoulder: Flexion, extension, adbuction, adduction, internal and external rotation **Elbow:** Supination	C5
Elbow: Pronation **Wrist:** Flexion	C6
Finger: Flexion at proximal joint, extension **Thumb:** Flexion, extension and abduction in plane of thumb	C7
Finger: Flexion at MCP joint **Thumb:** Opposition, adduction and abduction perpendicular to palm	C8
Finger: Abduction of the index finger	T1
Hip: Adduction	L2
Hip: External rotation	L3
Hip: Extension, abduction, internal rotation **Knee:** Flexion **Ankle:** Inversion and eversion **Toe:** MP and IP extension	L4
Hallux and Toe: DIP and PIP flexion and abduction	L5
Hallux: Adduction	S1

ASIA Impairment Scale (AIS)

A = Complete. No sensory or motor function is preserved in the sacral segments S4-5.

B = Sensory Incomplete. Sensory but not motor function is preserved below the neurological level and includes the sacral segments S4-5 (light touch or pin prick at S4-5 or deep anal pressure) AND no motor function is preserved more than three levels below the motor level on either side of the body.

C = Motor Incomplete. Motor function is preserved at the most caudal sacral segments for voluntary anal contraction (VAC) OR the patient meets the criteria for sensory incomplete status (sensory function preserved at the most caudal sacral segments S4-5 by LT, PP or DAP), and has some sparing of motor function more than three levels below the ipsilateral motor level on either side of the body. (This includes key or non-key muscle functions to determine motor incomplete status.) For AIS C – less than half of key muscle functions below the single NLI have a muscle grade ≥ 3.

D = Motor Incomplete. Motor incomplete status as defined above, with at least half (half or more) of key muscle functions below the single NLI having a muscle grade ≥ 3.

E = Normal. If sensation and motor function as tested with the ISNCSCI are graded as normal in all segments, and the patient had prior deficits, then the AIS grade is E. Someone without an initial SCI does not receive an AIS grade.

Using ND: To document the sensory, motor and NLI levels, the ASIA Impairment Scale grade, and/or the zone of partial preservation (ZPP) when they are unable to be determined based on the examination results.

ASIA — American Spinal Injury Association

INTERNATIONAL STANDARDS FOR NEUROLOGICAL CLASSIFICATION OF SPINAL CORD INJURY

ISCOS — International Spinal Cord Society

Page 2/2

Steps in Classification

The following order is recommended for determining the classification of individuals with SCI.

1. Determine sensory levels for right and left sides.
The sensory level is the most caudal, intact dermatome for both pin prick and light touch sensation.

2. Determine motor levels for right and left sides.
Defined by the lowest key muscle function that has a grade of at least 3 (on supine testing), providing the key muscle functions represented by segments above that level are judged to be intact (graded as a 5).
Note: in regions where there is no myotome to test, the motor level is presumed to be the same as the sensory level, if testable motor function above that level is also normal.

3. Determine the neurological level of injury (NLI).
This refers to the most caudal segment of the cord with intact sensation and antigravity (3 or more) muscle function strength, provided that there is normal (intact) sensory and motor function rostrally respectively.
The NLI is the most cephalad of the sensory and motor levels determined in steps 1 and 2.

4. Determine whether the injury is Complete or Incomplete.
(i.e. absence or presence of sacral sparing)
*If voluntary anal contraction = **No** AND all S4-5 sensory scores = **0** AND deep anal pressure = **No**, then injury is **Complete**.*
*Otherwise, injury is **Incomplete**.*

5. Determine ASIA Impairment Scale (AIS) Grade.
Is injury Complete? If YES, AIS=A
NO ↓
Is injury Motor Complete? If YES, AIS=B
NO ↓ (No=voluntary anal contraction OR motor function more than three levels below the motor level on a given side, if the patient has sensory incomplete classification)

Are at least half (half or more) of the key muscles below the neurological level of injury graded 3 or better?
NO ↓ AIS=C
YES ↓ AIS=D

If sensation and motor function is normal in all segments, AIS=E
Note: AIS E is used in follow-up testing when an individual with a documented SCI has recovered normal function. If at initial testing no deficits are found, the individual is neurologically intact and the ASIA Impairment Scale does not apply.

6. Determine the zone of partial preservation (ZPP).
The ZPP is used only in injuries with absent motor (no VAC) OR sensory function (no DAP, no LT and no PP sensation) in the lowest sacral segments S4-5, and refers to those dermatomes and myotomes caudal to the sensory and motor levels that remain partially innervated. With sacral sparing of sensory function, the sensory ZPP is not applicable and therefore "NA" is recorded in the block of the worksheet. Accordingly, if VAC is present, the motor ZPP is not applicable and is noted as "NA".

Fig. 3.5 Asia Impairment Scale © 2020 American Spinal Injury Association. (Reprinted with permission)

significant difference in functional motor and sphincter improvement between patients with complete and incomplete SCI. Van Middendorp et al. reported 91.7% negative predictive value in grade A patients for regaining ambulatory capability at 1 year, whereas grade D patients have a 97.3% positive predictive value for regaining independent ambulation at 1 year [80]. Similarly, others have shown a low probability for any significant improvement in grade A patients, as only 2.1% improved to grades B through E at 5 years [42]. In AIS, grade A, or complete SCI, is defined as the absence of all motor and sensory functions, including sacral roots, distal to the site of injury. Grades B through E are defined as incomplete injuries that retain some degree of motor or sensory function below the site of injury.

Nevertheless, the AIS scale does have some limitations that require attention. First, the injury level specified as a grade A lower lumbar injury could result in loss of bowel and bladder function and a foot drop, but the patient would still remain ambulatory; while a mid-cervical grade C or D patient could still be quadriparetic and dependent on significant assistance for activities of daily living and mobility. Second, AIS grades do not account for pain, spasticity, or dysesthesias that can still produce significant functional and mental disability for patients who are otherwise AIS grade E. Finally, no minimal clinically important difference has been defined in evaluation of patients in response to surgical or medical intervention, resulting in confusion with regard to defining thresholds for clinically significant changes for interventions.

Management Guidelines

Despite advances in protective safety equipment technology, an average of 7 catastrophic cervical spinal injuries with incomplete recovery and six quadriplegic events occurred in football alone in 2009 [66]. Surgical and medical treatments are available for the treatment of traumatic SCI, depending on the severity of injury, the anatomy of the structural spinal injury adjacent to the SCI, and the overall medical condition of the patient. Surgical intervention is generally indicated in the presence of ongoing spinal cord compression or unstable spinal fractures or ligamentous injuries. The exact timing of surgery and the effects of delays on neurologic outcome have historically been a point of controversy due to conflicting clinical [27] and animal data [31, 58]; however, more recent clinical data increasingly support the adoption of urgent or emergent surgical decompression paradigms based on both clinical series and prospective controlled trials [28].

Medical management begins with close monitoring for prevention of common cardiovascular and pulmonary complications of spinal shock, as well as optimization of various physiologic parameters for such perfusion, including maintenance of elevated mean arterial blood pressure. Neuroprotective or therapeutic agents for the treatment of acute spinal cord injury do not exist [81] and the use of high-dose steroids is contraindicated in these patients. Other potential treatments, such as induced hypothermia [19], stem cell therapy, biodegradable scaffolding [71], and endogenous growth factors, remain under active investigation [35]. For a full explanation of the current evidence-based medicine SCI recommendations, please refer to Chap. 5.

Conclusion

Athletics remains a common cause of spinal injuries worldwide, especially as sports participation increases. Although sports injuries often present with milder muscular strain or are nonstructural, they can also be a leading cause of catastrophic outcomes, such as acute SCI, depending on the activity. Early recognition of spinal injuries in various sports disciplines is vital to ensure proper medical and surgical management of both minor and more severe injuries. While minor issues mainly require symptomatic control and restriction from participation and activity limitation, major spine injuries should be approached in the same fashion as traumatic spinal injuries from other causes. Besides common clinical syndromes, standardized and validated systematic grading systems as well as severity scoring systems have been introduced for traumatic cervical, thoracic, and lumbar spinal injuries to assist the surgeon in deciding between initial medical vs surgical intervention.

References

1. Aarabi B, Walters BC, Dhall SS, Gelb DE, Hurlbert RJ, Rozzelle CJ, et al. Subaxial cervical spine injury classification systems. Neurosurgery. 2013;72(Suppl 2):170–86.
2. Allen BL Jr, Ferguson RL, Lehmann TR, O'Brien RP. A mechanistic classification of closed, indirect fractures and dislocations of the lower cervical spine. Spine (Phila Pa 1976).1982;7:1–27.
3. Anderson LD, D'Alonzo RT. Fractures of the odontoid process of the axis. J Bone Joint Surg Am. 1974;56(8):1663–74.
4. Anderson PA, Montesano PX. Morphology and treatment of occipital condyle fractures. Spine (Phila Pa 1976). 1988;13(7):731–6.
5. Ball JR, Harris CB, Lee J, Vives MJ. Lumbar spine injuries in sports: review of the literature and current treatment recommendations. Sports Med Open. 2019;5(1):26.
6. Baranto A, Hellström M, Cederlund CG, Nyman R, Swärd L. Back pain and MRI changes in the thoraco-lumbar spine of top athletes in four different sports: a 15-year follow-up study. Knee Surg Sports Traumatol Arthrosc. 2009;17(9):1125–34.
7. Barber HM. Horse-play: survey of accidents with horses. Br Med J. 1973;3:532–4.
8. Bellabarba C, Mirza SK, West GA, Mann FA, Dailey AT, Newell DW, et al. Diagnosis and treatment of craniocervical dislocation in a series of 17 consecutive survivors during an 8-year period. J Neurosurg Spine. 2006;4(6):429–40.
9. Boden BP. Direct catastrophic injury in sports. J Am Acad Orthop Surg. 2005;13(7):445–54.
10. Boden BP, Jarvis CG. Spinal injuries in sports. Neurol Clin. 2008;26(1):63–78.
11. Boden BP, Lin W, Young M, Mueller FO. Catastrophic injuries in wrestlers. Am J Sports Med. 2002;30:791–5.

12. Boden BP, Tacchetti R, Mueller FO. Catastrophic cheerleading injuries. Am J Sports Med. 2003;31(6):881–8.
13. Broe MP, Kelly JC, Groarke PJ, Synnott K, Morris S. Cycling and spinal trauma: a worrying trend in referrals to a national spine Centre. Surg J R Coll Surg Edinb Irel. 2017;16:202–6.
14. Brooks WH, Bixby-Hammett D. Head and spinal injuries associated with equestrian sports: mechanism and prevention. In: Torg JS, editor. Athletic injuries to the head, neck and face. St Louis, MO: Mosby; 1991. p. 133–41.
15. Castinel BH, Adam P, Prat C. A stress fracture of the lumbar spine in a professional rugby player. Br J Sports Med. 2007;41:337–8.
16. Chan CW, Eng JJ, Tator CH. Krassioukov a; spinal cord injury research evidence team. Epidemiology of sport-related spinal cord injuries: a systematic review. J Spinal Cord Med. 2016;39(3):255–64.
17. Denis F. The three column spine and its significance in the classification of acute thoracolumbar spinal injuries. Spine (Phila Pa 1976). 1983;8:817–31.
18. DePasse JM, Durand W, Palumbo MA, Daniels AH. Sex- and sport-specific epidemiology of cervical spine injuries sustained during sporting activities. World Neurosurg. 2019;122:e540–5.
19. Dididze M, Green BA, Dietrich WD, Vanni S, Wang MY, Levi AD. Systemic hypothermia in acute cervical spinal cord injury: a case-controlled study. Spinal Cord. 2013;51(5):395–400.
20. Divi SN, Schroeder GD, Oner FC, Kandziora F, Schnake KJ, Dvorak MF, et al. AOSpine-spine trauma classification system: the value of modifiers: a narrative review with commentary on evolving descriptive principles. Global Spine J. 2019;9(1 Suppl):77S–88S.
21. Dodwell ER, Kwon BK, Hughes B, Koo D, Townson A, Aludino A, et al. Spinal column and spinal cord injuries in mountain bikers: a 13-year review. Am J Sports Med. 2010;38(8):1647–52.
22. Donaldson LD. Spondylolysis in elite junior-level ice hockey players. Sports Health. 2014;6(4):356–9.
23. Drakos MC, Domb B, Starkey C, Callahan L, Allen AA. Injury in the national basketball association: a 17-year overview. Sports Health. 2010;2(4):284–90.
24. Dreisinger TE, Nelson B. Management of back pain in athletes. Sports Med. 1996;21:313–20.
25. Dunn IF, Proctor MR, Day AL. Lumbar spine injuries in athletes. Neurosurg Focus. 2006;21(4):E4.
26. Effendi B, Roy D, Cornish B, Dussault RG, Laurin CA. Fractures of the ring of the axis. A classification based on the analysis of 131 cases. J Bone Joint Surg Br. 1981;63-B:319–27.
27. Fehlings MG, Perrin RG. The timing of surgical intervention in the treatment of spinal cord injury: a systematic review of recent clinical evidence. Spine (Phila Pa 1976). 2006;31(11 Suppl):S28–35; discussion S36.
28. Fehlings MG, Vaccaro A, Wilson JR, Singh A, W Cadotte D, Harrop JS, et al. Early versus delayed decompression for traumatic cervical spinal cord injury: results of the Surgical Timing in Acute Spinal Cord Injury Study (STASCIS). PLoS One. 2012;7(2):e32037.
29. Firth JL. Equestrian injuries. In: Schneider RC, Kennedy JC, Plant ML (eds). Sports injuries. Mechanisms, prevention, and treatment. Baltimore, MD: Williams & Wilkins; 1985. pp. 431–449.
30. Francis WR, Fielding JW, Hawkins RJ, Pepin J, Hensinger R. Traumatic spondylolisthesis of the axis. J Bone Joint Surg Br. 1981;63-B(3):313–8.
31. Furlan JC, Noonan V, Cadotte DW, Fehlings MG. Timing of decompressive surgery of spinal cord after traumatic spinal cord injury: an evidence-based examination of pre-clinical and clinical studies. J Neurotrauma. 2011;28(8):1371–99.
32. Gerbino PG II, Micheli LJ. Back injuries in the young athlete. Clin Sports Med. 1995;14:571–90.
33. Gray BL, Buchowski JM, Bumpass DB, Lehman RA Jr, Mall NA, Matava MJ. Disc herniations in the National Football League. Spine (Phila Pa 1976). 2013;38(22):1934–8.
34. Hangai M, Kaneoka K, Hinotsu S, Shimizu K, Okubo Y, Miyakawa S, et al. Lumbar intervertebral disk degeneration in athletes. Am J Sports Med. 2009;37(1):149–55.
35. Hansebout RR, Kachur E. Acute traumatic spinal cord injury. UpToDate; 2018. Accessed 8 Jan, 2021.Available from: https://www.uptodate.com/contents/acute-traumatic-spinal-cord-injury.

36. Harris JH, Edeiken-Monroe B, Kopaniky DR. A practical classification of acute cervical spine injuries. Orthop Clin North Am. 1986;17:15–30.
37. Hu R, Mustard CA, Burns C. Epidemiology of incident spinal fracture in a complete population. Spine (Phila Pa 1976). 1996;21:492–9.
38. Jackson DW. Low back pain in young athletes: evaluation of stress reaction and discogenic problems. Am J Sports Med. 1979;7:364–6.
39. Jonasson P, Halldin K, Karlsson J, Thoreson O, Hvannberg J, Swärd L, et al. Prevalence of joint-related pain in the extremities and spine in five groups of top athletes. Knee Surg Sports Traumatol Arthrosc. 2011;19(9):1540–6.
40. Keene JS, Albert MJ, Springer SL, Drummond DS, Clancy WG Jr. Back injuries in college athletes. J Spinal Disord. 1989;2:190–5.
41. Kelly RP, Whitesides TE Jr. Treatment of lumbodorsal fracture-dislocations. Ann Surg. 1968;167:705–17.
42. Kirshblum S, Millis S, McKinley W, Tulsky D. Late neurologic recovery after traumatic spinal cord injury. Arch Phys Med Rehabil. 2004;85:1811–7.
43. Lee BB, Cripps RA, Fitzharris M, Wing PC. The global map for traumatic spinal cord injury epidemiology: update 2011, global incidence rate. Spinal Cord. 2014;52(2):110–6.
44. Lee JY, Vaccaro AR, Lim MR, Oner FC, Hulbert RJ, Hedlund R, et al. Thoracolumbar injury classification and severity score: a new paradigm for the treatment of thoracolumbar spine trauma. J Orthop Sci. 2005;10(6):671–5.
45. Levine AM, Edwards CC. The management of traumatic spondylolisthesis of the axis. J Bone Joint Surg Am. 1985;67(2):217–26.
46. Levy AS, Smith RH. Neurologic injuries in skiers and snowboarders. Semin Neurol. 2000;20:233–45.
47. Magerl F, Aebi M, Gertzbein SD, Harms J, Nazarian S. A comprehensive classification of thoracic and lumbar injuries. Eur Spine J. 1994;3(4):184–201.
48. Mall NA, Buchowski J, Zebala L, Brophy RH, Wright RW, Matava MJ. Spine and axial skeleton injuries in the National Football League. Am J Sports Med. 2012;40(8):1755–61.
49. McAfee PC, Yuan HA, Fredrickson BE, Lubicky JP. The value of computed tomography in thoracolumbar fractures. An analysis of one hundred consecutive cases and a new classification. J Bone Joint Surg Am. 1983;65(4):461–73.
50. Micheli LJ, Wood R. Back pain in young athletes. Significant differences from adults in causes and patterns. Arch Pediatr Adolesc Med. 1995;149:15–8.
51. Morrow PL, McQuillen EN, Eaton LA Jr, Bernstein CJ. Downhill ski fatalities: the Vermont experience. J Trauma. 1998;28:95–100.
52. Mueller FO, Cantu RC. National Center for catastrophic sports injury research: twentieth annual report, fall 1982–spring 2002. Chapel Hill: National Center for Catastrophic Sports Injury Research; 2002. p. 1–25.
53. Mundt DJ, Kelsey JL, Golden AL, Panjabi MM, Pastides H, Berg AT, et al. An epidemiologic study of sports and weight lifting as possible risk factors for herniated lumbar and cervical discs. The northeast collaborative group on low back pain. Am J Sports Med. 1993;21:854–60.
54. National Spinal Cord Injury Statistical Center (NSCISC), 2018 Annual statistical report for the spinal cord injur model systems. Accessed 22 March 2020. Available from: https://www.nscisc.uab.edu/public/2018%20Annual%20Report%20-%20Complete%20Public%20Version.pdf.
55. National Spinal Cord Injury Statistical Center (NSCISC), Recent Trends in Causes of Spinal Cord Injury. Birmingham, AL: University of Alabama at Birmingham, 2015. Accessed 30 Nov, 2020. Available from: https://www.nscisc.uab.edu/PublicDocuments/fact_sheets/Recent%20trends%20in%20causes%20of%20SCI.pdf.
56. National Spinal Cord Injury Statistical Center. Annual statistical report for the spinal cord injury model systems—complete public version. Spinal Cord Injury Model Systems, University of Alabama at Birmingham, Alabama; 2013. Accessed 8 Jan 2021. Available from: https://www.nscisc.uab.edu/PublicDocuments/reports/pdf/2013%20NSCISC%20Annual%20Statistical%20Report%20Complete%20Public%20Version.pdf.

57. Posner M, Cameron KL, Wolf JM, Belmont PJ Jr, Owens BD. Epidemiology of Major League Baseball injuries. Am J Sports Med. 2011;39(8):1676–80.
58. Rabinowitz RS, Eck JC, Harper CM Jr, Larson DR, Jimenez MA, Parisi JE, et al. Urgent surgical decompression compared to methylprednisolone for the treatment of acute spinal cord injury: a randomized prospective study in beagle dogs. Spine (Phila Pa 1976). 2008;33(21):2260–8.
59. Reckling Carlton W, Webb JK. Equestrian sports. In: Watkins RG, editor. The spine in sports. St Louis, MO: Mosby; 1996. p. 527–49.
60. Roberts DJ, Ouellet JF, Sutherland FR, Kirkpatrick AW, Lall RN, Ball CG. Severe street and mountain bicycling injuries in adults: a comparison of the incidence, risk factors and injury patterns over 14 years. Can J Surg. 2013;56(3):E32–8.
61. Roberts TT, Leonard GR, Cepela DJ. Classifications in brief: American spinal injury association (ASIA) impairment scale. Clin Orthop Relat Res. 2017;475(5):1499–504.
62. Scher AT. Rugby injuries to the cervical spine and spinal cord: a 10 year review. Clin Sports Med. 1998;17:195–206.
63. Schmitt H, Gerner HJ. Paralysis from sport and diving accidents. Clin J Sports Med. 2001;11:17–22.
64. Silver JR. Spinal injuries resulting from horse riding accidents. Spinal Cord. 2002;40(6):264–71.
65. Stone AT, Bransford RJ, Lee MJ, Vilela MD, Bellabarba C, Anderson PA, et al. Reliability of classification systems for subaxial cervical injuries. Evid Based Spine Care J. 2010;1:19–26.
66. Swartz EE, Boden BP, Courson RW, Decoster LC, Horodyski M, Norkus SA, et al. National athletic trainers' association position statement: acute management of the cervical spine-injured athlete. J Athl Train. 2009;44(3):306–31.
67. Tarazi F, Dvorak MF, Wing PC. Spinal injuries in skiers and snowboarders. Am J Sports Med. 1999;27:177–80.
68. Tator CH, Carson JD, Edmonds VE. Spinal injuries in ice hockey. Clin Sports Med. 1998;17:183–94.
69. Tator CH, Provvidenza C, Cassidy JD. Spinal injuries in Canadian ice hockey: an update to 2005. Clin J Sport Med. 2009;19(6):451–6.
70. Tawfik S, Phan K, Mobbs RJ, Rao PJ. The incidence of pars interarticularis defects in athletes. Global Spine J. 2020;10(1):89–101.
71. Theodore N, Hlubek R, Danielson J, Neff K, Vaickus L, Ulich TR, et al. First human implantation of a bioresorbable polymer scaffold for acute traumatic spinal cord injury: a clinical pilot study for safety and feasibility. Neurosurgery. 2016;79(2):E305–12.
72. Torg JS, Guille JT, Jaffe S. Current concepts review: injuries to the cervical spine in American football players. J Bone Joint Surg Am. 2002;84:112–22.
73. Torg JS, Vegso JJ, O'Neill MJ, Sennett B. The epidemiologic, pathologic, biomechanical, and cinematographic analysis of football-induced cervical spine trauma. Am J Sports Med. 1990;18(1):50–7.
74. Traynelis VC, Marano GD, Dunker RO, Kaufman HH. Traumatic atlanto-occipital dislocation. Case Report J Neurosurg. 1986;65(6):863–70.
75. United States Consumer Product Safety Commission summary reports. National Electronic Injuries Surveillance System [Internet]. Washington (DC): U.S. Consumer Safety Commission. Available from https://www.cpsc.gov.
76. Vaccaro AR, Hulbert RJ, Patel AA, Fisher C, Dvorak M, Lehman RA Jr, et al. The subaxial cervical spine injury classification system: a novel approach to recognize the importance of morphology, neurology, and integrity of the disco-ligamentous complex. Spine (Phila Pa 1976). 2007;32(21):2365–74.
77. Vaccaro AR, Koerner JD, Radcliff KE, Oner FC, Reinhold M, Schnake KJ, et al. AOSpine subaxial cervical spine injury classification system. Eur Spine J. 2016;25(7):2173–84.
78. Vaccaro AR, Lehman RA Jr, Hurlbert RJ, Anderson PA, Harris M, Hedlund R, et al. A new classification of thoracolumbar injuries: the importance of injury morphology, the integrity of the posterior ligamentous complex, and neurologic status. Spine (Phila Pa 1976). 2005;30:2325–33.

79. Vaccaro AR, Zeiller SC, Hulbert RJ, Anderson PA, Harris M, Hedlund R, et al. The thoracolumbar injury severity score: a proposed treatment algorithm. J Spinal Disord Tech. 2005;18:209–15.
80. van Middendorp JJ, Hosman AJ, Donders AR, Pouw MH, Ditunno JF Jr, Curt A, et al. A clinical prediction rule for ambulation outcomes after traumatic spinal cord injury: a longitudinal cohort study. Lancet. 2011;377:1004–10.
81. Walters BC, Hadley MN, Hurlbert RJ, et al. Guidelines for the management of acute cervical spine and spinal cord injuries: 2013 update. Neurosurgery. 2013;60(CN_suppl_1):82–91.
82. White AA, Panjabi MM, editors. Clinical biomechanics of the spine. 2nd ed. Philadelphia, PA: JB Lippincott; 1990.
83. Zahir U, Ludwig SC. Sports-related cervical spine injuries: on-field assessment and management. Semin Spine Surg. 2010;22(4):173–80.

Chapter 4
Neurosurgical Management of Spinal Cord Injuries in Athletes

Frank A. De Stefano, William J. Steele III, and Allan D. Levi

Epidemiology

Spinal cord injury (SCI) is a transient or permanent injury that affects sensory, motor, or autonomic function leading to neurological impairment or disability. SCI involving axon damage is mostly irreversible due to the non-regenerating properties of the central nervous system (CNS). Limited neuron growth, absence of neurotrophic factors, the involvement of CNS-related inhibitory factors, and glial scar development contribute to the poor prognosis of such injuries [2]. The United States reports the highest incidence of SCI with an estimated 906 cases per million. SCI is disproportionately more common in males below 30 years of age [3]. An estimated 7% of all new SCIs diagnosed each year are due to athletic activities in the United States [1]. Figure 4.1 demonstrates the percentage of SCI that occurs in each sport in comparison to the total sports-related SCI reported. Due to its higher level of interest, a common misconception exists that injuries of the spinal cord occur at a higher rate in organized sports, such as football, hockey, and rugby. Nonorganized sports, such as skiing and free-diving, have significantly higher rates of these injuries in comparison to organized sports [4]. In this section, we will discuss common injuries of the spine and spinal cord in athletes and their respective management.

F. A. De Stefano
School of Medicine, Kansas City University, Kansas City, MO, USA
e-mail: fdestefano@kansascity.edu

W. J. Steele III · A. D. Levi (✉)
Department of Neurosurgery, University of Miami Miller School of Medicine, Miami, FL, USA
e-mail: wjs98@med.miami.edu; alevi@med.maimi.edu

M. E. Oppenlander (ed.), *Neurosurgical Care of Athletes*, https://doi.org/10.1007/978-3-030-88227-3_4

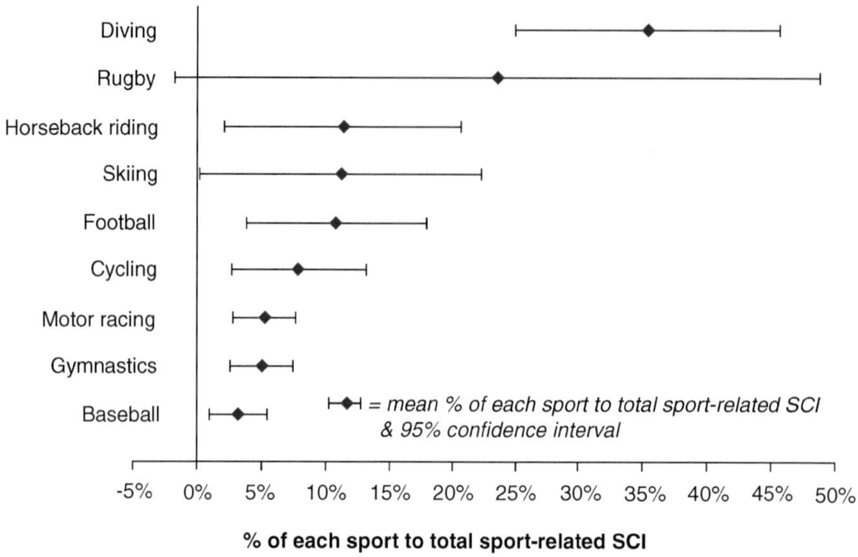

Fig. 4.1 Percentage of SCI as a percentage of all sports-related SCI reported worldwide. (Figured provided courtesy of Taylor and Francis Group [5])

Pathophysiology

Four main types of traumatic forces exist that can result in SCI: impact with persistent compression, impact with transient compression, distraction, and laceration/transection. Impact with persistent compression is most commonly seen in vertebral burst fractures or fractures resulting in dislocation. It is important to note that hyperextension forces typically result in an impact with transient compression. This type of force vector is a common cause of injury in contact sports [6, 7]. SCI occurs most often in the cervical region (53%), followed by thoracic (35%) and lumbosacral areas (11%). Concerning sports-related SCI, the cervical region is disproportionately affected in sports with the highest incidence of SCI [5]. Positioning of the cervical spine during impact is critical in its capability of dissipating axial forces applied at the head during impact. Flexion of the cervical spine during this force of impact is particularly vulnerable to fracture or dislocation, resulting in the most common cause of SCI [8]. The thoracic spine provides the highest structural integrity of the spinal column. High-impact forces are necessary to produce unstable injury. This integrity is, in part, due to support from costotransverse articulations and ligamentous attachments. In the thoracolumbar spine, the relatively narrow spinal canal and transition to more mobile vertebrae place the spinal cord at increased risk of injury with fracture/dislocation.

Two different pathomechanisms, primary and secondary injury, contribute to neurologic recovery and overall prognosis. The primary injury in SCI is a direct result of the mechanical forces applied to the cord during trauma. These forces disrupt vascular supply and directly damage neurons and supporting glia, resulting in cell dysfunction and possible death. The immediate cascade of pathologic events resulting from a primary injury is referred to as secondary injury. Cell dysfunction results in failure to maintain cell membrane integrity and metabolic requirements resulting in edema, inflammation, and apoptotic signaling pathways [9]. The resulting recruitment of inflammatory cells can lead to further permanent damage. It is critical to recognize and treat both pathomechanisms of SCI to improve neurologic recovery and prognostic outcomes.

Initial Evaluation and Management of Sports-Related Spinal Cord Injuries

The rapid, on-field assessment of the athlete suspected of traumatic SCI is strictly performed by qualified athletic staff or first responders. Trauma to multiple organ systems should be considered when evaluating suspected SCI due to the large impact forces needed to produce these injuries. The protocols for initial care in suspected SCI do not diverge from any other trauma scene. It is critical to assess the patient using Advanced Trauma Life Support (ATLS) guidelines, classically known as the ABCD's of trauma support: Airway maintenance, Breathing, Circulation, Disability (Neurologic Evaluation) [10]. Growing evidence suggests that up to 25% of SCI occur after the traumatic event, suggesting the spinal cord is extremely vulnerable to injury during transportation and medical care following suspected SCI [11]. Any patient with suspected SCI or injury that could potentially damage the spinal cord should be immobilized with a focus on moving the patient as minimal as possible. Steps to help with this include the immediate use of a rigid cervical collar, backboard with straps, and the log-roll method when transportation of the patient is necessary (Fig. 4.2) [12].

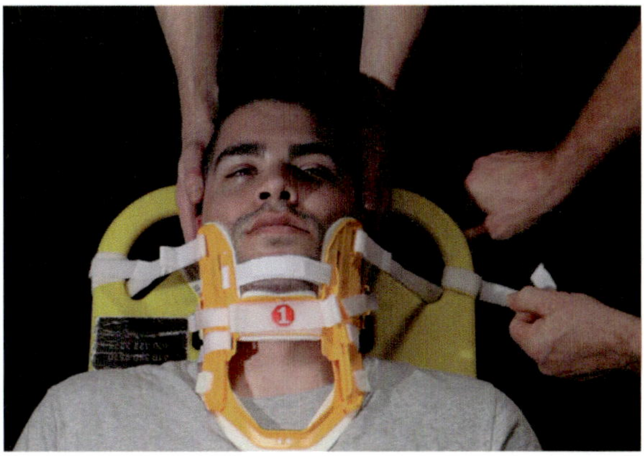

Fig. 4.2 Proper immobilization for suspected SCI. (Photo: XCollar Co. Ltd., all rights reserved)

In sports that require helmet and shoulder pads, it is advised to keep both pieces of equipment on the player until fracture can be ruled out with radiographic imaging [13]. If removing equipment from the player is necessary, removal of both pieces is recommended. Proper technique to remove equipment is critical to limit motion of the spine and prevent further injury. The chin strap and face mask should be removed first before removing the helmet. During removal of the helmet, manual inline stabilization of the cervical spine is necessary to restrict motion. Padding should be immediately placed under the athlete's head to decrease hyperextension during removal of the shoulder pads. Athletic trainers and medical staff are encouraged to practice equipment removal to better prepare for traumatic SCI during sporting events.

Classification of Spinal Cord Injuries

A full neurologic evaluation of the athlete with suspected SCI is critical in determining the course of acute medical management. Along with this, initial neurologic impairment is highly correlative with the degree of neurologic injury and prognostic outcome for the patient. Many classification tools have been proposed over time taking into consideration the anatomic location of the injury, initial neurologic deficits, and mental status at the time of injury. In 1984, the International Standards for Neurological Classification of Spinal Cord Injury (ISNSCI) produced a classification system for acute SCI to better assess neurological outcomes. The American Spinal Injury Association (ASIA) standard (Table 4.1) is a classification tool used to define neurologic levels of impairment and extent of injury in acute SCI. With its latest revision in 2013, this protocol is recommended in all patients with acute SCI at hospital admission. The ASIA Impairment Score (AIS) determines the level of neurological injury to be the most caudal spinal cord segment with intact motor and sensory function [14].

Table 4.1 American Spinal Injury Association (ASIA) assessment protocol

Grade	Impairment	Details
A	Complete	No sensory or motor function preserved in sacral segment S4–S5
B	Sensory incomplete	Sensory function is preserved below neurological level and includes sacral segments S4–S5. Motor function is not preserved
C	Motor incomplete	Motor function is preserved below the neurological level. Greater than 50% of key muscles below the neurological level have muscle grade < 3
D	Motor incomplete	Motor function is preserved below the neurological level. Greater than 50% of key muscles below the neurological level have muscle grade ≥ 3
E	Normal	Absence of any sensory or motor function deficit

Complete Spinal Cord Injury (AIS A)

Complete SCI results in both sensory and motor function deficits bilaterally below the level of the injury resulting from a complete disruption of the spinal cord pathways at any level. From 1973 to 2013, complete SCI composed 43.1% of all sports-related SCI in the United States [15]. Complete SCI illustrates the most severe level of injury and neurologic deficit. Depending on the neurological level, these patients can present with immediate death, respiratory failure (C3 and higher), autonomic instability, or bowel and bladder incontinence. Neurologic recovery and prognosis from complete SCI remains poor. Patients diagnosed with AIS A injuries have an 8.3% probability of walking independently at 1-year follow-up [16].

Incomplete Spinal Cord Injury (AIS B-D)

Injury resulting in any amount of preserved motor or sensory function below the neurologic level is classified as an incomplete SCI. An important diagnostic criterion differentiating incomplete from complete is the preservation of sensory function in sacral segments S4–S5. Several subtypes of incomplete SCI are described based on the anatomic location of injury: cervicomedullary syndrome, central cord syndrome, Brown–Séquard syndrome, anterior cord syndrome, and posterior cord syndrome. Each subtype of incomplete SCI varies greatly by the inflicting injury, typical neurologic deficit pattern, and prognosis. In clinical practice, patients typically present with mixed subtype presentations.

Early Medical Evaluation and Treatment

Management of patients with acute SCI is necessary in the neurologic intensive care unit (ICU) due to hemodynamic instability, need for continuous neurologic monitoring, and treatment for other injuries. Studies validate that early transfer to the ICU, rapid diagnosis, and management of systemic impairment mitigates further spinal cord damage due to secondary injury [17]. Interview of the patient and informants, physical examination, and vitals should be performed as soon as possible with great caution when moving or examining the patient. Physical examination should include a thorough inspection of the head, axial spine, and extremities. Documentation of any focal neurologic deficits, tenderness, structural abnormalities, or gross injuries is recommended. AIS grading, described earlier, is recommended in all patients with acute SCI within 72 h of admission. It is important to note that AIS grading may be unreliable up to 48 h postinjury due to transient manifestations of spinal shock [14]. Clinical factors that should raise suspicion of SCI include focal tenderness on the spinal column, weakness or numbness of the extremity, bowel or bladder incontinence, loss of consciousness during inciting event, or substance intoxication. It is important to note that 50% of patients with a Glasgow Coma Scale (GCS) less than 8 have been later found to have evidence of cervical spine injury [18]. Unfortunately, guidelines do not exist in the clearing of SCI in unconscious, sedated, or intubated patients and rely solely on radiographic imaging.

Neurogenic shock is a life-threatening sequela due to the disruption of autonomic innervation that maintains hemodynamic stability. Suspicion of neurogenic shock should be raised in injuries of the upper cord, with this form of shock occurring in 19.3% of cervical SCI and 7% of thoracic SCI [19]. It requires immediate recognition and should be distinguished from other causes of shock such as hypovolemic shock due to blood loss. Patients with neurogenic shock present with sudden hypotension, regular or irregular bradycardia, warm extremities, and possible priapism. Medical treatment should focus initially on blood pressure elevation utilizing intravenous fluids as first-line therapy followed by vasopressors for refractory cases [20]. Intravenous phenylephrine and norepinephrine have been described as viable options in the literature, although comparative data investigating outcomes has not been elucidated. Mean arterial pressure greater than 90 mm Hg for a minimum of 7 days post-injury is recommended to allow for adequate perfusion to the spinal cord [21]. Atropine in the treatment of bradycardia is recommended to improve bradycardia.

Respiratory complications are a major factor contributing to high morbidity and mortality in patients with SCI. The C3–C5 nerve roots are responsible for innervation of the diaphragm, the primary inspiratory muscle of the lungs. The diaphragm, along with the intercostal muscles, is the primary driver of inspiration. While expiration is primarily a passive movement, paralysis of the abdominal muscles in SCI can hinder full expiration cycles. Respiratory failure due to cervical SCI requires immediate intervention to establish an airway and support breathing. Flaccid paralysis of the intercostal muscles and diaphragm during spinal shock significantly reduces thoracic cavity volume and inspiratory drive resulting in an estimated 70% of forced vital capacity and 60% of maximal inspiratory force, respectively [22]. Fortunately, rebound spasticity allows for some return to baseline dynamics. Unopposed cholinergic activity resulting from neurogenic shock results in increased mucus production with ineffective clearance due to ciliary muscle paralysis. It is critical to take into consideration the many pathophysiologic factors that contribute to respiratory failure in patients with SCI to prevent hypoxemia and worsening of spinal cord ischemia.

Up to 84% of patients diagnosed with cervical SCI and 65% of patients with thoracic SCI experience respiratory complications post-injury, with atelectasis (36.4%), pneumonia (31.4%), and respiratory failure (22.6%) being the most common [23]. One-third of patients with cervical SCI will require endotracheal intubation with ventilator support. Indications for imminent respiratory failure include a reduction in respiratory vital capacity to less than 1 L, increasing respiratory rate, and a rising arterial PCO_2 [24]. Tracheal intubation techniques are variable in clinical practice and should take into consideration the instability of the spinal cord in patients with SCI. Traditional full extension of the atlanto-occipital and atlanto-axial joints has potential to cause iatrogenic injury to the spinal cord. A systematic review investigating outcomes of different intubation methods concludes that direct laryngoscopy results in increased adverse events and intubation should be performed utilizing a videolaryngoscope or fiberoptic assistance [25]. Ventilator-acquired pneumonia (VAP) is a common cause of mortality in patients requiring prolonged intubation. The risk of developing VAP increases by 1–3% per day of intubation with mortality as high as 43% due to the specific pathogen [26]. It is critical to start empiric antibiotic treatment in patients with new-onset fever, increased secretions, and leukocytosis. It is important to stress that critically-ill patients may have an equivocal presentation with VAP and should be monitored closely. Patients with SCI may require ventilator support for multiple weeks but should be weaned from ventilator support as soon as possible to reduce complication rates. Parameters suggestive of successful weaning include increased forced vital capacity, $FIO_2 < 50\%$, and minute ventilation <10 L [27].

Neurogenic bladder is a common sequela of spinal cord injury. Spinal shock following SCI results in inactivation of the parasympathetic nervous system efferents (S2–S4) with loss of the micturition reflex. Loss of innervation to the bladder results in detrusor muscle hypoactivity and urinary retention. Stasis of the bladder puts the patient at increased risk for renal failure, urinary tract infection (UTI), and urosepsis. Proper bladder management is critical to prevent these complications. Clean intermittent catheterization is recommended for urinary retention using hydrophilic-coated catheters to mitigate the risk of UTI [28]. The use of prophylactic antibiotics to prevent UTI has been debated in the literature. A recent meta-analysis investigating the risks and benefits of prophylactic antibiotics concluded there is insufficient evidence for their use in most patient groups [29].

The use of methylprednisolone sodium succinate (MPSS) in the management of acute phase SCI to prevent or reduce secondary injury is controversial and has been extensively debated. Studies have suggested its inefficacy as a treatment option for acute SCI when taking into consideration the complications that may arise from its use [30]. It is important to note that MPSS is used exclusively off-label as current FDA guidelines lack an indication for its use in the treatment of SCI. 2013 AANS/CNS guidelines do not recommend the use of MPSS in the treatment of acute SCI [31].

Systemic hypothermia is a modality recently proposed in the literature for acute management of cervical SCI with growing research for its use in all SCI. Systemic hypothermia involves cooling methods to reduce the intrathecal cerebrospinal fluid temperature. The use of hypothermia is implemented to reduce the damaging effects of both primary and secondary injuries. Preclinical and clinical data suggest the use of hypothermia playing an effective role in reducing vasogenic edema, excitotoxic metabolites, and decreasing the metabolic demand of the injured tissue. Earlier methods to induce hypothermia included surface cooling utilizing ice packs applied to the groin and axilla, cooling blankets, and lowering the environmental temperature of the patient. Newer methods have proposed intravenous infusion of chilled saline and intravascular heat exchange cooling catheters.

Preclinical data have demonstrated the following parameters produced favorable neurologic outcomes when initiating systemic hypothermia: modest targeted temperatures (32–34 °C), the onset of treatment to injury less than 8 h, treatment lasting 48 h, and gradual rewarming (0.5 °C/6 h) [32]. Levi et al. proposed an endovascular cooling procedure utilizing central venous femoral cooling catheters to achieve modest systemic hypothermia of 33 °C for an average of 47.6 h. Investigation of this method on 14 patients with cervical SCI found that 6 patients improved one AIS grade or greater at 1-year follow-up. Along with this, the study found no significant increase in complication rates in comparison to historical data, suggesting it is relatively safe to consider in patients [33]. A 2010 case report highlighting the use of systemic hypothermia in a professional football player suffering from complete (AIS A) cervical SCI showed rapid neurologic improvement and long-term recovery [34]. A multicenter trial to evaluate the safety and efficacy of systemic hypothermia for the acute treatment of cervical SCI is ongoing.

Imaging

Cervical plain film radiographs are still regarded as acceptable initial imaging when clinical suspicion of SCI is low. However, noncontrast-enhanced computed tomography (CT) has recently become the preferred initial imaging modality in patients with suspected SCI due to its availability, speed, and cost. CT dramatically outperforms plain film in detecting fracture or dislocation with a sensitivity of 100% and 63%, respectively [35]. CT is capable of detecting large soft tissue lesions such as disk herniation and epidural hematomas of considerable size. Unfortunately, CT lacks in delineating soft tissue structures or ligamentous injury in comparison to magnetic resonance imaging (MRI).

MRI is the superior imaging modality in the assessment of the spinal cord and soft tissue in comparison to plain film or CT. Due to the cost and time needed for acquisition, clinicians should have a high suspicion of ligamentous or neural damage before ordering and expect to gain valuable insight with this study. 2013 AANS/CNS guidelines suggest a level III recommendation for the use of MRI in the following scenarios: cervical fracture–dislocation injury that cannot be examined before closed reduction or failed closed reduction, decision-making to discontinue immobilization in awake, symptomatic patients or obtunded patients, diagnosis of atlanto-occipital dislocation or SCI with normal/equivocal findings on CT, evaluation of cord/nerve root compression and ligamentous injury, or predict outcomes in pediatric patients with SCI [36]. Spinal cord injury without radiographic abnormality (SCIWORA) is seen in up to 19% and 14% in children and adults, respectively. It is important to recognize the shortcomings in CT for the detection of SCI. Due to this, patients with focal neurologic deficits and negative or equivocal CT findings should undergo MRI as soon as possible for further work-up [37].

Typical MRI protocol for evaluating SCI includes T1-weighted, T2-weighted, and short tau inversion recovery (STIR)-weighted techniques. The presence of edema, hematoma, herniation, or loss of continuity should raise suspicion for

SCI. Findings supportive of urgent surgical intervention include ligamentous injury resulting in instability of the spinal column and reversible compressive forces such as disk herniation or hematoma. Operations to stabilize the spinal column or decompress the canal may result in immediate resolution of neurologic deficits and should be urgently considered. Sagittal T1-weighted MRI provides sufficient coverage for an overview of anatomical and structural findings of the spinal cord. Spinal cord edema and ligamentous injury are best visualized as hyperintensity foci on T2-weighted MRI with adequate fat suppression or STIR techniques. Evidence of hemorrhage is time-sensitive based on the hemosiderin composition of the hematoma at the time of imaging. Hematoma within 1 week of injury is best visualized on T2-weighted imaging and described as hypointense [35]. Although MRI is the preferred imaging modality in the detection of soft tissue injury and SCI, cases have been reported in the literature of MRI failing to detect these lesions. Diffusion-weighted imaging (DWI) and diffusion tensor imaging (DTI) are newer modalities shown to have higher sensitivity in detecting SCI and possible prognostic information. However, their use is limited in today's clinical practice.

Indication for Closed Reduction with Traction

Cervical facet dislocation is imperative to recognize early in the management of SCI and typically results from flexion–distraction forces. Failure of the posterior ligamentous structures and fracture of the vertebral articular processes are common radiographic findings in cervical facet dislocation. Both unilateral and bilateral cervical facet dislocation commonly result in complete and incomplete SCI. There is an ongoing debate regarding the method (open vs. closed) and the timing of reduction attempts in the current literature. However, closed reduction with traction is safe and effective for realignment of the spinal canal due to cervical fracture, dislocation, and subluxation [38]. Closed reduction can be successfully performed using Gardner-Wells tongs or halo ring. It is important to note that evidence of skull fracture or patients with altered mental status is an absolute contraindication for closed reduction. Weight recommendations for traction after reduction should take into consideration the severity of the dislocation, manufacturer recommendations, and the likelihood of subsequent open reduction interventions. It is also imperative that closed reduction be performed strictly at institutions capable of performing emergent surgery in case of patient deterioration or new-onset neurological deficits.

Surgical Considerations for Acute SCI

Surgical intervention may be a necessary treatment option for acute SCI to decompress the spinal cord, stabilize the spinal column, and reduce dislocations or fractures. A primary goal of surgical intervention is restoration of spinal canal anatomy by removal of bone, hematoma, or foreign bodies that may impinge the spinal cord.

Evidence-based guidelines for surgical management of acute SCI still are not fully established due to the multifactorial approach needed in patients with suspected SCI. Surgery should be considered on a case-by-case basis taking into account the patient's neurologic status, anatomic location of pathology, imaging findings, and other comorbidities. Optimal timing from injury to decompression and this timing's effect on prognostic outcomes remain elusive. A systematic review by Fehlings et al. found class II evidence supporting surgical decompression within 24 h of injury as safe and effective for the treatment of SCI. It was also found that urgent surgical intervention is recommended in all patients with SCI and neurologic deterioration or with cervical SCI and evidence of bilateral locked facets [39]. For other cases, it is important for the surgeon to have a clear benefit in pursuing surgery. Surgical considerations unique to the anatomic location of injury are discussed below.

It is practical to subdivide the cervical spine into upper (occiput-C2) and lower (C3-C7) when considering surgical intervention due to anatomic variation, degree of freedom, and intrinsic stability. The upper cervical spine allows high freedom of motion due to the lack of osseous restriction with stability achieved primarily through ligamentous support. The atlanto-occipital joint allows for up to 50% of flexion and extension in the cervical spine with stability achieved primarily by the anterior and posterior atlanto-occipital membranes. The atlantoaxial joint allows for up to 60% of cervical rotation with stability achieved through the transverse atlantal ligament. Injuries of the upper cervical spine rarely manifest with SCI due to the relatively large spinal canal space. Disruption of these ligaments can result in severe instability refractory to non-operative immobilization. Osseous architecture and ligamentous structure both contribute significantly to the stability of the lower cervical spine. The spinal canal narrows caudally resulting in a greater risk of spinal cord impingement with compressive or translational force. Due to the anatomical design, lower cervical spine injuries present with neurologic injury at far greater rates than the upper cervical spine.

Injuries resulting in occipitocervical dislocation present with severe instability and rapid fatality in some circumstances. Along with the neurologic injury, injury to the vertebral artery should be considered and investigated. Non-operative stabilization techniques in this region should not be considered due to the level of instability resulting from ligament disruption. A posterior approach for stabilization and fusion is recommended utilizing an occipitocervical arthrodesis with rigid internal fixation. The transverse atlantal ligament provides the most stability for the C1–C2 region. Forces result in disruption of the transverse atlantal ligament commonly present with fracture of the C1 or C2 vertebrae. The decision model for surgical treatment with this injury diverges on the location of disruption based on radiographic evidence. Type 1 injuries are described as purely ligamentous injury located at the midportion (IA) or laterally at the periosteal insertion (IB). Due to this, non-operative immobilization is not sufficient and stabilization via C1–C2 posterior arthrodesis is recommended. Type II injuries involve ligamentous injury along with evidence of comminuted fracture (IIA) or avulsion fracture (IIB) at the C1 lateral tubercle. Regarding type II injury, one study demonstrated a 75% healing rate using non-operative immobilization techniques using halo orthosis [40]. Nonoperative stabilization is a viable option that should be initially considered in patients with type II injuries.

Injuries of the lower cervical spine and their management are defined by the causative forces inflicted on the area. Forces seen most include compressive flexion, compressive extension, and distractive flexion. Compressive flexion injuries occur due to a combination of axial and flexile load applied through the head. Radiographic evidence suggesting subluxation, posterior ligament disruption, injury to the anterior column of the vertebral body, or facet injury suggests instability. Alignment in the sagittal plane is key in determining the surgical approach. The presence of alignment allows for an anterior approach with discectomy +/− corpectomy and fusion. In cases with malalignment or evidence of posterior facet damage, a posterior approach may be recommended. Distractive flexion injuries routinely present with serious neurologic deterioration and almost always require immediate surgical intervention. Such forces cause bilateral or unilateral facet dislocation with or without the presence of rotational forces. The severity of injury results from the failure of posterior ligamentous structures. Initial management of distractive flexion injuries is to restore alignment using closed reduction with traction. An anterior approach for decompression and stabilization is recommended if the proper alignment was attained following reduction attempts. In cases of failed alignment, a posterior approach may be necessary. Distractive extension injuries primarily occur due to disruption of the anterior longitudinal ligament, allowing for a widening of the anterior disk space resulting in a central cord syndrome. Patients without significant cervical stenosis tend to recover spontaneously, and surgical intervention is not required if stability is maintained. Evidence of instability should be treated surgically and focuses on restoring the anterior tension band through reconstruction and plating techniques.

The thoracolumbar junction (T10–L2) is a unique transition zone of the spinal column that is particularly vulnerable to SCI, occurring in 50% of all SCI [41]. Determination of complete or incomplete SCI is recommended initially. Surgical efficacy with complete SCI is minimal regarding future neurologic recovery and should generally be reserved to restore alignment or palliation [42]. In contrast, patients with incomplete SCI were found to have greater neurologic recovery when undergoing surgical decompression and stabilization [43]. Many classification systems have been proposed in the literature to categorize fractures of the thoracic and lumbar spine, although a single system is not universally accepted. Denis et al. constructed a system to classify thoracolumbar injuries by dividing the spine into three anatomical regions: anterior column (anterior longitudinal ligament and anterior two-thirds of the vertebral body), middle column (posterior longitudinal ligament, posterior one-third of the vertebral body, posterior vertebral wall), and posterior column (all ligaments and osseous structures posterior to the posterior longitudinal ligament). Surgical indication guidelines based on evidence of injury to these areas have been proposed and include injury to all three columns: 50% reduction in vertebral body height with evidence of posterior column ligamentous injury, any fracture–dislocation injury, and any indication of incomplete SCI [44, 45].

Table 4.2 Thoracolumbar Injury Classification and Severity (TLICS) score [46]

Injury parameter	Point value
Injury morphology	
Compression	1
Burst	2
Translation or rotation	3
Distraction	4
Posterior ligamentous complex integrity	
Intact	0
Injury suspected or indeterminate	2
Injured	3
Neurologic status	
Intact	0
Nerve root involvement	2
Spinal cord or conus medullaris injury	
Incomplete	3
Complete	2
Cauda Equina Syndrome	3
Score: 0–3 = Nonoperative, 4 = Surgeon choice, >4 = Operative candidate	

The thoracolumbar injury classification and severity (TLICS) score is an assessment tool proposed in 2005 by Vaccaro et al. to assist with the determination of surgical necessity in patients with thoracolumbar spinal injuries [46]. The TLICS score calculation takes into consideration clinical and radiologic features of the injury using three parameters: radiographic injury morphology, the integrity of the posterior ligamentous complex, and neurologic status. Table 4.2 provides the dependent values of the TLICS score and the associated decision model based on the total calculated score. A systematic review in 2016 evaluating the TLICS score in clinical practice concluded the assessment tool as safe with high concordance and validity [47]. The study did caution inconsistencies regarding the surgical treatment of stable burst fractures. Possibilities to suggest weakness in the TLICS score are due to lack of consideration in factors such as loss of vertebral height, segmental kyphosis, and canal compromise [48]. Although not validated, these findings are widely reported in the literature as important indications for surgery in this specific injury.

Considerations for Long-Term Hospitalization

During the hospital stay, complications may arise due to prolonged immobilization. Deep venous thrombosis (DVT), and potential pulmonary embolism (PE), is a common, serious issue in patients recovering from acute SCI. DVT was reported in greater than 50% of patients with acute SCI. Five percent of these patients experienced fatal pulmonary embolism. DVT prophylaxis with low-molecular-weight heparin is recommended in all patients with acute SCI for 8–12 weeks post-injury [49]. Joint contractures and stiffness are the most common complications during the acute treatment phase of SCI. Passive exercises in paraplegic and tetraplegic patients are recommended to prevent muscle atrophy, contractures, and pain [50]. Sandbags and pillows can be useful in proper positioning of joints, or, in severe cases, plaster splints and rigid orthotics. Decubitus ulcers commonly occur on the sacrum, trochanter, and ischium due to prolonged immobilization. Steps to avoid this should include position changes not exceeding every 2 h with proper hygienic attention to the at-risk area [51].

Secondary Complications Following Spinal Cord Injury

Post-traumatic deformities of the spine are common manifestations following SCI. Posttraumatic syringomyelia (PTS) is the development of fluid-filled cavities within the spinal cord following SCI. While PTS is radiographically present in up to 30% of cases, less than 10% present with clinical manifestations [52]. Timing of presentation varies widely. Some factors associated with early-onset PTS were advanced age, injuries at the cervical and upper thoracic levels, complete SCI, and patients who underwent surgical stabilization. These factors suggest that the early onset of PTS is in part due to the degree of cervical stenosis at injury as well as the severity of the injury [53]. Surgical intervention for PTS is reserved for patients with radiographic evidence of syrinx progression, neurologic deterioration, or increasing pain. Non-surgical treatment options include off-label pharmacotherapy targeting neuropathic pain including anticonvulsants, tricyclic antidepressants, and narcotic analgesics. Surgical options for the treatment of PTS reported in the literature include spinal decompression, syringostomy, and syringosubarachnoid shunting. Surgical guidelines for the treatment of PTS have not been established [53]. Treatment methods for PTS should be based on the individual's pathoanatomy, syrinx progression, and neurologic status at presentation.

Post-traumatic kyphotic deformity of the cervical spine is a common manifestation following traumatic SCI but can occur iatrogenically due to surgical intervention for the treatment of SCI. Progression of cervical kyphosis places the head in constant flexion leading to significant strain on the cervical musculature. Persistent head flexion can adversely affect vision, swallowing, and breathing. Maintaining forward head posture requires constant muscle contraction and significant force load on the cervical intervertebral discs [54]. Indications for surgical intervention in cervical kyphosis include neurologic deterioration and deformity progression. Evidence from the literature suggests that kyphosis progression of greater than 5 degrees in radiographic sagittal imaging is sufficient for surgical reconstruction [55, 56]. Strategies of surgical intervention remain controversial in the literature. Three main approaches for the treatment of cervical kyphosis are widely used: anterior, posterior, and combined. The main indications regarding the posterior surgical approach include the presence of flexible kyphosis. Anterior and combined methods differ in the degree of deformity correction and post-operative complications. A 2011 literature review found the combined method to produce a greater degree of correction but with higher rates of postoperative complications. The anterior approach alone produced less degrees of cervical lordosis correction but was associated with lower post-operative complication rates [57]. More evidence is needed to fully elucidate the efficacy of these procedure paradigms.

Acute and Long-Term Neurologic Outcomes

With the continued universal acceptance of the ASIA classification scheme, the scientific community is better able to investigate prognostic outcomes associated with the severity of the injury. Physicians are therefore better capable of discussing realistic expectations with patients on their road to recovery. While neurologic recovery can be assessed with many functional outcomes, the capability of ambulation is most studied. The probability of ambulation at 1 year post injury markedly decreases with the severity of injury, with AIS grades A and D found to be 8.3% and 97.3% ambulatory at 1 year, respectively. It is important to note the greatest variability of ambulation recovery occurs in patients with injury grades AIS B and C. Also, the conversion of AIS grades during recovery was poorly correlated to the ability to walk at a 6-month and 1-year follow-up [58]. A 2019 meta-analysis investigating neurologic outcomes of traumatic SCI found the AIS conversation rates of AIS grades A through D to be 19.3%, 73.8%, 87.3%, and 46.5%, respectively. The study also found the level of injury to be a significant predictor of neurologic recovery. Recovery rates based on anatomic location followed this descending order: lumbar, cervical and thoracolumbar, thoracic [59]. These findings demonstrate that recovery of neurologic function strongly depends on the severity of the injury, injury location, and mechanism of injury. Unfortunately, current medical therapies seem to play a lesser role in the prognostic outcomes of SCI in comparison to the inciting injury.

Conclusion

Trauma resulting in injury to the spine and spinal cord is a significant issue in many contact and noncontact sports. Spinal cord injury (SCI) is a medical emergency leading to neurological impairment and disability. Proper neurosurgical care is critical in the acute management of these injuries to reduce or prevent long-term disability.

Conflict of Interest The authors report no conflict of interest concerning the materials or methods used in this study or the findings specified in this paper.

Funding Source/Disclosure The authors have not received any funding for this work from any organization.

Works Cited

1. Boden BP, Tacchetti RL, Cantu RC, Knowles SB, Mueller FO. Catastrophic head injuries in high school and college football players. Am J Sports Med. 2007;35:1075–81.
2. Silver J, Schwab ME, Popovich PG. Central nervous system regenerative failure: role of oligodendrocytes, astrocytes, and microglia. Cold Spring Harb Perspect Biol. 2015; https://doi.org/10.1101/cshperspect.a020602.
3. Singh A, Tetreault L, Kalsi-Ryan S, Nouri A, Fehlings MG. Global prevalence and incidence of traumatic spinal cord injury. Clin Epidemiol. 2014;6:309–31.
4. Maroon JC, Bailes JE. Athletes with cervical spine injury. Spine. 1996;21:2294–9.
5. Chan CW, Eng JJ, Tator CH, Krassioukov A, Team SCIRE. Epidemiology of sport-related spinal cord injuries: a systematic review. J Spinal Cord Med. 2016;39:255–64.
6. Dumont RJ, Okonkwo DO, Verma S, Hurlbert RJ, Boulos PT, Ellegala DB, Dumont AS. Acute spinal cord injury, part I: pathophysiologic mechanisms. Clin Neuropharmacol. 2001;24:254–64.
7. Alizadeh A, Dyck SM, Karimi-Abdolrezaee S. Traumatic spinal cord injury: an overview of pathophysiology, models and acute injury mechanisms. Front Neurol. 2019;10:282.
8. Ackerman PD, Adelson PD, Anderson DE, et al. Neurosurgical Emergencies. 3rd ed; 2018. https://doi.org/10.1055/b-006-149754
9. Ahuja CS, Wilson JR, Nori S, Kotter MRN, Druschel C, Curt A, Fehlings MG. Traumatic spinal cord injury. Nat Rev Dis Primers. 2017;3:1–21.
10. Krost W, Mistovich J, Limmer D. Beyond the basics: trauma assessment. Emerg Med Serv. 2006;35:71–5; quiz 76
11. Theodore N, Hadley MN, Aarabi B, Dhall SS, Gelb DE, Hurlbert RJ, Rozzelle CJ, Ryken TC, Walters BC. Prehospital cervical spinal immobilization after trauma. Neurosurgery. 2013;72:22–34.
12. Cervical spine immobilization before admission to the hospital. Neurosurgery. 2002;50:S7–S17.
13. Walters BC, Hadley MN, Hurlbert RJ, Aarabi B, Dhall SS, Gelb DE, Harrigan MR, Rozelle CJ, Ryken TC, Theodore N. Guidelines for the management of acute cervical spine and spinal cord injuries: 2013 update. Neurosurgery. 2013;60:82–91.
14. Kirshblum SC, Waring W, Biering-Sorensen F, et al. Reference for the 2011 revision of the International Standards for Neurological Classification of Spinal Cord Injury. J Spinal Cord Med. 2011;34:547–54.
15. Organization WH, Society ISC. International perspectives on spinal cord injury. World Health Organization; 2013.
16. van Middendorp JJ, Goss B, Urquhart S, Atresh S, Williams RP, Schuetz M. Diagnosis and prognosis of traumatic spinal cord injury. Global Spine J. 2011;1:001–7.
17. Ahuja CS, Martin AR, Fehlings M. Recent advances in managing a spinal cord injury secondary to trauma [version 1; referees: 2 approved]. F1000Research. 2016; https://doi.org/10.12688/F1000RESEARCH.7586.1.
18. Morris CGT, McCoy E. Clearing the cervical spine in unconscious polytrauma victims, balancing risks and effective screening. Anaesthesia. 2004;59:464–82.
19. Taylor MP, Wrenn P, O'Donnell AD. Presentation of neurogenic shock within the emergency department. Emerg Med J. 2017;34:157–62.
20. Resnick DK. Updated guidelines for the management of acute cervical spine and spinal cord injury. Neurosurgery. 2013;72:1–1.
21. Jia X, Kowalski RG, Sciubba DM, Geocadin RG. Critical care of traumatic spinal cord injury. J Intensive Care Med. 2011;28:12–23.
22. McMichan JC, Michel L, Westbrook PR. Pulmonary dysfunction following traumatic quadriplegia: recognition, prevention, and treatment. JAMA. 1980;243:528–31.
23. Jackson AB, Groomes TE. Incidence of respiratory complications following spinal cord injury. Arch Phys Med Rehabil. 1994;75:270–5.

24. Fehlings MG, Vaccaro AR, Boakye M. Essentials of spinal cord injury: basic research to clinical practice. New York: Thieme; 2012.
25. Cabrini L, Baiardo Redaelli M, Filippini M, et al. Tracheal intubation in patients at risk for cervical spinal cord injury: a systematic review. Acta Anaesthesiol Scand. 2020;64:443–54.
26. Craven DE. Epidemiology of ventilator-associated pneumonia. Chest. 2000;117:S186.
27. Ball PA. Critical care of spinal cord injury. Spine. 2001;26:S27–30.
28. De Ridder DJMK, Everaert K, Fernández LG, Valero JVF, Durán AB, Abrisqueta MLJ, Ventura MG, Sotillo AR. Intermittent catheterisation with hydrophilic-coated catheters (SpeediCath) reduces the risk of clinical urinary tract infection in spinal cord injured patients: a prospective randomised parallel comparative trial. Eur Urol. 2005;48:991–5.
29. Morton SC, Shekelle PG, Adams JL, Bennett C, Dobkin BH, Montgomerie J, Vickrey BG. Antimicrobial prophylaxis for urinary tract infection in persons with spinal cord dysfunction. Arch Phys Med Rehabil. 2002;83:129–38.
30. Hurlbert RJ. Methylprednisolone for acute spinal cord injury: an inappropriate standard of care*. J Neurosurg (Spine 1). 2000;93:1–7.
31. Hurlbert RJ, Hadley MN, Walters BC, Aarabi B, Dhall SS, Gelb DE, Rozzelle CJ, Ryken TC, Theodore N. Pharmacological therapy for acute spinal cord injury. Neurosurgery. 2013;72:93–105.
32. Ahmad FU, Wang MY, Levi AD. Hypothermia for acute spinal cord injury—a review. World Neurosurg. 2014;82:207–14.
33. Levi AD, Green BA, Wang MY, Dietrich WD, Brindle T, Vanni S, Casella G, Elhammady G, Jagid J. Clinical application of modest hypothermia after spinal cord injury. J Neurotrauma. 2009;26:407–15.
34. Cappuccino A, Bisson LJ, Carpenter B, Marzo J, Dietrich WDI, Cappuccino H. The use of systemic hypothermia for the treatment of an acute cervical spinal cord injury in a professional football player. Spine. 2010;35:E57–62.
35. Parizel PM, Van der Zijden T, Gaudino S, Spaepen M, Voormolen MHJ, Venstermans C, De Belder F, Van Den Hauwe L, Van Goethem J. Trauma of the spine and spinal cord: imaging strategies. Eur Spine J. 2010;19:8–17.
36. Ryken TC, Hadley MN, Walters BC, Aarabi B, Dhall SS, Gelb DE, Hurlbert RJ, Rozzelle CJ, Theodore N. Radiographic assessment. Neurosurgery. 2013;72:54–72.
37. Szwedowski D, Walecki J. Spinal cord injury without radiographic abnormality (SCIWORA)–clinical and radiological aspects. Pol J Radiol. 2014;79:461.
38. Bransford RJ, Stevens DW, Uyeji S, Bellabarba C, Chapman JR. Halo vest treatment of cervical spine injuries: a success and survivorship analysis. Spine. 2009;34:1561–6.
39. Furlan JC, Noonan V, Cadotte DW, Fehlings MG. Timing of decompressive surgery of spinal cord after traumatic spinal cord injury: an evidence-based examination of pre-clinical and clinical studies. J Neurotrauma. 2009;28:1371–99.
40. Dickman CA, Greene KA, Sonntag VKH. Injuries involving the transverse atlantal ligament: classification and treatment guidelines based upon experience with 39 injuries. Neurosurgery. 1996;38:44–50.
41. Singh K, Erdos J, Sah A, Vaccaro AR, McLain RF. The value of surgical intervention in spinal trauma. In: Spine surgery. Elsevier; 2005. p. 1367–72.
42. Fehlings MG, Tator CH. An evidence-based review of decompressive surgery in acute spinal cord injury: rationale, indications, and timing based on experimental and clinical studies. J Neurosurg Spine. 1999;91:1–11.
43. Mumford J, Weinstein JN, Spratt KF, Goel VK. Thoracolumbar burst fractures. The clinical efficacy and outcome of nonoperative management. Spine. 1993;18:955–70.
44. Denis F. The three column spine and its significance in the classification of acute thoracolumbar spinal injuries. Spine. 1983;8:817–31.
45. Cantor JB, Lebwohl NH, Garvey T, Eismont FJ. Nonoperative management of stable thoracolumbar burst fractures with early ambulation and bracing. Spine. 1993;18:971–6.

46. Vaccaro AR, Lehman RA Jr, Hurlbert RJ, Anderson PA, Harris M, Hedlund R, Harrop J, Dvorak M, Wood K, Fehlings MG. A new classification of thoracolumbar injuries: the importance of injury morphology, the integrity of the posterior ligamentous complex, and neurologic status. Spine. 2005;30:2325–33.
47. Joaquim AF, de Almeida Bastos DC, Jorge Torres HH, Patel AA. Thoracolumbar injury classification and injury severity score system: a literature review of its safety. Global Spine J. 2016;6:80–5.
48. Joaquim AF, Patel AA. Thoracolumbar spine trauma: evaluation and surgical decision-making. J Craniovertebr Junction Spine. 2013;4:3.
49. Teasell RW, Hsieh JT, Aubut J-AL, Eng JJ, Krassioukov A, Tu L. Venous thromboembolism after spinal cord injury. Arch Phys Med Rehabil. 2009;90:232–45.
50. Diong J, Harvey LA, Kwah LK, Eyles J, Ling MJ, Ben M, Herbert RD. Incidence and predictors of contracture after spinal cord injury - a prospective cohort study. Spinal Cord. 2012;50:579–84.
51. Kruger EA, Pires M, Ngann Y, Sterling M, Rubayi S. Comprehensive management of pressure ulcers in spinal cord injury: current concepts and future trends. J Spinal Cord Med. 2013;36:572–85.
52. Carroll ÁM, Brackenridge P. Post-traumatic syringomyelia: a review of the cases presenting in a regional spinal injuries unit in the north east of England over a 5-year period. Spine. 2005;30:1206–10.
53. Vannemreddy S, Rowed DW, Bharatwal N. Posttraumatic syringomyelia: predisposing factors. Br J Neurosurg. 2002;16:276–83.
54. Katsuura A, Hukuda S, Imanaka T, Miyamoto K, Kanemoto M. Anterior cervical plate used in degenerative disease can maintain cervical lordosis. J Spinal Disord. 1996;9:470–6.
55. Woodworth RS, Molinari WJ, Brandenstein D, Gruhn W, Molinari RW. Anterior cervical discectomy and fusion with structural allograft and plates for the treatment of unstable posterior cervical spine injuries. J Neurosurg Spine. 2009;10:93–101.
56. Koivikko MP, Myllynen P, Karjalainen M, Vornanen M, Santavirta S. Conservative and operative treatment in cervical burst fractures. Arch Orthop Trauma Surg. 2000;120:448–51.
57. Han K, Lu C, Li J, Xiong G-Z, Wang B, Lv G-H, Deng Y-W. Surgical treatment of cervical kyphosis. Eur Spine J. 2011;20:523–36.
58. van Middendorp JJ, AJF H, Pouw MH, Van de Meent H, EM-SCI Study Group. ASIA impairment scale conversion in traumatic SCI: is it related with the ability to walk? A descriptive comparison with functional ambulation outcome measures in 273 patients. Spinal Cord. 2009;47:555–60.
59. Khorasanizadeh MH, Yousefifard M, Eskian M, et al. Neurological recovery following traumatic spinal cord injury: a systematic review and meta-analysis. J Neurosurg Spine. 2019;30:683–99.

Chapter 5
Evaluation and Management of Cervical Radiculopathy in Athletes

Steve Monk, David Peters, and Tim Adamson

Abbreviations

ACDF	anterior discectomy and fusion
ASD	adjacent segment disease
CDR	cervical disc replacement
MED	microendoscopic
PCF	posterior cervical foraminotomy

Introduction

Cervical radiculopathy is a common source of pain and impairment in the general population. For athletes in particular, it provides challenges in diagnosis and management. One large population-based study reported an estimated incidence of 107.3 per 100,000 men and 63.5 per 100,000 for women [1]. The C6–7 level is by far the most frequently affected level, with C5–6 following as a distant second [2]. Although no population-based studies have examined incidence among athletes, a study of military patients found an incidence of 1.79 per 1000 person-years [3]. Analysis of a National Football League (NFL) database revealed an incidence of

S. Monk (✉) · D. Peters
Atrium Health Carolinas Medical Center, Department of Neurosurgery, Charlotte, NC, USA
e-mail: Steve.Monk@CNSA.com; David.Peters@CNSA.com

T. Adamson
Carolina Neurosurgery & Spine Associates, Charlotte, NC, USA
e-mail: Tim.Adamson@CNSA.com

M. E. Oppenlander (ed.), *Neurosurgical Care of Athletes*,
https://doi.org/10.1007/978-3-030-88227-3_5

2208 spine injuries over 10 years, 987 of which affected the cervical spine [4]. This study did not isolate cervical radiculopathy, but of these 987 cervical spine injuries, 5.8% were disc herniations, 4.7% were impingement, and 45.9% were nerve injuries, commonly referred to as "stingers" or "burners." Notably, upper cervical sources of radiculopathy involving C2–3 and C3–4 are exceedingly rare in the general population, but are much more common in athletes, particularly those participating in high-velocity contact sports [5]. A study of 40 NFL players found that 37.5% had degenerative changes at C2–3 (1) or C3–4 (14) [6].

Cervical radiculopathy is a major concern among athletes and the medical staff that provide care for them, especially in high-velocity contact sports. Proper diagnosis and management of each individual athlete is critically important given the potential for catastrophic injury and potentially career-ending decisions if not managed appropriately. Decisions are frequently made during competition, and confirming a diagnosis of radiculopathy is crucial in order to eliminate the much more serious cervical myelopathy, or the less serious brachial plexus "stinger." Once a diagnosis is made, the severity of signs and symptoms often dictates early management and the need for radiographic work-up. The majority of these cases can be managed with conservative therapy measures, including physical therapy, chiropractic care, anti-inflammatories, and targeted cervical steroid injections. In cases refractory to conservative measures, the decision to proceed to surgical intervention poses significant challenges. Although outcomes from single-level cervical surgery in the general population are excellent, with 90–95% patient satisfaction [7], the decision process in athletes is complicated by timing of return to competition and possible career-ending factors. Cervical fusion limits segmental motion, flexibility, and strength, which can significantly impact sport-specific performance in high-level and professional athletes. At a minimum, it can often leave players with a psychological barrier from perceived limited ability, which can in turn impact time to return, intensity of play, and stoke fears of catastrophic spinal cord injury [8]. The type of surgical intervention can significantly impact these factors. An anterior cervical fusion, posterior cervical foraminotomy, or cervical disc arthroplasty can all be effective in managing cervical radiculopathy, but each has its own nuances regarding proper patient selection and timing of return to play. The following chapter covers the diagnosis, conservative management, operative management, and return-to-play decisions encountered when managing cervical radiculopathy in athletes.

Diagnosis

Clinical History

Cervical radiculopathy can often be diagnosed from the clinical history and physical examination alone. It is important to determine the nature of onset and the pattern of symptoms. For example, did the pain start suddenly during a game or insidiously over days to weeks? Does the pain stop in the shoulder or radiate to the hand? Does the athlete notice any numbness or weakness? Do any positions improve or worsen the symptoms? How much of the pain is in the neck versus the arm? Classic symptoms include burning, shooting pain, and paresthesia in a dermatomal distribution based on the affected nerve root. Neck and shoulder pain may be present, particularly with disc herniations in the upper cervical spine (e.g., C2–3, C3–4, C4–5). It is also extremely important to determine if there are any bilateral arm symptoms, leg symptoms, alterations of gait, or bowel/bladder changes, as these symptoms suggest cervical myelopathy over radiculopathy and can have significant implications on subsequent management decisions.

Physical Examination

A complete neurological evaluation should be completed on every athlete presenting with cervical radiculopathy symptoms. The confirmation of specific myotome, dermatome, and reflex changes frequently allows identification of the specific root involved. No myelopathic findings should be present, and the lower extremity examination should be normal in the absence of a concomitant thoracic or lumbar spine injury. If greater than one ipsilateral nerve root or bilateral nerve roots are found to be involved, then this must be presumed to be myelopathy until proven otherwise, especially during competition. Provocative tests such as Spurling's maneuver can be helpful if present but are not highly sensitive. Upper cervical radiculopathies are much harder to diagnose on examination, but the pattern of pain radiation can be very helpful. This pattern of pain is generally suboccipital in C2 or C3 and to the top of the shoulder in C4.

Imaging Studies

MRI is readily available and is frequently the initial source of imaging for evaluating cervical radiculopathy. It provides detailed visualization of the cervical anatomy and allows for assessment of nerve root or spinal cord compression. In the setting of a competition injury, CT scans of the cervical spine may be indicated to rule out a fracture, as they are preferable for the evaluation of bony anatomy. CT scans also provide a clearer view of the foraminal anatomy and are often helpful for clarifying the etiology of foraminal nerve root compression, specifically a disc herniation versus spondylotic foraminal narrowing. Disc herniations and spondylosis are equally common causes of radiculopathy, even in younger athletes (Fig. 5.1). Cervical x-rays with flexion and extension views are helpful in assessing the stability of the spine. Occasionally, in more challenging cases, cervical myelography with CT evaluation can be helpful.

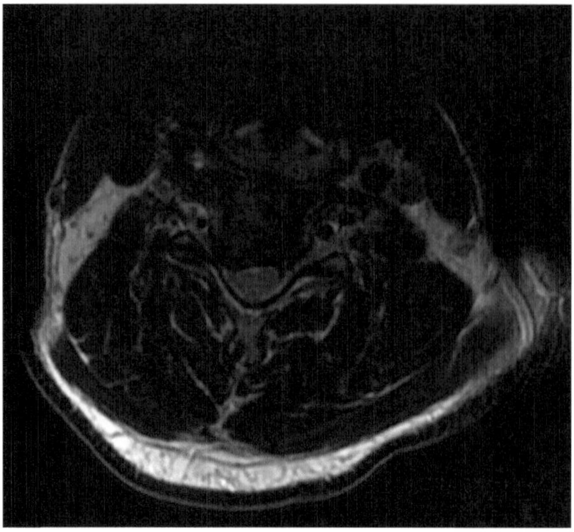

Fig. 5.1 Cervical spondylosis causing unilateral severe foraminal narrowing and right-sided radiculopathy

Ancillary Testing

Electrodiagnostic evaluation including electromyography (EMG) and nerve conduction velocity (NCV) can also play a role in the diagnosis of cervical radiculopathy, particularly in cases with an atypical history and/or examination. Their utility is limited in the setting of acute nerve injury, however, due to a high false-negative rate in the first 3 to 4 weeks after injury [9]. Positive results on these tests can help make the diagnosis, but many cases of painful and acute radiculopathy will be negative due to the low sensitivity in the acute period.

Differential Diagnosis

The variety of cervical radiculopathy syndromes can make diagnosis and management challenging, especially when considering return-to-play decisions and the role of surgical intervention. It is important and sometimes challenging to differentiate a radiculopathy from a "stinger" or "burner" and the more serious "spinal cord concussion," also known as cervical cord neuropraxia. A stinger or burner is a common injury seen in collision and contact sports characterized by unilateral burning and lancinating dysesthesia radiating down an upper extremity with variable motor and sensory changes [10]. The purported etiology is a traction injury to the upper brachial plexus from forced depression of the shoulder or from lateral hyperflexion of the head to the contralateral side. Symptoms usually resolve in minutes to hours. Cervical spine imaging should be obtained in the setting of prior episodes or persistent symptoms. Foraminal stenosis and congenital spinal stenosis are risk factors for stingers.

A cervical cord concussion, also known as cervical cord neuropraxia, represents a transient spinal cord injury [11]. It can usually be distinguished from stingers and radiculopathy by the presence of bilateral symptoms and/or involvement of the lower extremities. Patients are frequently observed to have quadriparesis, paresthesia, and dysesthesias, which may resolve over minutes to hours. Urgent medical evaluation and imaging are indicated to assess for congenital or acquired spinal stenosis. A small percentage of these patients will have no significant structural abnormality, and the mechanism of injury in this subset of patients is presumed to be transient cord compression secondary to a supraphysiologic range of motion.

Management

Nonsurgical

The benign natural history of cervical radiculopathy has been consistently reported in the general population, with over 90% of patients achieving complete symptom resolution within a few months [12, 13]. Consequently, nonoperative management is the initial treatment of choice in the vast majority of cases. Interventions that fall under this umbrella include activity modification, analgesia (NSAIDs, steroids, narcotics), epidural steroid injections, and physical therapy.

Nonoperative management is likewise the initial standard of care for cervical radiculopathy in athletes. Physical therapy plays a crucial role in this population, as complete symptom resolution, full range of motion, and full strength are required for return to play. Epidural steroids are safe and effective in this population [14]. It is worth noting, however, that multiple series report a lower return-to-play rate in athletes treated nonoperatively versus operatively. In Hsu's series of 99 NFL players, 72% (38 of 53) of players who underwent surgery returned to play, compared to just 46% (21 of 46) treated nonoperatively [15]. Moreover, athletes treated surgically went on to have longer and more productive careers than those treated nonoperatively. Similarly, Roberts' report of MLB pitchers showed an 88% (7 of 8) return-to-play rate in players treated surgically versus 33% (1 of 3) in those treated nonoperatively [16].

Surgical

Operative intervention is indicated for patients who fail initial nonoperative management, have significant motor deficits, cord signal change, or intractable, life-altering pain on presentation. There are three surgical techniques that can be used to address cervical radiculopathy: anterior cervical discectomy and fusion (ACDF), posterior cervical foraminotomy (PCF), and cervical disc replacement (CDR). The following pages discuss each of these procedures specifically in athletes, including their effectiveness, complications, and return-to-play considerations.

Effectiveness

Anterior Cervical Discectomy and Fusion

Anterior cervical discectomy and fusion (ACDF) is the most common surgical intervention for cervical radiculopathy. First described by Smith and Robinson in 1955, it has a long track record of proven success for treating a variety of cervical spine pathologies with good clinical outcomes and a favorable safety profile. ACDF similarly has become the workhorse operation for cervical radiculopathy in athletes. Among the three surgical options for cervical radiculopathy, ACDF has the strongest evidence base to support its safety and efficacy in professional athletes, even those who play high-velocity collision sports.

Andrews et al. were the first to report the use of ACDF for cervical radiculopathy in professional athletes [17]. Their retrospective review of 19 professional rugby players found that radicular pain was eradicated in 15 patients and improved in 2 patients, while neck pain was eradicated in 8 patients and improved in 9 patients. Thirteen of the cohort returned to their previous level of play.

A landmark paper by Hsu et al. first reported the use of ACDF for surgical management of cervical disc herniation in National Football League players [15]. In their cohort of 99 players, 53 underwent operative treatment—single-level ACDF in 32 cases, PCF in 3 cases, and an undetermined procedure in 18 cases. Those treated surgically were significantly more likely to return to play (72% vs. 46%), play more games (29.3 vs. 14.7), and have longer careers (2.8 years vs. 1.5 years) than those treated nonoperatively. Moreover, those who successfully returned to play had no significant difference in performance outcomes, and none suffered a subsequent spinal cord injury. Given that the average NFL career is 3.5 years and the average retirement age is 27 years [18], these results directly refuted the popular belief that a cervical disc herniation represented a devastating injury to a player's professional career.

Roberts et al. reported a series of 40 Major League Baseball (MLB) pitchers with cervical (11) or lumbar (29) disc herniations [16]. Of those with a cervical disc herniation, 8 underwent operative treatment—7 with single-level ACDF and 1 with cervical disc replacement. Overall, 88% (7/8) of those treated surgically returned to play, compared to 33% (1/3) of those treated nonoperatively. Surgical patients returned to play an average of 11.6 months postoperatively and pitched an average of 63 games over 3.7 years. Although these players pitched less innings per season, their performance status was not statistically different than before surgery.

Maroon et al. reported the experience of 15 professional football players and wrestlers who underwent ACDF for cervical radiculopathy (8) or neuropraxia (7) [19]. Thirteen (87%) returned to play on average 6 months after surgery, including all 8 who were treated for a cervical radiculopathy. In sum, these studies in high-level athletes demonstrate that the well-known efficacy and safety of ACDF in the general population has good generalizability to athletes.

Posterior Cervical Foraminotomy

The use of a posterior approach for surgical management of cervical radiculopathy was introduced over 70 years ago. The initial experience by Semmes and Murphy

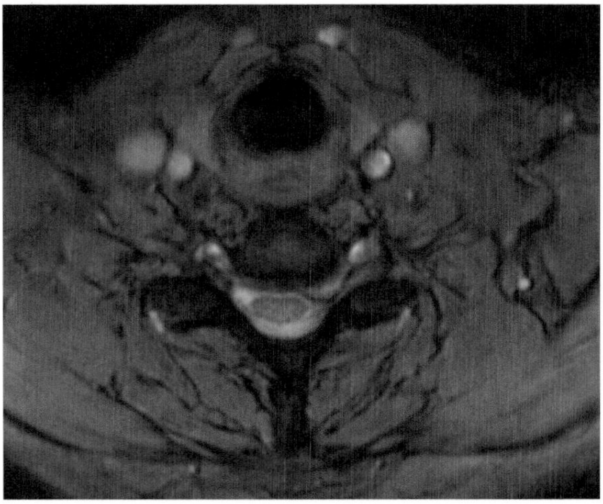

Fig. 5.2 Left paracentral cervical disc herniation causing foraminal stenosis and left-sided radiculopathy. This disc was removed by a PCF and symptoms resolved

[20] and Frykholm [21] described creation of a small laminoforaminotomy to treat lateral or foraminal disc herniations and spondylotic foraminal narrowing with good outcomes (Fig. 5.2). Although the anterior approach has largely supplanted posterior cervical foraminotomy for the surgical management of cervical disc herniation, concern over adjacent segment disease and recent advances in microendoscopic (MED) techniques make PCF a better alternative for appropriately selected patients. Contraindications to the approach include spinal deformity, instability, myelopathy, or bilateral disc herniation.

Adamson pioneered the use of microendoscopic (MED) techniques for the treatment of cervical radiculopathy nearly 20 years ago. In his first report of 100 consecutive patients, 97 achieved excellent or good outcome and were able to return to their previous employment and level of physical activity [22]. Only 3 patients experienced a surgical complication. Multiple other authors have reported similarly excellent outcomes [23, 24].

The efficacy, safety, and quick return-to-activity afforded by MED-PCF make it an attractive option for athletes who require surgical management of cervical radiculopathy. Adamson reported the first series in this population with encouraging results [25]. Ten athletes (8 professional football players and 2 professional race car drivers) were treated. Seven of the 8 football players returned to play after resolution of preoperative motor deficits. The one who did not return to play had a C5 motor deficit that never fully recovered. Both race car drivers were treated in the offseason and returned to driving within 4 weeks.

Adamson's personal series of over 1600 MED-PCFs performed since 1997 contains 22 athletes, including the 10 in the study cited above (unpublished data). The current series includes 16 collegiate or professional football players and 6 professional race car drivers. Fifteen of the 16 football players returned to play by the next season (10 in the same season, 5 in the next season), and all 6 race car drivers returned to competition after the off-season. One of the football players required additional surgery 1.5 years later for multilevel spondylotic disease.

In the aforementioned study by Hsu et al. [15], 3 of the 53 NFL players who underwent surgical treatment for cervical radiculopathy were treated with a

PCF. The reported outcomes did not stratify patients by surgical approach, but overall 72% of patients returned to play for an average of 29.3 games over a 2.8-year period. Notably, 5.3% of players required another operation at the index or an adjacent level during the study period.

Cervical Disc Replacement

Cervical disc replacement (CDR) was developed as alternative to ACDF with the goal of preserving motion at the index level and decreasing the rate of adjacent segment disease. The safety and efficacy of CDR has been consistently demonstrated in multiple FDA investigational device exemption (IDE) studies [26]. Currently, the FDA-approved indications for CDR include 1- and 2-level central and/or paracentral soft disc herniation from C3 to C7 for patients with radiculopathy with or without neck pain. Multiple studies have demonstrated a lower rate of adjacent-level reoperation in the long-term compared to ACDF [26–29].

Despite the abundance of literature evaluating CDR in the general population, there are few studies that specifically address the safety and efficacy of CDR for the treatment of cervical radiculopathy in athletes. Although not involving athletes, Tumialan et al.'s report of CDR in a military population shows good results in high-activity patients [30]. In their series, 12 patients underwent CDR for cervical radiculopathy. All 12 returned to full active duty at an average of 10.3 weeks after surgery with no complications.

The aforementioned study of MLB pitchers by Roberts et al. reported the first known case of a professional athlete who underwent CDR [16]. Eight of 11 patients with a cervical disc herniation were treated surgically, of which 1 was treated with CDR and successfully returned to play. More granular data concerning this patient were not provided. Reinke et al. evaluated return to play after CDR in 50 athletes, the majority of whom were semiprofessional or hobby athletes in noncontact sports [31]. All patients returned to some level of activity at a median of 4 weeks and to their preoperative level of activity at a median of 12 weeks postoperatively. Notably, there were only two professional athletes in the study (luge) and only two patients that participated in contact sports (martial arts).

Complications

ACDF has long been the gold-standard surgery for cervical radiculopathy due to its widespread use, efficacy, and safety. Even so, complications unique to the anterior approach (e.g., neck hematoma, esophageal injury, recurrent nerve palsy), concerns about adjacent segment degeneration (ASD), and limits to segmental motion and flexibility caused by fusion have increased interest in alternative options. Both PCF and CDR are motion-sparing alternatives to ACDF that have been consistently shown to have similar efficacy and safety to ACDF in the treatment of cervical radiculopathy [26, 32–36], and may be a better option for select patients. An area of intense study is the rate of index- and adjacent-level reoperation after these three procedures.

Index-Level Reoperation

Due to the focus on adjacent segment disease, few studies specifically report rates of index-level reoperation after ACDF. A recent meta-analysis comparing ACDF to PCF found a lower overall reoperation rate following ACDF (4.1% vs. 7.6%) [32]. Although no discrete data were provided, the authors stated that most of the reoperations after ACDF were at the adjacent level, while most of the reoperations after PCF were at the index level. These findings echo a common sentiment that unfortunately has little evidence basis. In their review of 303 patients who underwent single-level PCF for cervical radiculopathy, Clarke et al. found that only 10 patients developed index-level disease and required reoperation [37]. Estimated rates of index-level reoperation were 2.2%, 3.2%, and 5.0% at 1, 5, and 10 years, respectively. This contrasts with an 8.1% rate of index-level reoperation after single-level ACDF at 5 years in a recent meta-analysis [36]. Data from our unpublished series of PCF (8.3% at 15 years) support the findings of Clarke et al. and refute the notion that PCF results in a higher rate of index-level reoperation than ACDF.

There are scant data comparing reoperation rates following ACDF and PCF in athletes. Mai et al. reported the only known direct comparison in their analysis of 101 professional athletes treated over a 25-year span [38]. Six of 13 (46.2%) athletes who underwent PCF required index-level reoperation compared to 1 of 86 (1.1%) who underwent ACDF. There was notably a higher proportion of NFL players in the PCF (77.0%) versus the ACDF group (68.6%). In our unpublished series of 22 collegiate and professional athletes who underwent PCF, none required reoperation at the index level.

Numerous FDA-IDE studies have demonstrated a lower index-level reoperation rate after CDR than ACDF. A recent meta-analysis found a significantly lower 7-year index-level reoperation after CDR (5.2%) versus ACDF (12.7%) [36]. Similar findings were reported by Zhang et al. in their meta-analysis of 13 RCTs [26].

The paucity of studies examining CDR in athletes limits comparison to ACDF in this patient population. In the study by Mai et al., only two athletes underwent CDR, so they were excluded from the data analysis and their outcomes were not reported [40].

Adjacent-Level Reoperation

Arthrodesis, by definition, sacrifices motion at the index level, subsequently increasing stress on adjacent levels. Hilibrand et al. articulated the clinical consequences of this phenomenon in their landmark paper [39]. Fifty-five of 374 patients (14.7%) developed symptomatic adjacent segment degeneration during the study period. This occurred at a relatively constant rate of 2.9% per year, with an estimated risk of 25% within 10 years of surgery. Twenty-seven (7.2%) required an operation at the adjacent level.

In response to this study, the following decades saw an explosion of interest in motion-sparing alternatives to ACDF, with the goal of limiting the development of

Table 5.1 Estimates of index-level and adjacent-level reoperation rates at 5 years post-op

	Index-level reoperation	Adjacent-level reoperation
ACDF	8%	7 to 8%
PCF	5%	2 to 3%
CDR	5%	2 to 3%

adjacent segment degeneration and additional surgery. PCF represents one motion-sparing alternative to ACDF as it does not involve arthrodesis or instrumentation. Clarke et al. found that 15 of 303 patients (5.0%) developed symptomatic adjacent segment degeneration after single-level PCF, of which nine (3.0%) required surgery [37]. Estimated rate of development was 0.7% per year and 6.7% within 10 years of surgery. As mentioned previously, the meta-analysis by Fang et al. reported a lower rate of adjacent-level reoperation after PCF compared to ACDF, although no granular data were provided [32].

In Mai et al.'s study of ACDF vs. PCF in athletes, 4 (4.7%) patients developed ASD after ACDF and required reoperation [38]. No patients who underwent PCF developed ASD. Similarly, none of the 22 athletes in our unreported series developed ASD after PCF.

CDR is another motion-sparing alternative to ACDF that has gained popularity in recent decades. There is overwhelming evidence from numerous randomized controlled trials for lower rates of adjacent segment reoperation following CDR compared to ACDF. A recent meta-analysis reported a 4.3% adjacent-level reoperation rate after CDR compared to 10.8% after ACDF at 7 years [36]. Similar findings were corroborated by a subsequent meta-analysis [26]. Unfortunately, there is no literature directly comparing these techniques in athletes (Table 5.1).

Return to Play

Return to play after ACDF is a controversial topic with no consensus guidelines. Current recommendations are based on the few aforementioned studies and expert opinion. The decision-making process involves a number of variables including the extent of initial injury, number of instrumented levels, resolution of symptoms, quality of fusion, and type of sport. In general, athletes who undergo a single-level ACDF with radiographic evidence of fusion and complete resolution of symptoms without motor deficit can safely return to play, including collision and contact sports [40, 41]. Common scenarios are briefly reviewed below.

Two-level ACDF has generally been viewed as a contraindication to return to play, especially for collision and contact sports, despite limited data to support this recommendation. The major underlying concern is an increased risk of adjacent segment degeneration for which surgical management (i.e., three-level ACDF) would unequivocally preclude return to play. Current expert opinion supports return to play in noncontact sports but is mixed for collision and contact sports, with some experts allowing return to football after a fully healed two-level ACDF [41].

The management of pseudarthrosis after ACDF poses a significant challenge that requires case-by-case evaluation. In general, all symptomatic patients should be considered for operative intervention regardless of sport. If a patient is asymptomatic, the sport type becomes crucial. Noncontact athletes can safely return to play, whereas contact or collision athletes require operative intervention with either a revision anterior procedure or a posterior procedure.

Myelomalacia represents another variable that requires nuanced decision making. While most experts prohibit return to play even after successful treatment, some allow return to play if there is a normal canal diameter and adequate cord decompression [41].

Athletes can return to play after PCF once soreness has resolved and any preoperative motor deficits have completely recovered. In our experience, this ranges from 2.5 to 6 weeks. Athletes with persistent symptoms should be held out of competition and considered for ACDF.

The paucity of literature evaluating the efficacy and safety of CDR in athletes limits return-to-play recommendations. CDR should be viewed as a contraindication to return to play in collision and contact sports. Although Reinke et al. reported a return to activity in two martial arts athletes [31], the sample size is small, and level of contact these athletes experienced was unclear. Thus, this study should not be used to validate return to play in contact sports. Return to play in noncontact sports appears acceptable. In Tumialan et al.'s study of military patients, those who underwent CDR returned to full active duty without complication significantly sooner than those who underwent ACDF (10.3 vs. 16.5 weeks) [30]. Return to duty required complete resolution of preoperative symptoms.

Conclusion

Cervical radiculopathy, whether from disc herniation or spondylosis, is a relatively common problem for athletes. The work-up and management of these cases require careful history taking, physical examination, and often imaging in order to adequately determine the differential diagnosis and eliminate the potentially catastrophic spinal cord concussion and myelopathy patients. Multimodal conservative therapy is very helpful in the majority of cases. However, there is a growing body of evidence that even professional athletes in collision and contact sports can safely return to play after operative intervention and might even perform better than those who are treated nonoperatively. Of the three surgical options, ACDF has the longest track record and most evidence to support its use, but PCF has been shown to be an equally effective alternative with the potential for a quicker return to play, no loss of motion, and much less risk of adjacent segment disease compared to ACDF. CDR is an emerging, motion-preserving technique that has been very effective in the general population as well as an initial experience in the military, but there has been limited experience in athletes, especially American football. Overall management and return-to-play considerations are nuanced decisions that must be individualized with input from the athlete, team, and surgeon.

References

1. Radhakrishnan K, Litchy WJ, O'Fallon WM, Kurland LT. Epidemiology of cervical radiculopathy: a population-based study from Rochester, Minnesota, 1976 through 1990. Brain. 1994;117(Pt 2):325–35.
2. Yoss RE, Corbin KB, Maccarty CS, Love JG. Significance of symptoms and signs in localization of involved cervical disk protrusion. Neurology. 1957;7(10):673.
3. Schoenfeld AJ, George AA, Bader JO, Caram PM Jr. Incidence and epidemiology of cervical radiculopathy in the United States military: 2000 to 2009. J Spinal Disord Tech. 2012;25(1):17–22.
4. Mall NA, Buchowski J, Zebala L, et al. Spine and axial skeleton injuries in the National Football League. Am J Sports Med. 2012;40:1755–61.
5. Gray BL, Buchowski JM, Bumpass DB, et al. Disc herniations in the National Football League. Spine (Phila Pa 1976). 2013;38:1934–8.
6. Mai HT, Burgmeier RJ, Mitchel SM, et al. Does the level of cervical disc herniation surgery affect performance-based outcomes in national football league athletes? Spine (Phila Pa 1976). 2016;41(23):1785–9.
7. Bohlman HH, Emery SE, Goodfellow DB, et al. Robinson anterior cervical discectomy and arthrodesis for cervical radiculopathy: long-term follow-up of one hundred and twenty-two patients. J Bone Joint Surg Am. 1993;75:1298–307.
8. Preston M. Rolle warns about sticking your neck out. The Baltimore Sun. 2009. Accessed 4 Nov 2020.
9. Shin AY, Spinner RJ, Steinmann SP, Bishop AT. Adult traumatic brachial plexus injuries. J Am Acad Orthop Surg. 2005;13(6):382–96.
10. Dossett AB. Stingers and burners. In: Hecht A, editor. Spine injuries in athletes. Philadelphia: Wolters Kluwer; 2017. p. 86–91.
11. Valone FH, Riew KD. Cervical cord neurapraxia. In: Hecht A, editor. Spine injuries in athletes. Philadelphia: Wolters Kluwer; 2017. p. 92–9.
12. Lees F, Turner JW. Natural history and prognosis of cervical spondylosis. Br Med J. 1963;2(5373):1607–10.
13. Dillin W, Booth R, Cuckler J, et al. Cervical radiculopathy. A review. Spine (Phila Pa 1976). 1986;11(10):988–91.
14. Clark R, Doyle M, Sybrowsky C, Rosenquist R. Epidural steroid injections for the treatment of cervical radiculopathy in elite wrestlers: case series and literature review. Iowa Orthop J. 2012;32:207–14.
15. Hsu WK. Outcomes following nonoperative and operative treatment for cervical disc herniations in National Football League athletes. Spine. 2011;36(10):800–5.
16. Roberts DW, Roc GJ, Hsu W. Outcomes of cervical and lumbar disk herniations in Major League Baseball pitchers. Orthopedics. 2011;34(8):602–9.
17. Andrews J, Jones A, Davies PR, et al. Is return to professional rugby union likely after anterior cervical spinal surgery? J Bone Joint Surg (Br). 2008;90-B(5):619–21.
18. Schwarz A. Concussions tied to depression in ex-NFL players. The New York Times. 2007. Accessed 4 Nov 2020.
19. Maroon JC, Bost JW, Petraglia AL, et al. Outcomes after anterior cervical discectomy and fusion in professional athletes. Neurosurgery. 2013;73(1):103–12.
20. Semmes RE, Murphy F. Syndrome of unilateral rupture of the sixth cervical intervertebral disc, with compression of the seventh cervical nerve root. Report of four cases with symptoms simulating coronary disease. JAMA. 1943;121:1209–14.
21. Frykholm R. Cervical root compression resulting from disc degeneration and root sleeve fibrosis. Acta Chir Scand. 1951;160:1–149.
22. Adamson T. Microendoscopic posterior cervical laminioforaminotomy for unilateral radiculopathy: results of a new technique in 100 cases. J Neurosurg Spine. 2001;95:51–7.

23. Coric D, Adamson T. Minimally invasive cervical microendoscopic laminoforaminotomy. Neurosurg Focus. 2008;25(2):E2.
24. Kim KT, Kim YB. Comparison between open procedure and tubular retractor assisted procedure for cervical radiculopathy: results of a randomized controlled study. J Korean Med Sci. 2009;24(4):649–53.
25. Adamson TE. Posterior cervical endoscopic laminoforaminotomy for the treatment of radiculopathy in the athlete. Oper Tech Sports Med. 2005;13:96–100.
26. Zhang Y, Lv N, He F, Pi B, Liu H, et al. Comparison of cervical disc arthroplasty and anterior cervical discectomy and fusion for the treatment of degenerative disease on the basis of more than 60 months of follow-up: a systematic review and meta-analysis. BMC Neurol. 2020;20(143) https://doi.org/10.1186/s12883-020-01717-0.
27. Burkus JK, Traynelis VC, Haid RW Jr, et al. Clinical and radiographic analysis of an artificial cervical disc: 7-year follow-up from the prestige prospective randomized controlled clinical trial. J Neurosurg Spine. 2014;21(4):516–28.
28. Lanman TH, Burkus JK, Dryer RG, et al. Long-term clinical and radiographic outcomes of the prestige LP artificial cervical disc replacement at 2 levels: results from a prospective randomized controlled clinical trial. J Neurosurg Spine. 2017;27(1):1–19.
29. Radcliff K, Davis RJ, Hisey MS, et al. Long-term evaluation of cervical disc arthroplasty with the Mobi-C© cervical disc: a randomized, prospective, multicenter clinical trial with severy-year follow-up. Int J Spine Surg. 2017;11(4) https://doi.org/10.14444/4031.
30. Tumialan LM, Ponton RP, Garvin A, Gluf WM. Arthroplasty in the military: a preliminary experience with ProDisc-C and ProDisc-L. Neurosurg Focus. 2010;28(5):E18.
31. Reinke A, Behr M, Preuss A, et al. Return to sports after cervical total disc replacement. World Neurosurg. 2017;97:241–6.
32. Fang W, Huang L, Feng F, et al. Anterior cervical discectomy and fusion versus posterior cervical foraminotomy for the treatment of single-level unilateral cervical radiculopathy: a meta-analysis. J Orthop Surg and Res. 2020;15(202):1–12.
33. Alvin MD, Lubelski D, Abdullah KG, et al. Cost-utility analysis of anterior cervical discectomy and fusion with plating (ACDFP) versus posterior cervical foraminotomy (PCF) for patients with single-level cervical radiculopathy at 1-year follow-up. Clin Spine Surg. 2016;29:E67–72.
34. Dunn C, Moore J, Sahai N, et al. Minimally invasive posterior cervical foraminotomy with tubes to prevent undesired fusion: a long-term follow-up study. J Neurosurg Spine. 2018;29:358–64.
35. Ruetten S, Komp M, Merk H, et al. Full endoscopic cervical posterior foraminotomy for the operation of lateral disc herniations using 5.9-mm endoscopes: a prospective, randomized, controlled study. Spine (Phila Pa 1976). 2008;33:940–8.
36. Badhiwala JH, Platt A, Witiw CD, Traynelis VC. Cervical disc arthroplasty versus anterior cervical discectomy and fusion: a meta-analysis of rates of adjacent-level surgery to 7-year follow-up. J Spine Surg. 2020;6(1):217–32. https://doi.org/10.21037/jss.2019.12.09.
37. Clarke MJ, Ecker RD, Krauss WE, et al. Same-segment and adjacent-segment disease following posterior cervical foraminotomy. J Neurosurg Spine. 2007;6:5–9.
38. Mai HT, Chun DS, Schneider AD, et al. The difference in clinical outcomes after anterior cervical fusion, disk replacement, and foraminotomy in professional athletes. Clin Spine Surg. 2018;31(1):1–5.
39. Hilibrand AS, Carlson GD, Palumbo MA, et al. Radiculopathy and myelopathy at segments adjacent to the site of a previous anterior cervical arthrodesis. J Bone Joint Surg Am. 1999;81:519–28.
40. Hecht AC, McAnany S, Qureshi S. Cervical disk herniation in athletes. In: Hecht A, editor. Spine injuries in athletes. Philadelphia: Wolters Kluwer; 2017. p. 100–11.
41. Hecht AC, Vaccaro AR, Hsu W, et al. Spine and sports: a roundtable discussion. In: Hecht A, editor. Spine injuries in athletes. Philadelphia: Wolters Kluwer; 2017. p. 278–84.

Chapter 6
Return to Play After Spinal Injury

Daipayan Guha and David O. Okonkwo

An estimated 9–15% of spine injuries and 8% of spinal cord injuries (SCI) in the United States are attributable to participation in sports [1–6]. Among elite or professional athletes involved in collision sports, studies suggest 7–10% of injuries in college-level or National Football League (NFL)-level athletes involve the spine, of which 35–49% affect the cervical spine [1, 3, 7–9]. While formal return-to-play (RTP) guidelines have been, or are currently being developed for, concussion, anterior cruciate ligament injury with reconstruction, and other musculoskeletal injuries, consensus protocols for RTP in elite athletes following a spinal injury remain lacking, due in part to anatomic complexity as well as heterogeneity of injury patterns [10–12]. A classification of spinal injuries relevant to athletes is discussed in Chap. 3, and the definitive management of associated SCI and peripheral nerve injuries is reviewed in Chaps. 4, 8, and 9. The aim of this chapter is therefore to provide a framework for decision making for RTP after common spinal injuries encountered in the care of the elite athlete.

In general, return to play following spinal injury requires an asymptomatic patient with an intact neurological examination, along with the radiologic absence of pathologic spinal segmental motion or ongoing spinal cord compression. The nuances of RTP decision making for cervical and brachial plexus injuries along with lumbar spinal injuries, following either operative or nonoperative management, are discussed herein.

D. Guha
Department of Neurological Surgery, University of Pittsburgh Medical Center, Pittsburgh, PA, USA
e-mail: guhad@upmc.edu

D. O. Okonkwo (✉)
UPMC/University of Pittsburgh, Department of Neurological Surgery, Pittsburgh, PA, USA
e-mail: okonkwodo@upmc.edu

M. E. Oppenlander (ed.), *Neurosurgical Care of Athletes*, https://doi.org/10.1007/978-3-030-88227-3_6

Cervical Spine and Brachial Plexus Injuries

Cervical Stingers

Traumatic upper trunk brachial plexopathy, also known as a cervical 'stinger' or 'burner', is characterized by transient burning pain down a unilateral upper extremity, often associated with paresthesias/numbness and/or motor deficits, after a significant contact injury to the neck or upper extremity [13, 14]. The pain typically resolves in seconds to minutes, with motor weakness lasting up to 24 h though in severe cases persisting up to 6 weeks [1, 15, 16]. While commonly thought to occur from traction injury to the brachial plexus following ipsilateral shoulder depression and contralateral lateral neck flexion, injury to the upper trunk is also possible via direct mechanical compression from contact to Erb's point, while cervical root compression may occur within the intervertebral foramina from ipsilateral lateral neck flexion coupled with hyperextension [13]. The severity of an acute injury, and therefore the natural history and prognosis for motor recovery, is categorized as per either the Seddon or Sunderland classification systems.

While athletes may be prone to underreporting stingers due to the transient nature of the injury, as well as the potential playing-time and career implications, it is nonetheless well known that the likelihood of sustaining a cervical stinger is considerably higher among rugby and American football players, though also among boxers, ice hockey players, and gymnasts [13, 17, 18]. At the collegiate level, a survey of National Collegiate Athletic Association (NCAA) football players revealed a cervical stinger rate of 1.87 per 10,000 athlete exposures [5], with a 50.3% lifetime prevalence among high-school-, collegiate-, and professional-level players [19], and an increased risk of recurrent stingers among those experiencing a single event [20, 21].

Algorithms for the sideline diagnosis and initial management of stingers, along with the role of subsequent imaging and/or electrodiagnostic studies, are discussed thoroughly in other chapters. In general, the vast majority of stingers are managed nonsurgically. Nonoperative management consists predominantly of rest and analgesia and, if persistent, physical therapy targeting postural correction and normalizing flexibility and strength imbalances in the cervicothoracic spine as well as scapular and core stabilizers [22, 23]. MRI is indicated if a stinger does not resolve within 24 h, or if the athlete has a history of repeated stingers.

While there are no standardized RTP guidelines for stingers managed nonoperatively, athletes with a first-time stinger, in whom symptoms resolve completely within 1 h, with normal painless cervical range of motion and normal neurovascular examinations, may RTP within the same or subsequent games [13, 24]. In a modified-Delphi survey of spine surgeon members of the Cervical Spine Research Society (CSRS), Schroeder et al. found 84.5% agreement among members that athletes with stinger symptoms for <5 min should be allowed to RTP, with a case-by-case evaluation for anyone with symptoms lasting >5 min [25]. In general, first-time stingers with symptoms lasting >1 h, involving more than a unilateral upper extremity, associated with persistent neck pain, or recurrent stingers within the same game or season, mandate removal from competition and workup with cervical radiographs and magnetic resonance imaging [26]. Athletes with persistent symptoms beyond 1 week are often investigated with electrodiagnostic studies to assess the severity of nerve injury. While electromyographic (EMG) changes may persist after the resolution of clinical symptoms, and hence alone are not a reason to prohibit RTP, a plan for return to competition in athletes with electrodiagnostic evidence of denervation should commence only after the absence of spontaneous fibrillation potentials, and the emergence of polyphasic potentials indicative of larger motor unit recruitment as part of reinnervation [22]. In those athletes investigated with cervical radiographs or MRI, spinal cord parenchymal signal changes, or persistent root/cord compression in the presence of ongoing symptoms, are traditional contraindications to safe RTP. Bowles et al. have recently summarized the literature evidence on RTP recommendations after cervical stingers, encapsulated in Table 6.1 [13].

Table 6.1 Summary of RTP criteria following cervical stingers

	Clinical	Radiologic
Absolute contraindications	Second stinger in the same game	Cervical spine fracture
	Persistent neurological deficits	Ligamentous injury
	Bilateral or multiple extremity symptoms	Cervical spinal cord edema or intramedullary abnormality
	Persistent neck pain	Active neural element compression
	Diminished cervical range of motion	Evidence of spear-tackler's spine
		Multilevel fusion from Klippel–Feil syndrome
		Ankylosing spondylitis or diffuse idiopathic skeletal hyperostosis
		Evidence of rheumatic arthritis
Relative contraindications	Persistent symptoms >1 h	
	Second stinger in the same season	
	Three or more prior stingers with full return to baseline neurological function and cervical range of motion	
No contraindications	First-time stinger, with symptoms <1 h, followed by complete resolution	Single-level Klippel–Feil anomaly, without involvement of C0–C1
	Second-time stinger not in the same game or season, with symptoms <1 h, followed by complete resolution	Spina bifida occulta
	Less than three prior stingers each lasting <24 h, with no neurological deficit or diminished cervical range of motion	Torg ratio <0.8 and asymptomatic

Cervical Nerve Root Injuries

Cervical nerve root avulsion injuries represent the most severe end of the spectrum of traumatic brachial plexopathy. These are extremely rare, in the context of the far more common transient neurapraxia or 'stinger', with only case series of functional root avulsion described in rugby and collegiate-level American football players [27, 28]. Following electrodiagnostic and/or magnetic resonance imaging (MRI) evidence of nerve functional transection (Seddon Grade 3), these severe injuries are often treated surgically with delayed nerve transfers and/or grafts primarily to restore stability of the shoulder girdle and re-animate shoulder abduction and elbow flexion, depending on the specific deficits. Injuries of this nature, with or without surgical reconstruction, are typically career-ending from competitive sport.

Congenital Cervical Stenosis

The incidence of osseous cervical canal stenosis has been estimated in cadaveric studies to be 4.9% of the adult North American population; when soft-tissue canal encroachment is accounted for on MRI, this number rises to as high as 24% in susceptible Asian populations [29, 30]. Cervical stenosis has historically been defined on plain radiographs by the segmental sagittal canal diameter (Fig. 6.1), with diameters of <14 mm at any level considered stenotic. On MRI, a sagittal canal diameter of <10 mm at any level has been considered as 'absolute' stenosis, with 'relative' stenosis defined as <13 mm [31–33]. To account for differences in XR magnification, Torg and Pavlov defined an eponymous ratio of the sagittal canal diameter to vertebral body diameter (Fig. 6.1), with a ratio of <0.8 portending an increased risk of cervical cord neurapraxia in the initial study, and reflecting the current literature definition of cervical stenosis [34]. Among athletes, a Torg ratio <0.8 in a retrospective study was 93% sensitive for those suffering a transient cervical neurapraxia, however with a positive predictive value of only 0.2 in predicting future injury [35]. This is due in part to the Torg ratio perhaps being not as accurate in elite athletes in high-impact sports, due to their larger vertebral bodies. Various measurements of functional reserve on MRI have therefore been proposed, reflecting the available cerebrospinal fluid (CSF) cushion around the cord (Fig. 6.2) [36–38].

Injuries typically associated with cervical stenosis include cervical cord neurapraxia, as well as cervical spinal cord injury (SCI), of which traumatic central cord syndrome is a subset. RTP recommendations after injuries associated with cervical stenosis are discussed in the subsequent sections. For athletes with an incidental discovery of radiographic cervical stenosis, 'functional' stenosis, defined as a complete obliteration of the CSF space or frank cord deformation on MRI, is typically considered a contraindication to RTP [24, 39]. It follows therefore that while

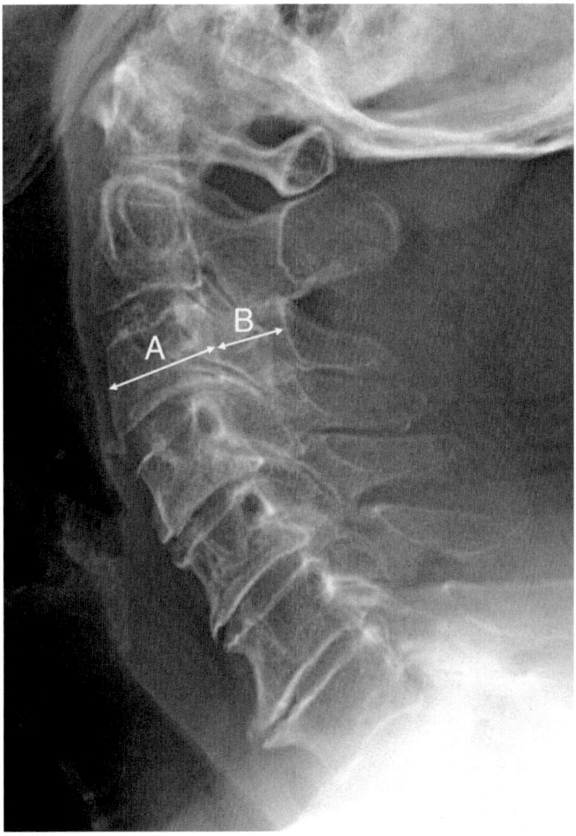

Fig. 6.1 Demonstration of calculation of Torg ratio on lateral cervical spine x-ray. *A*—vertebral body width. *B*—segmental sagittal canal diameter. Torg–Pavlov ratio = B/A. A Torg ratio <0.8 is indicative of congenital spinal stenosis and increased risk of a cervical neuropraxic event

incidental stenosis on radiographs or computed tomography (CT) imaging is not, in the absence of overt mechanical instability, an indication for surgical intervention, functional stenosis on MRI for an elite athlete in a collision sport may warrant consideration for surgical decompression in order to preserve the possibility of a playing career. This is borne out in the potentially increased risk for cervical SCI if the CSF space around the cord is obliterated, and the greater risk for symptom recurrence following cervical cord neurapraxia in the context of congenital stenosis rather than spondylosis [40, 41].

Cervical Cord Neurapraxia

Cervical cord neurapraxia is defined as a transient posttraumatic cervical neurologic deficit, occurring most frequently in professional American football and soccer players, with an estimated incidence of 1.3–6 per 10,000 exposures [42]. Cervical stenosis is a predominant risk factor, with up to 86–93% of cervical cord

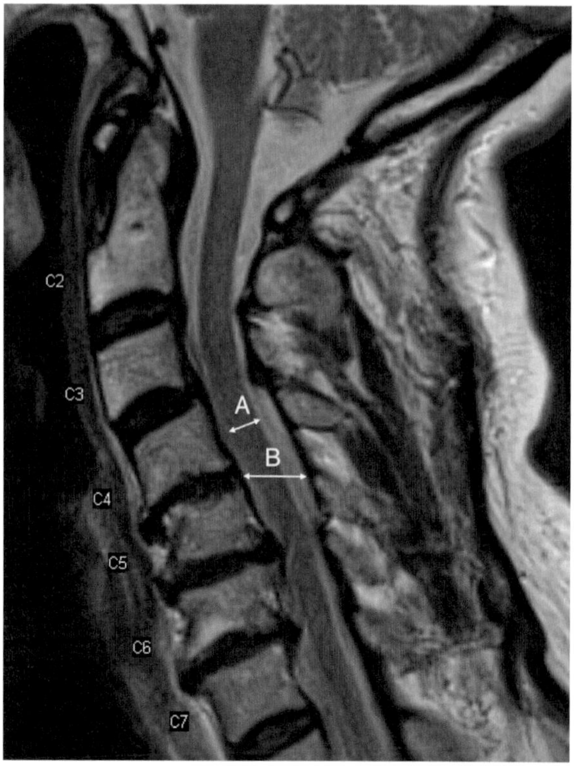

Fig. 6.2 Measurement of spinal canal functional reserve on MRI, reflecting the available cerebrospinal fluid cushion around the spinal cord. Mid-sagittal T2-weighted cervical spine MRI. *A*—spinal cord diameter. *B*—Adjacent disc-level spinal canal diameter. "Space available for cord" (SAC) = (B-A). "Functional reserve" = A/B

neurapraxia cases associated with a Torg ratio <0.8 [35, 38], though with poor positive predictive value for future recurrence [43]. MRI measurements of functional reserve, or space available for cord (SAC) (Fig. 6.2), may have better predictive value for the future risk of developing cervical cord neurapraxia [44].

Prognostication, and therefore RTP recommendations, following cervical cord neurapraxia in the current era is predicated on MRI measurements of the extent of cervical stenosis, as well as the presence of intramedullary T2 hyperintensity. While the literature on elite athletes with cervical cord neurapraxia consists entirely of case series, no athlete who returned to play following cervical cord neurapraxia without functional stenosis, that is, without complete obliteration of the CSF space around the cord, has been documented to have suffered from recurrent cord symptoms [34, 38, 40, 45–47]. Tempel et al. retrospectively reviewed the impact of intramedullary T2 hyperintensity in four National Football League players and one professional wrestler with cervical cord neurapraxia, of which four were ultimately cleared for RTP. In three of these four, RTP preceded complete resolution of MRI intramedullary T2 hyperintensity, with no subsequent neurologic symptoms in all, suggesting that functional canal reserve rather than intramedullary T2 hyperintensity is a predominant prognosticator for future injury [48]. This is captured in a recent Delphi survey of CSRS members, which provides strong consensus (71–94% agreement) for the following recommendations [25]:

1. Following an episode of transient paralysis, asymptomatic athletes with no T2 intramedullary signal change and no absolute cervical stenosis (canal diameter >10 mm on MRI) are allowed to RTP, but those with absolute stenosis (canal diameter <10 mm) should be evaluated on a case-by-case basis.
2. Following an episode of transient paralysis, asymptomatic athletes with resolved T2 intramedullary signal change and no relative cervical stenosis (canal diameter >13 mm on MRI) are allowed to RTP; those with a canal diameter 10–13 mm should be evaluated on a case-by-case basis; those with canal diameter <10 mm should not RTP.

This survey also provides weak consensus (60–70% agreement) for the following recommendation:

1. Following an episode of transient paralysis, asymptomatic athletes with continued T2 intramedullary signal change and no relative cervical stenosis (canal diameter >13 mm on MRI) should be evaluated on a case-by-case basis; those with canal diameter <13 mm should not RTP.

Cervical Disc Herniation

Asymptomatic cervical disc herniations are estimated to occur in approximately 25% of the general population under 40 years of age, unsurprisingly with a greater incidence in professional football players given prolonged exposures to repetitive axial loading [11, 49]. Asymptomatic cervical disc herniations, discovered incidentally, do not preclude RTP as long as the abovementioned criteria for preservation of CSF signal surrounding the cord on MRI are met [50, 51].

Symptomatic disc herniations, on the other hand, whether manifesting as radiculopathy and/or myelopathy, represent a consensus absolute contraindication to RTP due to the risk of worsening nerve root or cord injury with further impact [24, 52]. Surgery for an acute disc herniation is typically reserved for symptoms of myelopathy or progressive neurological deficits with ongoing radiographic cord compression or intramedullary T2 signal change on MRI. Conservative management is generally attempted as first-line for radicular-only symptoms, or for cord deficits with preserved surrounding CSF space on MRI [41].

Multiple authors have investigated RTP outcomes for elite athletes in the National Football League (NFL), Major League Baseball (MLB), and professional rugby, with generally >65% of athletes returning to play following cervical disc herniation treated either operatively or nonsurgically [53–57]. RTP rates in the literature have been equivalent among athletes treated operatively vs. conservatively [41], with the exception of one study by Hsu et al. suggesting increased RTP among surgically treated NFL players along with longer careers post treatment, perhaps reflective of athletes more advanced in their careers opting to retire rather than undergo surgery [54]. Sport-specific performance metrics in those NFL and MLB athletes who do RTP following cervical disc herniation have been equivalent among those treated operatively vs. conservatively [54, 56, 57].

Return-to-Play Recommendations Following Cervical Spine Surgery

The specific indications for surgical intervention following cervical spinal injuries have been discussed briefly here and more thoroughly in other chapters. Broadly, surgical options include anterior cervical discectomy with fusion (ACDF), cervical arthroplasty, posterior cervical decompression with fusion (PCDF), and posterior cervical foraminotomy +/– discectomy. RTP following operative cervical intervention has been most widely studied for ACDF; in studies of cervical injuries in athletes in the four major North American professional sporting leagues (NFL, MLB, NBA, NHL), 75–85% underwent ACDF, with 15–20% undergoing posterior cervical foraminotomy and a small minority cervical arthroplasty [41, 47, 48, 54–56, 58, 59].

Among elite athletes undergoing ACDF, RTP rates following a single-level ACDF range from 68% to 100% [53–55, 57–59]. To our knowledge, there are no literature reports to date of successful RTP in a professional athlete following 2+-level ACDF. In fact, in two studies by Maroon et al. evaluating ACDF in predominantly NFL players and professional wrestlers, 3 of 20 combined patients suffered adjacent-level disc herniation, with two requiring re-operation and none returning to play after their second injury [55, 58]. Similarly, in a series by Mai et al., four NFL athletes suffered adjacent segment disease after returning to play following single-level ACDF, with all undergoing reoperation and none returning to play thereafter [59]. Among those athletes returning successfully after single-level ACDF, RTP occurred within 6–12 months postsurgery [53, 55, 58–60]. The level of ACDF does not appear to impact the ability to RTP, with equivalent RTP rates and postsurgery career lengths in NFL players undergoing a 'high-cervical' (C2–4) ACDF vs. 'low-cervical' (C4–T1) [61].

RTP following posterior cervical foraminotomy has been compared to ACDF in only one recent retrospective series by Mai et al., encompassing 101 professional athletes in one of the four major North American sporting leagues, with 86 undergoing ACDF, 13 foraminotomies, and 2 arthroplasties [59]. In this series, RTP following single-level posterior cervical foraminotomy (PCF) was 92.3%, compared with 70.9% for the ACDF cohort; these data are consistent with the >90% return-to-duty rate following PCF in a military cohort with presumably similar increased mechanical stresses as athletes [62]. While the time to return following PCF was markedly shorter than ACDF (238 vs. 367 d), the rate of reoperation was substantially higher (46.2% vs. 5.8%), with all reoperations following PCF occurring at the index level versus the majority following ACDF occurring at adjacent segments [59, 61].

Cervical arthroplasty, while studied extensively and with long-term follow-up in the general population, has been described infrequently in athletes, and at the professional level only in MLB players [57, 59]. All players were able to RTP in these series, with none of the two in the series by Mai et al. requiring reoperation at a follow-up of 6 years, with preserved or improved performance metrics postoperatively. To our knowledge, there have been no reports of elite athletes returning to play following posterior cervical decompression with fusion.

Sport-specific performance outcomes in those athletes returning to play after ACDF, foraminotomy and cervical arthroplasty have been evaluated by numerous authors. Among NFL players suffering a cervical disc herniation, there was no difference in position-specific performances scores among those treated operatively or nonoperatively, though with a slight decline in performance score among both groups [54]. In a retrospective review by Mai et al., of 101 professional athletes across the NFL, NBA, MLB, and NHL, only MLB players experienced a statistically -significant decline in performance after surgery (−14%) [59]. However, Roberts et al. found no change in performance metrics in MLB pitchers following ACDF, with respect to time-averaged metrics such as earned-run average (ERA) and walks + hits per inning pitched (WHIP), though with a significant decline in the number of innings pitched postsurgery and an increase in the rate of conversion of starting pitchers to relievers [57].

While formal RTP criteria have not been published or identified clearly in the majority of series of surgical intervention for cervical disease, in all cases the general rules of a neurologically intact patient with no neck pain and full painless cervical range of motion apply, along with the absence of radiographic spinal cord compression and pathologic vertebral motion. Following ACDF, Maroon et al. permitted the progressive return to full aerobic activity and 50% of weight-training capacity by 4 weeks postsurgery, with flexion-extension X-rays performed at 8 weeks. Return to full conditioning and subsequent contact was permitted if there was no motion on dynamic X-rays, therefore as early as 8 weeks postoperatively [55]. Formal radiographic criteria for RTP after posterior cervical foraminotomy or cervical arthroplasty have not yet been outlined in the literature.

The latest guidance for RTP after cervical surgery, from the CSRS survey by Schroeder et al., provide strong consensus for the following recommendations [25]:

1. Asymptomatic athletes with no T2-signal change after a solid 1-/2-level ACDF are allowed to RTP, but a 3-level ACDF should not RTP.
2. Asymptomatic athletes with continued T2-signal change after a solid 2-/3-level ACDF should not RTP, but a 1-level ACDF should be taken on a case-by-case basis.
3. Asymptomatic athletes with a solid fusion after a compression fracture, burst fracture, or facet fracture with no instability and no T2-signal change are allowed to RTP.
4. Following an episode of transient paralysis, asymptomatic athletes with no T2-signal change following a 1-/2-level ACDF are allowed to RTP, but following a corpectomy or posterior cervical surgery RTP should be taken on a case-by-case basis.

Lumbar Injuries

Lumbar Disc Herniation

The lifetime prevalence of radiographic lumbar degenerative disc disease has been reported to range from 33% to 84% in a variety of North American professional athletes, with increased rates in collision relative to noncontact sports [63–66]. Symptomatic lumbar herniations, as in the general population, occur most frequently at the L4/5 and L5/S1 levels [67].

The management of lumbar disc herniations is fairly consistent between the general population and elite athletes, with perhaps a lower threshold for surgical intervention for subtle motor deficits that might be tolerable for the average individual, but have an appreciable impact on performance for an elite athlete [68]. As with the general population, >90% of athletes with symptomatic lumbar disc herniations will recover within 6 weeks [69]. In a large study of 342 professional players across the four major North American leagues, Hsu et al. demonstrated RTP rates of 82% after symptomatic lumbar disc herniation, comparable between those treated surgically vs. conservatively [69]. A noticeable drop in sport-specific performance scores, ranging from 64% to 104% of baseline, was seen in both operatively and nonoperatively treated patients, with no significant differences between groups [70, 71].

Surgical treatment for lumbar disc herniations typically consists of a laminotomy with discectomy, with 75%–100% of athletes returning successfully to play after this procedure at a mean of 2.8–8.7 months postoperatively [70]. Percutaneous discectomy may have slightly lower RTP rates (70%) relative to traditional microdiscectomy (85%) or conservative therapy (79%) [72]. Revision decompression for re-herniation has been reported to occur in approximately 13%, comparable to the general population, with similar RTP rates of 85% following a revision procedure [73]. RTP outcomes may differ between sports, with higher rates seen among MLB players (96%) and lower among NFL players (70%). RTP after posterolateral fusion in professional athletes has been described to date only for NHL players, with 8 of 8 returning to play after a single-level posterolateral fusion [74].

Lumbar Isthmic Spondylolisthesis

The incidence of isthmic spondylolisthesis with spondylolysis is estimated to be 15–47% in young athletes with low back pain, a significantly greater rate than in the general population [75]. Spondylolysis is seen most frequently in wrestlers, weightlifters, gymnasts, and divers, than athletes in other sports [76]. The initial management of symptomatic spondylolysis is nonsurgical, with sport activity cessation for up to 3–6 months, bracing with limitation of hyperextension, and subsequently targeted physical therapy [77]. RTP rates in a cohort of adolescent soccer players were shown to be significantly greater among those who ceased sport activity for 3 months relative to those who continued to play [78].

Surgical intervention is considered typically after failure of a trial of conservative therapy for at least 6 months, or with persistent neurological symptoms or progressive radiographic spondylolisthesis. For young patients with minimal spondylolisthesis, preserved disc height, and no neurological symptoms, direct pars repair through a variety of lag screw, pedicle screw-sublaminar hook or wiring constructs, may be performed. Direct pars repair in adolescent athletes has been reported in a number of studies to have excellent outcomes, with RTP rates from 80% to 100% to a variety of sports in amateur competition [79–91]. In patients with Grade 1–2 isthmic spondylolisthesis, surgical treatment generally involves an L5–S1 fusion with interbody grafting, with or without decompression. An anterior lumbar interbody fusion with percutaneous backup theoretically preserves lumbar paraspinal muscle integrity and provides a stronger foundation for rehabilitation and return to competition, though this has not been compared directly to traditional posterior approaches. While RTP after lumbar interbody fusion procedures is less well studied, they have been described for athletes returning to elite levels of competition, including Olympic equestrian [92].

RTP criteria following lumbar fusion are less well defined than in the cervical spine, owing in part to their relatively lower frequency. While RTP to elite competition in noncollision sports is documented, return to sports with greater axial loads remains a case-by-case determination. Literature surveys cite only 27–36% of surgeons permitting return to collision sports at 1 year post lumbar fusion, with half forbidding return to collision sports for low-grade spondylolisthesis, and 60% disallowing return for high-grade slips [93]. Among the four professional North American leagues, RTP after lumbar fusion has been described to date in only eight NHL players [74].

Conclusion

Return to play after spinal injuries remains a highly individualized discussion between the athlete and treatment team, taking into account sport-specific loads, pretreatment performance levels, and anticipated realistic career prospects and goals. RTP after cervical injuries, treated nonoperatively or with single-level procedures, is feasible with a high degree of safety given appropriate clinical and radiographic clearance. RTP after lumbar disc herniation is common and safe. Further study is needed to assess the safety of return to play after lumbar fusion and following emerging techniques, including cervical arthroplasty.

References

1. Schroeder GD, Vaccaro AR. Cervical spine injuries in the athlete. J Am Acad Orthop Surg. 2016;24(9):e122–33. https://doi.org/10.5435/JAAOS-D-15-00716.
2. Hachem LD, Ahuja CS, Fehlings MG. Assessment and management of acute spinal cord injury: from point of injury to rehabilitation. J Spinal Cord Med. 2017;40(6):665–75. https://doi.org/10.1080/10790268.2017.1329076.

3. Puvanesarajah V, Qureshi R, Cancienne JM, Hassanzadeh H. Traumatic sports-related cervical spine injuries. Clin Spine Surg. 2017;30(2):50–6. https://doi.org/10.1097/BSD.0000000000000441.
4. Deckey DG, Makovicka JL, Chung AS, et al. Neck and cervical spine injuries in National College Athletic Association Athletes: a 5-year epidemiologic study. Spine (Phila Pa 1976). 2020;45(1):55–64. https://doi.org/10.1097/BRS.0000000000003220.
5. Chung AS, Makovicka JL, Hassebrock JD, et al. Epidemiology of cervical injuries in NCAA football players. Spine (Phila Pa 1976). 2019;44(12):848–54. https://doi.org/10.1097/BRS.0000000000003008.
6. The University of Alabama at Birmingham. Spinal cord information network - facts and figures at a glance. National Spinal Cord Injury Statistical Center (NSCISC). https://www.nscisc.uab.edu/. Published 2020. Accessed 24 Jan 2021.
7. Lawrence DW, Hutchison MG, Comper P. Descriptive epidemiology of musculoskeletal injuries and concussions in the national football league, 2012-2014. Orthop J Sports Med. 2015;3(5) https://doi.org/10.1177/2325967115583653.
8. Mall NA, Buchowski J, Zebala L, Brophy RH, Wright RW, Matava MJ. Spine and axial skeleton injuries in the national football league. Am J Sports Med. 2012;40(8):1755–61. https://doi.org/10.1177/0363546512448355.
9. Beaulieu-Jones BR, Rossy WH, Sanchez G, et al. Epidemiology of injuries identified at the NFL scouting combine and their impact on performance in the national football league: evaluation of 2203 athletes from 2009 to 2015. Orthop J Sports Med. 2017;5(7) https://doi.org/10.1177/2325967117708744.
10. Dingenen B, Gokeler A. Optimization of the return-to-sport paradigm after anterior cruciate ligament reconstruction: a critical step back to move forward. Sports Med. 2017;47(8):1487–500. https://doi.org/10.1007/s40279-017-0674-6.
11. Huang P, Anissipour A, McGee W, Lemak L. Return-to-play recommendations after cervical, thoracic, and lumbar spine injuries: a comprehensive review. Sports Health. 2016;8(1):19–25. https://doi.org/10.1177/1941738115610753.
12. Ukogu C, Bienstock D, Ferrer C, et al. Physician decision-making in return to play after cervical spine injury: a descriptive analysis of survey data. Clin Spine Surg. 2020;33(7):E330–6. https://doi.org/10.1097/BSD.0000000000000948.
13. Bowles DR, Canseco JA, Alexander TD, Schroeder GD, Hecht AC, Vaccaro AR. The prevalence and management of stingers in college and professional collision athletes. Curr Rev Musculoskelet Med. 2020;13(6):651–62. https://doi.org/10.1007/s12178-020-09665-5.
14. Ahearn BM, Starr HM, Seiler JG. Traumatic brachial plexopathy in athletes: current concepts for diagnosis and management of stingers. J Am Acad Orthop Surg. 2019;27(18):677–84. https://doi.org/10.5435/JAAOS-D-17-00746.
15. Thomas BE, McCullen GM, Yuan HA. Cervical spine injuries in football players. J Am Acad Orthop Surg. 1999;7(5):338–47. https://doi.org/10.5435/00124635-199909000-00006.
16. Green J, Zuckerman SL, Dalton SL, Djoko A, Folger D, Kerr ZY. A 6-year surveillance study of "Stingers" in NCAA American Football. Res Sports Med. 2017;25(1):26–36. https://doi.org/10.1080/15438627.2016.1258642.
17. Meron A, McMullen C, Laker SR, Currie D, Comstock RD. Epidemiology of cervical spine injuries in high school athletes over a ten-year period. PM R. 2018;10(4):365–72. https://doi.org/10.1016/j.pmrj.2017.09.003.
18. Steiner ME, Berkstresser BD, Richardson L, Elia G, Wang F. Full-contact practice and injuries in college football. Sports Health. 2016;8(3):217–23. https://doi.org/10.1177/1941738115626689.
19. Starr HM, Anderson B, Courson R, Seiler JG. Brachial plexus injury: a descriptive study of American football. J Surg Orthop Adv. 2014;23(2):90–7. https://doi.org/10.3113/JSOA.2014.0090.
20. Sarac N, Haynes W, Pedroza A, Kaeding C, Borchers J. Lifetime prevalence of injuries in incoming division I collegiate football players. Phys Sportsmed. 2017;45(4):458–62. https://doi.org/10.1080/00913847.2017.1386068.

21. Charbonneau RME, McVeigh SA, Thompson K. Brachial neuropraxia in Canadian Atlantic University sport football players: what is the incidence of "stingers"? Clin J Sport Med. 2012;22(6):472–7. https://doi.org/10.1097/JSM.0b013e3182699ed5.
22. Weinstein SM. Assessment and rehabilitation of the athlete with a "stinger.". Clin Sports Med. 1998;17(1):127–35. https://doi.org/10.1016/S0278-5919(05)70067-3.
23. Hartley RA, Kordecki ME. Rehabilitation of chronic brachial plexus neuropraxia and loss of cervical extension in a high school football player: a case report. Int J Sports Phys Ther. 2018;13(6):1061–72. https://doi.org/10.26603/ijspt20181061.
24. Cantu RC, Li YM, Abdulhamid M, Chin LS. Return to play after cervical spine injury in sports. Curr Sports Med Rep. 2013;12(1):14–7. https://doi.org/10.1249/JSR.0b013e31827dc1fb.
25. Schroeder GD, Canseco JA, Patel PD, et al. Updated return-to-play recommendations for collision athletes after cervical spine injury: a modified Delphi consensus study with the cervical spine research society. Neurosurgery. 2020;87(4):647–54. https://doi.org/10.1093/neuros/nyaa308.
26. Vaccaro AR, Klein GR, Ciccoti M, et al. Return to play criteria for the athlete with cervical spine injuries resulting in stinger and transient quadriplegia/paresis. Spine J. 2002;2(5):351–6. https://doi.org/10.1016/S1529-9430(02)00202-4.
27. Daly CA, Payne SH, Seiler JG. Severe brachial plexus injuries in American football. Orthopedics. 2016;39(6):e1188–92. https://doi.org/10.3928/01477447-20160721-03.
28. Altaf F, Mannan K, Bharania P, Sewell MD, Di Mascio L, Sinisi M. Severe brachial plexus injuries in rugby. Injury. 2012;43(3):272–3. https://doi.org/10.1016/j.injury.2011.04.001.
29. Lee MJ, Cassinelli EH, Riew KD. Prevalence of cervical spine stenosis. Anatomic study in cadavers. J Bone Joint Surg Am. 2007;89(2):376–80. https://doi.org/10.2106/JBJS.F.00437.
30. Nagata K, Yoshimura N, Muraki S, et al. Prevalence of cervical cord compression and its association with physical performance in a population-based cohort in Japan: the Wakayama Spine Study. Spine (Phila Pa 1976). 2012;37(22):1892–8. https://doi.org/10.1097/BRS.0b013e31825a2619.
31. Prasad SS, O'Malley M, Caplan M, Shackleford IM, Pydisetty RK. MRI measurements of the cervical spine and their correlation to Pavlov's ratio. Spine (Phila Pa 1976). 2003;28(12):1263–8. https://doi.org/10.1097/01.brs.0000065570.20888.aa.
32. Bajwa NS, Toy JO, Young EY, Ahn NU. Establishment of parameters for congenital stenosis of the cervical spine: an anatomic descriptive analysis of 1066 cadaveric specimens. Eur Spine J. 2012;21(12):2467–74. https://doi.org/10.1007/s00586-012-2437-2.
33. Jenkins TJ, Mai HT, Burgmeier RJ, Savage JW, Patel AA, Hsu WK. The triangle model of congenital cervical stenosis. Spine (Phila Pa 1976). 2016;41(5):E242–7. https://doi.org/10.1097/BRS.0000000000001227.
34. Torg JS, Pavlov H, Genuario SE, et al. Neurapraxia of the cervical spinal cord with transient quadriplegia. J Bone Joint Surg Am. 1986;68(9):1354–70.
35. Torg JS, Naranja RJ, Pavlov H, Galinat BJ, Warren R, Stine RA. The relationship of developmental narrowing of the cervical spinal canal to reversible and irreversible injury of the cervical spinal cord in football players. An epidemiological study. J Bone Jt Surg Ser A. 1996;78(9):1308–14. https://doi.org/10.2106/00004623-199609000-00003.
36. Muhle C, Metzner J, Weinert D, et al. Classification system based on kinematic MR imaging in cervical spondylitic myelopathy. AJNR Am J Neuroradiol. 1998;19(9):1763–71.
37. Kang Y, Lee JW, Koh YH, et al. New MRI grading system for the cervical canal stenosis. Am J Roentgenol. 2011;197(1):134–40. https://doi.org/10.2214/AJR.10.5560.
38. Torg JS, Corcoran TA, Thibault LE, et al. Cervical cord neurapraxia: classification, pathomechanics, morbidity, and management guidelines. J Neurosurg. 1997;87(6):843–50. https://doi.org/10.3171/jns.1997.87.6.0843.
39. Cantu RC. Functional cervical spinal stenosis: a contraindication to participation in contact sports. Med Sci Sports Exerc. 1993;25(3):316–7. https://doi.org/10.1249/00005768-199303000-00003.
40. Bailes JE. Experience with cervical stenosis and temporary paralysis in athletes. J Neurosurg Spine. 2005;2(1):11–6. https://doi.org/10.3171/spi.2005.2.1.0011.

41. Joaquim AF, Hsu WK, Patel AA. Cervical spine surgery in professional athletes: a systematic review. Neurosurg Focus. 2016;40(4):1–8. https://doi.org/10.3171/2016.1.FOCUS15560.
42. Clark A, Auguste K, Sun P. Cervical spinal stenosis and sports-related cervical cord neurapraxia in children. Neurosurg Focus. 2011;31(5):2709–12; discussion 2713. https://doi.org/10.1097/00007632-200112150-00015.
43. Herzog RJ, Wiens JJ, Dillingham MF, Sontag MJ. Normal cervical spine morphometry and cervical spinal stenosis in asymptomatic professional football players. Plain film radiography, multiplanar computed tomography, and magnetic resonance imaging. Spine (Phila Pa 1976). 1991;16(6 Suppl):S178–86.
44. Presciutti SM, DeLuca P, Marchetto P, Wilsey JT, Shaffrey C, Vaccaro AR. Mean subaxial space available for the cord index as a novel method of measuring cervical spine geometry to predict the chronic stinger syndrome in American football players. J Neurosurg Spine. 2009;11(3):264–71. https://doi.org/10.3171/2009.3.SPINE08642.
45. Nagoshi N, Tetreault L, Nakashima H, Nouri A, Fehlings MG. Return to play in athletes with spinal cord concussion: a systematic literature review. Spine J. 2017;17(2):291–302. https://doi.org/10.1016/j.spinee.2016.09.013.
46. Torg JS, Sennett B, Pavlov H, Leventhal MR, Glasgow SG. Spear tackler's spine: an entity precluding participation in tackle football and collision activities that expose the cervical spine to axial energy inputs. Am J Sports Med. 1993;21(5):640–9. https://doi.org/10.1177/036354659302100502.
47. Brigham CD, Adamson TE. Permanent partial cervical spinal cord injury in a professional football player who had only congenital stenosis: a case report. J Bone Jt Surg Ser A. 2003;85(8):1553–6. https://doi.org/10.2106/00004623-200308000-00018.
48. Tempel ZJ, Bost JW, Norwig JA, Maroon JC. Significance of T2 hyperintensity on magnetic resonance imaging after cervical cord injury and return to play in professional athletes. Neurosurgery. 2015;77(1):23–30. https://doi.org/10.1227/NEU.0000000000000728.
49. Zmurko MG, Tannoury TY, Tannoury CA, Anderson DG. Cervical sprains, disc herniations, minor fractures, and other cervical injuries in the athlete. Clin Sports Med. 2003;22(3):513–21. https://doi.org/10.1016/S0278-5919(03)00003-6.
50. Kepler CK, Vaccaro AR. Injuries and abnormalities of the cervical spine and return to play criteria. Clin Sports Med. 2012;31(3):499–508. https://doi.org/10.1016/j.csm.2012.03.005.
51. Torg JS, Ramsey-Emrhein JA. Cervical spine and brachial plexus injuries: return-to-play recommendations. Phys Sportsmed. 1997;25(7) https://doi.org/10.3810/psm.1997.07.1487.
52. Ellis JL, Gottlieb JE. Return-to-play decisions after cervical spine injuries. Curr Sports Med Rep. 2007;6(1):56–61. https://doi.org/10.1007/s11932-007-0013-z.
53. Andrews J, Jones A, Davies PR, Howes J, Ahuja S. Is return to professional rugby union likely after anterior cervical spinal surgery? J Bone Jt Surg Ser B. 2008;90(5):619–21. https://doi.org/10.1302/0301-620X.90B5.20546.
54. Hsu WK. Outcomes following nonoperative and operative treatment for cervical disc herniations in national football league athletes. Spine (Phila Pa 1976). 2011;36(10):800–5. https://doi.org/10.1097/BRS.0b013e3181e50651.
55. Maroon JC, Bost JW, Petraglia AL, et al. Outcomes after anterior cervical discectomy and fusion in professional athletes. Neurosurgery. 2013;73(1):103–12. https://doi.org/10.1227/01.neu.0000429843.68836.91.
56. Meredith DS, Jones KJ, Barnes R, Rodeo SA, Cammisa FP, Warren RF. Operative and nonoperative treatment of cervical disc herniation in national football league athletes. Am J Sports Med. 2013;41(9):2054–8. https://doi.org/10.1177/0363546513493247.
57. Roberts DW, Roc GJ, Hsu WK. Outcomes of cervical and lumbar disk herniations in major league baseball pitchers. Orthopedics. 2011;34(8):602–9. https://doi.org/10.3928/01477447-20110627-23.
58. Maroon JC, El-Kadi H, Abla AA, et al. Cervical neurapraxia in elite athletes: evaluation and surgical treatment. J Neurosurg Spine. 2007;6:356–63. https://doi.org/10.3171/spi.2007.6.4.356.

59. Mai HT, Chun DS, Schneider AD, Hecht AC, Maroon JC, Hsu WK. The difference in clinical outcomes after anterior cervical fusion, disk replacement, and foraminotomy in professional athletes. Clin Spine Surg. 2018;31(1):E80–4. https://doi.org/10.1097/BSD.0000000000000570.
60. Robertson PA, Novotny JE, Grobler LJ, Agbai JU. Reliability of axial landmarks for pedicle screw placement in the lower lumbar spine. Spine (Phila Pa 1976). 1998;23(1):60–6.
61. Mai HT, Burgmeier RJ, Mitchell SM, et al. Does the level of cervical disc herniation surgery affect performance-based outcomes in national football league athletes? Spine (Phila Pa 1976). 2016;41(23):1785–9. https://doi.org/10.1097/BRS.0000000000001868.
62. Tumialán LM, Ponton RP, Gluf WM. Management of unilateral cervical radiculopathy in the military: the cost effectiveness of posterior cervical foraminotomy compared with anterior cervical discectomy and fusion. Neurosurg Focus. 2010;28(5):1–6. https://doi.org/10.3171/2010.1.FOCUS09305.
63. Farahbakhsh F, Rostami M, Noormohammadpour P, et al. Prevalence of low back pain among athletes: a systematic review. J Back Musculoskelet Rehabil. 2018;31(5):901–16. https://doi.org/10.3233/BMR-170941.
64. Rajeswaran G, Turner M, Gissane C, Healy JC. MRI findings in the lumbar spines of asymptomatic elite junior tennis players. Skelet Radiol. 2014;43(7):925–32. https://doi.org/10.1007/s00256-014-1862-1.
65. Trompeter K, Fett D, Platen P. Prevalence of back pain in sports: a systematic review of the literature. Sports Med. 2017;47(6):1183–207. https://doi.org/10.1007/s40279-016-0645-3.
66. Mundt DJ, Kelsey JL, Golden AL, et al. An epidemiologic study of sports and weight lifting as possible risk factors for herniated lumbar and cervical discs. Am J Sports Med. 1993;21(6):854–60. https://doi.org/10.1177/036354659302100617.
67. Lawrence JP, Greene HS, Grauer JN. Back pain in athletes. J Am Acad Orthop Surg. 2006;14(13):726–35. https://doi.org/10.5435/00124635-200612000-00004.
68. Yamaguchi JT, Hsu WK. Intervertebral disc herniation in elite athletes. Int Orthop. 2019;43(4):833–40. https://doi.org/10.1007/s00264-018-4261-8.
69. Hsu WK, McCarthy KJ, Savage JW, et al. The professional athlete spine initiative: outcomes after lumbar disc herniation in 342 elite professional athletes. Spine J. 2011;11(3):180–6. https://doi.org/10.1016/j.spinee.2010.12.009.
70. Nair R, Kahlenberg CA, Hsu WK. Outcomes of lumbar discectomy in elite athletes: the need for high-level evidence. Clin Orthop Relat Res. 2015;473(6):1971–7. https://doi.org/10.1007/s11999-014-3762-z.
71. Earhart JS, Roberts D, Roc G, Gryzlo S, Hsu W. Effects of lumbar disk herniation on the careers of professional baseball players. Orthopedics. 2012;35(1):43–9. https://doi.org/10.3928/01477447-20111122-40.
72. Iwamoto J, Sato Y, Takeda T, Matsumoto H. The return to sports activity after conservative or surgical treatment in athletes with lumbar disc herniation. Am J Phys Med Rehabil. 2010;89(12):1030–5. https://doi.org/10.1097/PHM.0b013e3181f71044.
73. Weistroffer JK, Hsu WK. Return-to-play rates in national football league linemen after treatment for lumbar disk herniation. Am J Sports Med. 2011;39(3):632–6. https://doi.org/10.1177/0363546510388901.
74. Schroeder GD, McCarthy KJ, Micev AJ, Terry MA, Hsu WK. Performance-based outcomes after nonoperative treatment, discectomy, and/or fusion for a lumbar disc herniation in National Hockey League athletes. Am J Sports Med. 2013;41(11):2604–8. https://doi.org/10.1177/0363546513499229.
75. Brooks BK, Southam SL, Mlady GW, Logan J, Rosett M. Lumbar spine spondylolysis in the adult population: using computed tomography to evaluate the possibility of adult onset lumbar spondylosis as a cause of back pain. Skelet Radiol. 2010;39(7):669–73. https://doi.org/10.1007/s00256-009-0825-4.
76. Rossi F, Dragoni S. Lumbar spondylolysis: occurrence in competitive athletes. Updated achievements in a series of 390 cases. J Sports Med Phys Fitness. 1990;30(4):450–2.

77. Hsu WK, Jenkins TJ. Management of lumbar conditions in the elite athlete. J Am Acad Orthop Surg. 2017;25(7):489–98. https://doi.org/10.5435/JAAOS-D-16-00135.
78. El Rassi G, Takemitsu M, Woratanarat P, Shah SA. Lumbar spondylolysis in pediatric and adolescent soccer players. Am J Sports Med. 2005;33(11):1688–93. https://doi.org/10.1177/0363546505275645.
79. Hardcastle PH. Repair of spondylolysis in young fast bowlers. J Bone Jt Surg Ser B. 1993;75(3):398–402. https://doi.org/10.1302/0301-620x.75b3.8496207.
80. Debnath UK, Freeman BJC, Gregory P, de la Harpe D, Kerslake RW, Webb JK. Clinical outcome and return to sport after the surgical treatment of spondylolysis in young athletes. J Bone Jt Surg Ser B. 2003;85(2):244–9. https://doi.org/10.1302/0301-620X.85B2.13074.
81. Menga EN, Kebaish KM, Jain A, Carrino JA, Sponseller PD. Clinical results and functional outcomes after direct intralaminar screw repair of spondylolysis. Spine (Phila Pa 1976). 2014;39(1):104–10. https://doi.org/10.1097/BRS.0000000000000043.
82. Brennan RP, Smucker PY, Horn EM. Minimally invasive image-guided direct repair of bilateral L-5 pars interarticularis defects: technical note. Neurosurg Focus. 2008;25(2) https://doi.org/10.3171/FOC/2008/25/8/E13.
83. Widi GA, Williams SK, Levi AD. Minimally invasive direct repair of bilateral lumbar spine pars defects in athletes. Case Rep Med. 2013;2013 https://doi.org/10.1155/2013/659078.
84. Ranawat VS, Dowell JK, Heywood-Waddington MB. Stress fractures of the lumbar pars interarticularis in athletes: a review based on long-term results of 18 professional cricketers. Injury. 2003;34(12):915–9. https://doi.org/10.1016/S0020-1383(03)00034-2.
85. Reitman CA, Esses SI. Direct repair of spondylolytic defects in young competitive athletes. Spine J. 2002;2(2):142–4. https://doi.org/10.1016/S1529-9430(02)00179-1.
86. Linte CA, Davenport KP, Cleary K, et al. On mixed reality environments for minimally invasive therapy guidance: systems architecture, successes and challenges in their implementation from laboratory to clinic. Comput Med Imaging Graph. 2013;37(2):83–97. https://doi.org/10.1016/j.compmedimag.2012.12.002.
87. Bozarth GR, Fogel GR, Toohey JS, Neidre A. Repair of pars interarticularis defect with a modified cable-screw construct. J Surg Orthop Adv. 2007;16(2):79–83.
88. Noggle JC, Sciubba DM, Samdani AF, Anderson DG, Betz RR, Asghar J. Minimally invasive direct repair of lumbar spondylolysis with a pedicle screw and hook construct. Neurosurg Focus. 2008;25(2) https://doi.org/10.3171/FOC/2008/25/8/E15.
89. Nozawa S, Shimizu K, Miyamoto K, Tanaka M. Repair of pars interarticularis defect by segmental wire fixation in young athletes with spondylolysis. Am J Sports Med. 2003;31(3):359–64. https://doi.org/10.1177/03635465030310030601.
90. Hioki A, Miyamoto K, Sadamasu A, et al. Repair of pars defects by segmental transverse wiring for athletes with symptomatic spondylolysis: relationship between bony union and postoperative symptoms. Spine (Phila Pa 1976). 2012;37(9):802–7. https://doi.org/10.1097/BRS.0b013e318232303a.
91. Sutton JH, Guin PD, Theiss SM. Acute lumbar spondylolysis in intercollegiate athletes. J Spinal Disord Tech. 2012;25(8):422–5. https://doi.org/10.1097/BSD.0b013e318236ba6c.
92. Burgmeier RJ, Hsu WK. Spine surgery in athletes with low back pain-considerations for management and treatment. Asian J Sports Med. 2014;5(4) https://doi.org/10.5812/asjsm.24284.
93. Rubery PT, Bradford DS. Athletic activity after spine surgery in children and adolescents: results of a survey. Spine (Phila Pa 1976). 2002;27(4):423–7. https://doi.org/10.1097/00007632-200202150-00019.

Chapter 7
Chiropractic: An Integrative Approach to the Evaluation and Treatment of Elite Athletes Utilizing Spinal Manipulation

Michael A. Miller

Introduction

> "The doctor of the future will give no medication, but will interest his patients in the care of the human frame, diet and in the cause and prevention of disease."—Thomas A. Edison

Chiropractic, derived from the Greek words cheir/praktos, is essentially interpreted as "the practice by hand." Merriam-Webster dictionary defines it as, "a system of noninvasive therapy which holds that certain musculoskeletal disorders result from nervous system dysfunction arising from misalignment of the spine and joints and that focuses treatment especially on the manual adjustment or manipulation of the spinal vertebrae." Daniel David Palmer, the founder of Palmer College of Chiropractic in Davenport, Iowa in 1895, introduced the world to chiropractic. Through his innovative thoughts and pioneering spirit, chiropractic evolved into a science, art, and philosophy. Misalignments of the spine, referred to as vertebral subluxations, were considered to be the cause of disease. Hippocrates, the father of modern medicine, reportedly stated, "Look well to the spine for the cause of disease." In its present-day form, chiropractic searches for the cause of the patient's symptom complex rather than treating the symptoms. This is the art of chiropractic which involves both static and motion palpation of the spine to identify misalignments or subluxations. The term *subluxation* refers to the altered position of the vertebral segment and its subsequent hypomobility or loss of normal function and biomechanical motion. The practitioner or chiropractor learns palpation skills in chiropractic technique classes and becomes efficient in palpating the vertebral column searching for signs of misalignment including muscle spasm or hypertonicity, muscle weakness or inhibition, anatomical alignment and tenderness, and/or temperature changes in the surrounding tissues. Throughout this chapter, I will attempt

M. A. Miller (✉)
Palmer College of Chiropractic, Professional Football Chiropractic Society Hall of Fame, Norwood, MA, USA

M. E. Oppenlander (ed.), *Neurosurgical Care of Athletes*,
https://doi.org/10.1007/978-3-030-88227-3_7

to focus on spinal manipulation and the most common chiropractic techniques used especially as it relates to care of the professional athlete with emphasis on NFL (National Football League) players and the concomitant conditions that lead them to seek chiropractic services. My experience is derived from thirty eight years (38) as the chiropractic physician to the New England Patriots football team.

Indications for Spinal Manipulation

1. *Pain*—This is the most common symptom prompting an athlete or individual to seek chiropractic care. Due to the most recent opioid epidemic in our country, spinal manipulation offers a natural, health care alternative to the dependency of pain-killers.
2. *Decreased range of motion*—Musculoskeletal stiffness or lack of motion in the cervical, thoracic, lumbar, pelvic, sacroiliac, and/or extremities.
3. *Posture*—This is associated with mechanical problems such as those encountered with scoliosis or curvature of the spinal column. Postural analysis can evaluate multidimensional factors including head tilt or forward head carriage, elevated shoulders, scapular positioning, hypolordosis or hyperlordosis in the cervical and lumbar spine, kyphosis in the thoracic spine, and pelvic imbalance. Postural screenings are usually a component of an examination that can detect muscular imbalances and/or gait disturbances.
4. *Neurological or nerve root entrapment*—One of the most commonly encountered problems seen with football players are "burners" or "stingers." The player will complain of an electrical sensation radiating into their trapezius muscle or arm, which is typically caused by tractioning of nerve roots when the head is hyperflexed or hyperextended with forces seen during collisions or tackling. This is compounded by the weight of the helmet which can weigh up to six to eight pounds. We refer to this medically as neuropraxia when a player experiences a transient or temporary loss of motor and sensory function due to blockage of nerve conduction. Depending upon how long this sensation lasts (seconds vs. minutes vs. hours) determines the extent of injury to the nerve and the recovery period. Brachial plexus injuries can affect nerves exiting the spinal cord. Since it is formed from the anterior rami of the lower four cervical nerves (C5, C6, C7, C8) and the first thoracic nerve (T1), spinal manipulation can be beneficial to remove the nerve interference and alleviate radicular complaints into the upper extremities. Another commonly treated complaint is sciatica or inflammation of the sciatic nerve which is the longest nerve in the human body. The player will describe this condition as a "hot poker sensation" radiating into the leg or buttock region. It is usually unilateral. We see these conditions usually as a result of low back injuries when a disc can either bulge or herniate, causing the disc material to contact the nerve and create an inflammatory reaction. If symptoms persist without abatement over a course of several weeks, it is advisable to perform an MRI examination to confirm your suspicion.

Practice Pearl: Another condition that can mimic sciatica is called piriformis syndrome. The piriformis muscle is located behind the gluteus maximus in the buttock and the sciatic nerve is sandwiched between the piriformis layers. When the piriformis muscle spasms it compresses the sciatic nerve and can be confused with sciatica resulting from a herniated disc. Piriformis syndrome is considered a pseudo-sciatica or false sciatica. Trigger point therapy applied to the piriformis muscle with either percussive massage or direct acupressure seems to relax the muscle and alleviate the symptoms.

5. *Sacroiliac disorders*—These are another common entity encountered in football collisions especially from impact to the artificial playing field surfaces when hitting the ground. Direct impact to the hip, referred to as "hip pointers," occurs from an impact force to the iliac crest or greater trochanter. When the sacroiliac joints misalign, the most prevalent finding on exam is a shortened appearance of the affected leg length when the patient is lying on a table in the prone position, since the SI joint most commonly moves posterior and inferior, raising the acetabular region. Chiropractic technique utilizes a leg check test called the Derifield leg length test to determine if the patient has a functional leg length discrepancy caused by misalignment. When the SI joint misaligns posteriorly and inferiorly, it lifts the femur head causing the involved side to appear shorter. This should not be confused with an anatomical short leg which can be caused from prior injuries or surgeries to the foot, ankle or leg or congenital anomalies. When spinal manipulation is used in these functional leg discrepancies, the leg length can be restored to normal.

During clinical practice, I have found a common thread with players who have sacroiliac injuries or pelvic disorders. Oftentimes they will complain of groin pain. Other than initially suspecting a sports hernia, and after medical examination rules this out as a possibility, I have proposed that these symptoms emanate from taut ilioinguinal ligaments that are strained as a result of these types of injuries involving misalignment of the sacroiliac joints. After the SI joints are manipulated, the ligament relaxes and the pain subsides.

6. *Headaches*— One of the most studied areas in sports medicine is the effects of concussion injuries and symptoms attributable to postconcussion syndromes. The concussion protocol involves a multidimensional approach to minimizing symptoms and allowing the athlete to return to play once he passes a battery of tests. The headaches that a chiropractor may treat can be:

    - Cervicogenic (resulting from problems in the cervical spine)
    - Migraine
    - Vascular
    - Occipital (arising from tension in the occipital fibers)

Since football is a direct contact sport, the likelihood of head and neck injuries is high. Present day research is focusing on the advent and creation of newly designed helmets that can more accurately dissipate forces and minimize concussion type injuries. Players are trained with respect to proper tackling skills in attempts to minimize their exposure to these head and neck injuries.

7. *Vertigo/equilibrium/balance problems*—These symptoms can occur from a variety of sources including inner ear problems which involve the movement of tiny particles in the ear called otoconia that break loose. These can be repositioned by centrifugal force exercises or require more intensive therapy. Most of the dizziness or lightheadedness that chiropractors treat originates from a condition known as benign positional vertigo (BPV). Another common cause in the sports arena for athletes involves dehydration of the athlete. These symptom complexes are also associated with whiplash injuries of the neck seen in cervical acceleration–deceleration injuries and postconcussion injuries.

Practice Pearl: When a player presents to me with vertigo and equilibrium problems and after he has been cleared medically, I have found a relationship between these symptoms and temporomandibular (TMJ) joint dysfunction. The TMJ can be misaligned from face mask injuries, direct contact injuries or even from grinding the teeth during sleep. Often overlooked, when an extremity adjustment is performed to the TMJ, resolution of these symptoms occurs and many other symptoms including jaw discomfort, headaches, lightheadedness, earaches, clicking, or crepitus in the jaw and even shoulder pain may disappear.

8. *Whiplash*—Commonly occurring as a result of collision whether it be helmet to helmet during football or related to motor vehicle crashes (CAD), these injuries present themselves with cervical spine pain, limited range of motion and a myriad of secondary symptoms. The player will usually develop tightness or spasm in the trapezius and cervical musculature and may or may not experience radicular complaints. For players who have suffered prior whiplash injuries, neck collars can be fitted to their shoulder pads that prevent the head from hyperextension movements.
9. *Concussion*—When a player suffers a concussion and after appropriate neurological and orthopedic testing including SCAT testing (Standardized Concussion Assessment Tool) has been performed, spinal manipulation has been found to decrease many associated symptoms and allow the player to return to play with diminished repercussions both physically and cognitively.

Practice Pearl: Recent developments in the NFL over the last few years have mandated that each of the 32 teams has a board licensed medical neurologist in the stands or football facilities on game day to assess and grade concussions of the injured player(s). Although the medical team and the trainers have shared input with regards to evaluation techniques, this individual has the responsibility of deciding whether the player can return to active play, avoiding conflict of interest disputes. With the recent developments and research into chronic traumatic encephalopathy (CTE), this topic is being actively debated as to the long-term effects of head injuries from cumulative microtrauma to the brain. Since the CTE diagnosis can only be made during postmortem brain studies, there is no other way to diagnose this condition in living athletes. There are new tests being developed to determine if CTE can be evaluated through blood testing that may identify certain markers associated with the Tau proteins which ultimately cause brain cell death and problems with dementia.

10. *Degenerative disc disease (DDD)*—This condition is often diagnosed by plain film radiographs or MRI testing. It relates to diminished interosseous disc spacing and is usually associated with degenerative changes or desiccation within the disc. Early degenerative disc changes can be detected in athletes that have had cumulative microtrauma to different parts of their spines. They are mostly asymptomatic and may not contribute to the etiology of pain. Sometimes, if there is a known disc degeneration, MRI examination will interpret it as a protruding or herniated disc. Since the MRI attracts hydrogen ions (water) when there is less fluid or gel in the disc, the diagnosis of herniated disc is prevalent. When a radiological interpretation of a sequestered or fragmented disc is made that demonstrates a free-floating fragment, it has been my policy to refer these cases out for neurosurgical review and possible surgical intervention. Research has shown that the precise cause of low back pain can be determined in less than 50% of cases and some studies have shown little to no relationship to the severity of the MRI findings and the actual perceived pain.
11. *Degenerative joint disease (DJD)*—These conditions correspond to degenerative or arthritic changes seen in the spine and its contiguous structures and usually occur with arthritic conditions. They are more likely to be seen in athletes that have sustained repetitive stress injuries. There are also genetic predispositions to different forms of arthritis.
12. *Extremity injuries*—Chiropractic physicians trained in extremity adjusting techniques are able to manipulate the TMJ (temporomandibular joint), shoulders, acromioclavicular and sternoclavicular joints, elbows, wrists, fingers, ribs, knees, ankles, feet, and toes. NFL players are constantly misaligning these extremities and joints and feel immediate gratification when these are corrected. Extremity adjustments fire mechanoreceptors which cause an inhibition of nociceptors which are considered to be the primary interpreters of pain.

Practice Pearl: When a player complains of elbow pain and does not respond to treatment, look at the wrist or lower hand. Sometimes the radius and ulnar torque and can cause pain into the next proximal joint. Likewise, an athlete can complain of knee pain emanating from misalignment of the lower foot involving the tibia and fibula. You must explore other options instead of fixating solely on the area of complaint. Chiropractic is an evidence-based science. You need to approach searching the cause as if you are a forensic detective.

13. *Overall performance*—This is by far the greatest reason that spinal manipulation and chiropractic care has earned its spot in the sports arena. It is my contention that pain and limited range of motion cause a distraction to the player as they try to determine what is causing their discomfort. This distraction interferes with their focus. During professional sports, this can alter their response rate by microseconds and make the difference of interfering with their optimal performance.

14. *Proactive care*—We have been able to educate professional teams as to the benefit of chiropractic care as a preventative type of health care. Rather than just treat musculoskeletal injuries, we attempt to align the spine by removing vertebral subluxations to minimize any nerve interference. By doing this, we can minimize injuries, prolong playing time and reduce disability associated with injuries. We can also hopefully prolong their playing careers. The mindset that has been the established norm of seeking care only when pain occurs first has to be reevaluated. The Professional Football Chiropractic Society presently encompasses chiropractors from all 32 NFL teams with the intent of educating other physicians through our annual symposiums as to advanced techniques in spinal manipulation and extremity adjusting, concussion forums and treatment protocols.

Contraindications for Spinal Manipulation

- Any patient that has had a history of prior cerebrovascular hemorrhages or strokes and/or vertebral artery dissection should be considered high risk for cervical rotational manipulation.
- Fractures
- Tumors
- Ankylosing spondylitis
- History of malignancies or cancers
- Moderate to severe osteoporosis
- Cauda equina syndrome
- Fragmented disc

Although each case has to be individually evaluated, these are conditions that warrant additional investigative work by the treating physician.

What Is an Adjustment?

An adjustment refers to a spinal manipulation in which a force is applied equal and opposite to the side of misalignment. When a vertebral segment is adjusted, there is usually a sound or audible that is produced which is referred to as cavitation. The sound has been described by different researchers as carbon dioxide gases released due to a hydrostatic pressure change in the joint surface during this maneuver. One must understand the principles of physics to analyze force vectors, lines of drive and acceleration or thrust. The thrust or force is produced by taking the involved vertebral segment to tension or end point range and then applying additional pressure known in the literature as "peak force." Most spinal manipulation performed by chiropractors is referred to as high-velocity, low-amplitude thrust (HVLA). According to research done in a paper titled, "Physiological Responses to Spinal

Manipulation Therapy: between Electromyographic Responses and Peak Force" [2], it was determined that the manipulative force caused an increase in paraspinal EMG activity during both the thrust phase and immediately following the thrust. They concluded that "local mechanical changes induced by spinal manipulation technique may lead to both instantaneous and long-lasting neurophysiological changes at the spinal and supraspinal levels." In another article titled, "The biomechanics of spinal manipulation" [1], the authors suggest that chiropractic manipulation was a mechanical event. They also determined that spinal manipulation of the cervical spine caused less tension to the vertebral artery than those produced by diagnostic orthopedic testing and passive range of motion.

Chiropractic spinal manipulation is an art and many research studies have demonstrated a disparity among practitioners in both the preload and thrust phase of the adjustment. Some of this can be attributable to different techniques utilized as well as the expertise and clinical experience of the practitioner. In an article entitled "Establishing force and speed training targets for lumbar spine high velocity, low amplitude chiropractic adjustments" [3], the authors concluded that "peak loads ranged from 100 to 1400 N" and that the average thrust rate averaged 3 N/ms. Their studies also revealed that male practitioners on the average had higher rates of thrust than their female counterparts.

Prior to performing a spinal manipulation, I will usually take a case history and either do a problem-focused exam or specialized orthopedic and neurological examination to determine if additional testing or x-rays are required. Although the X-ray findings represent a structural or mechanical representation of the spine, they are useful to determine conditions of pathology or curvatures in the spine such as scoliosis. There are also radiographic line drawings used on the X-rays to determine hypolordotic or hyperlordotic cervical and lumbar spines, rotational misalignments (rotational malposition subluxations), pelvic level and areas demonstrating foraminal encroachment or pinched nerves. No examination of the patient is complete without a thorough examination of the spine utilizing both static and motion palpation. If a vertebra is restricted or fixated, motion will be introduced in the form of a chiropractic manipulative thrust. By tracking the patient's subluxation or misalignments on a weekly basis, we are able to determine if the patient is responding favorably to chiropractic care. In more chronic cases, the rotation tends to shift from different directions and side to side until the body comes to an equilibrium. Since muscles move bone it takes a period of time, usually 4 to 6 weeks, to retrain the muscle to accept the desired position. The first direction of misalignment in most vertebra(e) is posterior. When the vertebra misaligns, the spinous process comes closer to the surface of the skin and feels sensitive to palpation due to a multitude of sensory nerve fibers that become irritated. The vertebra(e) can then either rotate or laterally flex to one side. The remaining chapter will discuss the most common chiropractic techniques and their methods.

As a chiropractic team physician, you should acquire strength in the ability of differential diagnosis. Not all pain is attributable to spinal misalignment. When an athlete complains of headaches, there can be other causes to consider. Was there a traumatic head or neck injury? Is the player dehydrated? Could it be related to eye strain? Is it cervicogenic in origin from tension in the occipital fibers? Your skills have to be compared to a detective searching for clues. Is it related to TMJ disorders? Can it be a side effect from prescribed medications? It is important to understand referred pain patterns especially with low back complaints. Oftentimes a patient can complain of severe low back pain and it is the result of a kidney stone in the ureter causing spasm as the stone descends the tract. Pain below the right scapula can cause thoracic pain and may be caused by a gallstone. Ultrasound studies may need to be performed to rule out this cause. If a player reports numbness in one of his upper extremities, is it caused by brachial radiculitis or can it be a cardiac or circulatory origin? Have you performed a thorough extremity examination to rule out a subluxed shoulder or impingement syndrome? Is there a carpal tunnel syndrome caused by misalignment of the carpal bones that could be affecting the median nerve? If your athlete is complaining of buttock pain, is it merely sciatica or could it be piriformis syndrome which mimics these symptoms? Is it radicular pain caused from disc material pressing on the exiting nerve root? A common complaint in my sports practice is from players that complain of groin pain. It could be a sports hernia or strained abdominal oblique muscles. It could also be originating from a misalignment of the sacroiliac joint when it moves posterior and inferior causing traction or stretching of the ilioinguinal ligament.

The Effects of Spinal Misalignments (See Fig. 7.1)

When a vertebra or vertebrae misalign, they can cause symptoms that involve irritation or dysfunction to organs in the human body. Neurologically it can be traced to a compressed nerve from the spinal column that causes interference to an organ system. We refer to this phenomenon as a somatovisceral response. We can also understand that if an organ becomes irritated it can reflex to the area of the spine that controls its function and this is called a viscerosomatic reflex. Understanding the autonomic nervous system helps to visualize how pathology can develop. The autonomic nervous system controls bodily functions that are not directed by conscious thought such as breathing, heartbeat, digestion, papillary response, and urination to name a few. It is divided into two systems known as the sympathetic and parasympathetic systems. They act as regulators for each other and maintain balance or homeostasis in the body. For example, if an athlete gets too hot while competing during a game, the autonomic or involuntary nervous system causes increased blood circulation to the skin which induces the sweating process to cool down their bodies. A good analogy is to think of the sympathetic nervous system as excitatory since it is involved in the fight or flight response when the body is subjected to

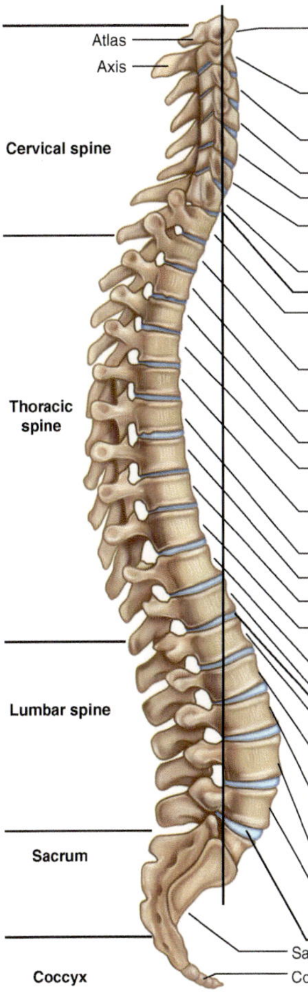

Vertebrae	Areas	Effects
1C	Blood supply to the head, pituitary gland, Scalp, bones of the face, brain, inner & middle ear, sympathetic nervous system	Headaches, nervousness, insomnia, head colds, high blood pressure, migraine headaches, nervous breakdowns, amnesia. chronic tiredness, dizziness
2C	Eyes, optic nerves, auditory nerves, sinuses, mastoid bones, tongue, forehead	Sinus trouble, allergies, crossed eyes, deafness, eye troubles, earache, fainting spells, certain cases of blindness
3C	Cheeks, outer ear, face bones, teeth, trifacial nerve	Neuralgia, neuritis, acne or pimples, eczema
4C	Nose, lips, mouth, eustachian tube	Hay fever, catarrh, hearing loss, adenoids
5C	Vocal cords, neck glands, pharynx	Laryngitis, hoarseness, throat conditions
6C	Neck muscles. shoulders, tonsils	Sliff neck, pain in upper arms, tonsillitis, whooping cough, croup
7C	Thyroid gland, bursae in shoulders, elbows	Bursitis, colds, thyroid conditions
1T	Arms from the elbow down; including hands, wrists and fingers; esophagus and trachea	Asthma, cough, difficult breathing, shortness of breath, pain in lower arms and hands
2T	Heart; valves and coverings, coronary arteries	Functional heart conditions and certain chest conditions
3T	Lungs, bronchial tubes, pleura, chest, breast	Bronchitis, pleurisy, pneumonia, congestion, influenza
4T	Gall bladder, common duct	Gall bladder conditions, jaundice, shingles
5T	Liver, solar plexus, circulation	Liver conditions, fevers, low blood pressure, poor circulation, arthritis
6T	Stomach	Stomach trouble; nervous stomach, indigestion, heartburn, dyspepsia
7T	Pancreas, duodenum	Ulcers, gastritis
8T	Spleen	Lowered resistance
9T	Adrenal and supra-renal glands	Allergies, hives
10T	Kidneys	Kidney troubles, hardening of the arteries, chronic tiredness, nephritis, pyelitis
11T	Kidneys, ureters	Skin conditions: acne, pimples, eczema, or boils
12T	Small intestines, lymph circulation	Rheumatism, gas pains, certain types of sterility
1L	Large intestines, inguinal ring	Constipation, colitis, dysentery, diarrhea, some ruptures or hernias
2L	Appendix, abdomen, upper leg	Cramps, difficult breathing, acidosis, varicose veins
3L	Sex organs, uterus, bladder, knees	Bladder troubles, menstrual troubles: painful or irregular periods, miscarriages, bed wetting, impotency, change in life symptoms, many knee pains
4L	Prostate gland, muscles of lower back, sciatic nerve	Sciatica, lumbago, difficult/painful or too frequent urination, backaches
5L	Lower legs, ankles, feet	Poor circulation in the legs, swollen ankles, weak ankles and arches, cold feet, weakness in the legs, leg cramps
Sacrum	Hip bones, buttocks	Sacro-iliac conditions, spinal curvatures
Coccyx	Rectum, anus	Hemorrhoids (piles), pruritis (itching), pain at end of spine on sitting

For further explanation of the conditions shown above and information about those not shown ask your Doctor of Chiropractic.

Fig. 7.1 Chart of effects of spinal misalignments

extreme stress and the parasympathetic nervous system as inhibitory or lessening the effect. A study published in the *Journal of Chiropractic Medicine* [4] determined that cervical manipulations result in parasympathetic responses, whereas thoracic manipulations influence sympathetic responses. “Autonomic mediated reflex responses including change in heart rate, blood pressure, papillary diameter and distal skin temperature, as well as, endocrine and immune system effects have been clearly demonstrated” as they are linked to spinal corrective manipulation (see Fig. 7.2).

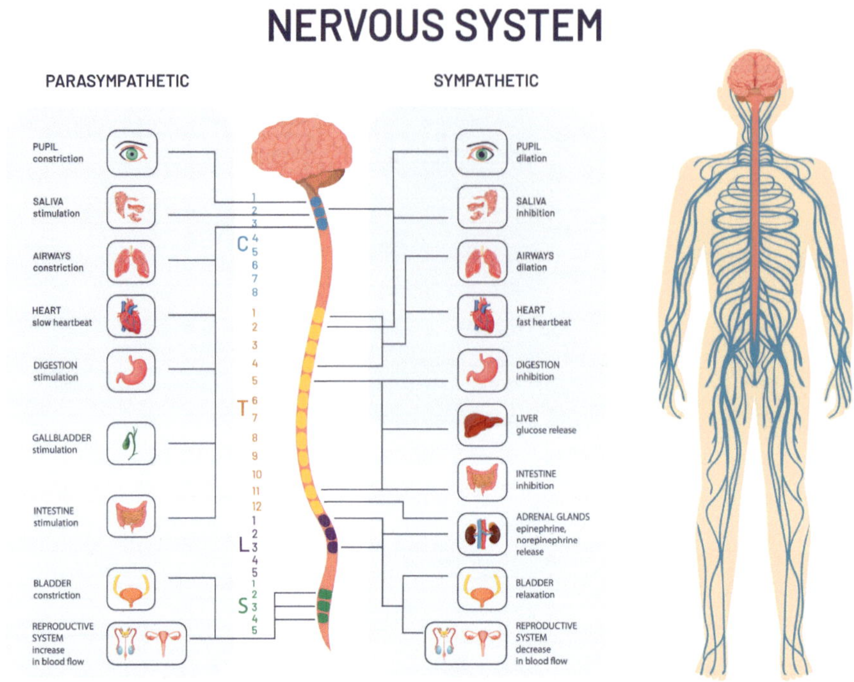

Fig. 7.2 Autonomic nervous system

Commonly Utilized Chiropractic Techniques

Diversified technique is the most commonly used technique by chiropractors. It is used by approximately 90% to 95% of the profession. It is essentially an integration of several techniques that encompass adjustments of the full spine and extremities after identifying subluxations through palpation, X-ray findings, leg length checks, and examination findings. Spinal dysfunction is the tenet of the technique. Some practitioners incorporate postural analysis and gait analysis during evaluation. It is characterized by a high-velocity, low-amplitude (HVLA) thrust. The main objective is to restore joint motion and free the vertebral column from fixation or misalignment.

Extremity adjusting is another specialized skill utilized by approximately 90% of chiropractors. Some of these procedures are taught at chiropractic colleges or as post graduate training. With many chiropractic sports physicians, this is an essential part of their evaluation protocols.

Gonstead technique is used by 55% to 58% of the chiropractic profession. Its premise centers around the belief that a vertebra subluxates posteriorly in relationship to the segment below with the exception of the atlas (first cervical vertebra). Dr. Gonstead, the originator of the technique, theorized that the “spinal range C5-occiput and below L5 governed the parasympathetic nervous system and C6-L5 the sympathetic nervous system." He believed that "subluxation evolved in stages, beginning with fixations, progressing to misalignment and cumulative damage leading to disc disease and finally nerve interference." The concept also believed that the thrust mechanism of the adjustment would cause the vertebral body to create a more normal weight bearing position on the disc. The Gonstead technique uses a specific X-ray analysis with regards to the classification of subluxation. Most practitioners take full spine X-rays and use line drawings to determine malposition of the spine. The practitioners may adjust the cervical spine in a seated chair position and the thoracic spine on a knee chest table specifically manufactured by Gonstead technique. It is also an HVLA technique.

Receptor tonus technique also known as *Nimmo technique*, founded by Dr. Raymond Nimmo, is used by approximately 40% of the practitioners. It is a technique focused on identifying myofascial trigger points in the musculoskeletal system and uses ischemic compression for 6–10 s by applying pressure with the examiner's hands into the musculature to release lactic acid deposits and break up adhesions. The pressure applied is directly proportional to the patient's tolerance level. Its philosophy is predicated upon the theory that dysfunctional muscles result in joint restriction or subluxation as well as creating abnormal visceral function.

Thompson technique created by Dr. Clay Thompson is another commonly practiced technique that uses drop pieces on a chiropractic designed segmental table to impart generated forces to the vertebrae being mobilized using less torque. It is based on Newton's Law of Physics. It also uses leg length analysis in determining the outcome of the adjustment to differentially diagnose the difference between cervical and pelvic involvement. Like other chiropractic techniques it is considered an HVLA technique with somewhat lower forces attributable to the spring-loaded drop pieces absorbing some of the thrust.

Palmer package is a subset of techniques taught at Palmer College of Chiropractic and incorporates Diversified, Gonstead, and Thompson techniques. The practitioner can use a combination of different techniques to establish their own method that they feel most comfortable with while adjusting their patients.

Graston technique is referred to as an Instrument Assisted Soft Tissue Mobilization (I.A.S.T.M.) technique designed to break up scar tissue and adhesions in either acute, chronic, or postsurgical conditions. It incorporates specialized stainless-steel instruments that are designed to restore mobility and function and reduce pain. It attempts to break down collagen cross-links found in adhesions and scar tissue. Practitioners must be trained and certified before they are allowed to practice this technique. There are sometimes small petechiae or capillary hemorrhages that occur as a result of the mechanical rubbing of the instrument against the skin surfaces, but these are transient in nature. Patients who have bleeding disorders or those who are taking blood thinners should be carefully evaluated prior to this technique (see Fig. 7.3).

A.R.T. refers to *active release technique* and is another soft tissue approach to injury. It is advantageous as a precursor to spinal manipulation. The technique relies

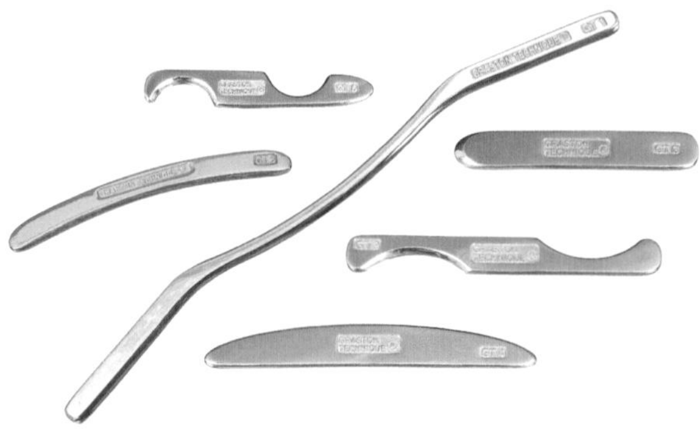

Fig. 7.3 Specialized stainless-steel instruments for Graston technique

on the palpation skills of the clinician as a stretch is applied to the involved muscles in the direction of venous and lymphatic flow. According to the literature, "The A.R.T. practitioner combines low compression, high tension muscle stripping with a variety of active patient motions using antagonist muscles to the ones being treated." By removing fibrous adhesions, biomechanical function is thought to be restored to a normal state.

Conclusion

This chapter was intended to offer insight into how chiropractic relates to treating many musculoskeletal injuries with emphasis on spinal misalignments, referred to as subluxations, and the relationship to the nervous system. I have attempted to incorporate some of my observations as it relates to treatment of professional athletes with respect to my experience over the past 38 years with the New England Patriots. The team approach to injury control has been the most effective with evaluation and treatment protocols. The entire medical team including physicians, trainers, physical therapists, nutritionists, massage therapists, and allied health professionals understand their role as specialists designed to foster optimum performance from the athlete. We also understand our limitations and realize we are all team members dependent upon each other's expertise. The players' confidence in our skills allows them to perform at their maximum potential and creates an environment of trust that we will maintain their health and if injuries occur we will design an appropriate rehabilitation and strengthening program customized to allow them to return to play. Chiropractic has proven its efficacy in treating these sport-related injuries and has gained national recognition among all 32 teams in the National Football League.

References

1. Herzog W. The biomechanics of spinal manipulation. J Bodyw Mov Ther. 2010;14:280–6.
2. Nougarou, Francois Dugas, Claude et al, Physiological responses to spinal manipulation therapy: investigation of the relationship between electromyographic responses and peak force, J Manipulative Physiol Ther 2013 36(9):557–563.
3. Owens E Jr, et al. Establishing force and speed training targets for lumbar spine high-velocity, low-amplitude chiropractic adjustments. J Chiropr Educ. 2016;30(1):7–13.
4. Welch A, Boone R. Sympathetic and parasympathetic responses to specific diversified adjustments to chiropractic vertebral subluxation of the cervical and thoracic spine. J Chirop Med. 2008;7(3):86–93.

Chapter 8
Diagnosis of Sports-Related Peripheral Nerve Injury

Nicholas F. Hug, Michael Jensen, David A. Purger, and Thomas J. Wilson

Introduction

Overview

Peripheral nerve injuries resulting from sports, exercise, or recreation, while rarer than other sports-related injuries, can cause significant functional impairment, with lengthy and variable degrees of recovery. Broadly, the causes of sports-related nerve injuries (SRNIs) can be characterized as acute trauma (e.g., a fall or blindside tackle) versus subacute/chronic trauma. The latter is due to overuse causing repetitive microtrauma on the musculature and nerve, which results in entrapment and progressive nerve injury. These categories encompass the wide range of possible mechanisms of injury, including contact-related trauma, acute and chronic stretch, and tissue swelling. Inadequate protective equipment, overtraining, and use of improper technique or positioning are all factors that increase an athlete's risk for developing an SRNI, as are preexisting stresses on the nerve, such as cysts or tumors [1, 2].

Epidemiology

Reports characterizing the incidence of SRNIs compared to all sports-related injuries have been few and far between. In 1983, Hirasaw and Sakakida reported that 5.7% of all peripheral nerve injury cases seen over the course of 18 years were

N. F. Hug · M. Jensen · D. A. Purger · T. J. Wilson (✉)
Department of Neurosurgery, Stanford University, Stanford, CA, USA
e-mail: wilsontj@stanford.edu

M. E. Oppenlander (ed.), *Neurosurgical Care of Athletes*,
https://doi.org/10.1007/978-3-030-88227-3_8

sports-related. In their analysis, SRNIs accounted for 0.5% of sports-related injuries [3]. A more recent report by Li et al. found that from 2009 to 2018, 21.9% of peripheral nerve injuries presenting to the emergency department (ED) were sports-related. Interestingly, they also found that the incidence of SRNIs increased over this time period [4]. Other studies have also reported that SRNIs account for more sports-related injuries than described by Hirasaw and Sakakida [5–8]. For high school athletes, the estimated incidence of peripheral nerve injuries is approximately 1.5 per 100,000 athlete-exposures, but this may represent a gross underestimation. Boys' football likely has the highest incidence, accounting for over 70% of the injuries in the study by Zuckerman and colleagues [9]. Other sports with higher incidence of SRNIs include baseball, volleyball, cycling, mountain climbing, and gymnastics [2, 3]. The lack of robust and granular data on this topic precludes reliable estimation of the true incidence and prevalence of SRNIs and of high-risk demographics.

Pathophysiology

A thorough knowledge of the pathophysiology underlying nerve damage is necessary for any clinician to understand the diagnosis, prognosis, and treatment of these injuries. Briefly, nerves comprise a bundle of fascicles, which in turn are bundles of many axons, with each axon arising from a single neuron. Each of these structures is surrounded by a sheath of connective tissue known as the endoneurium for axons, perineurium for fascicles, and epineurium for the entire nerve. Nerve injuries have been classically described by either the Seddon or Sunderland classification system [10, 11]. Seddon described three types of injuries—neurapraxia, axonotmesis, and neurotmesis—which Sunderland expanded based on the degree of injury to axons and surrounding connective tissue [10, 11]. Of note, recent advances in peripheral nerve magnetic resonance imaging (MRI) have led to proposals of novel MRI-based classification systems [12–14]. Neurapraxic injury, which is equivalent to Sunderland grade 1, describes injuries limited to damage of the myelin sheath, sparing the axon itself and surrounding connective tissue, with nerve enlargement and hyperintensity on T2-weighted MRI. The next category is axonotmesis, which is split into 3 grades by Sunderland and broadly consists of injuries in which the axon is disrupted but the epineurium and other supporting structures are spared. Sunderland's expanded grading details stepwise increases in damage to the axon (Grade 3), as well as surrounding structures including the endo- (Grade 4) and perineurium (Grade 5), and accounts for different clinical presentations and imaging findings. Finally, neurotmesis, or Sunderland grade 5, describes disruption of the entire nerve, including the epineurium [10, 11].

Recovery and Prognosis

The degree of nerve injury determines whether spontaneous recovery is possible, if surgical intervention is necessary, and the athlete's prognosis. The extent of axon loss and demyelination directly impacts recovery, which relies on effective reinnervation of the nerve's end-organ. Effective reinnervation is determined by axon regeneration, recovery of axonal flow, remyelination, and collateral reinnervation [15]. The proximity of the injury to the end-organ is also key to prognosis. Axonal regeneration occurs at an approximate rate of 1 inch per month. Thus, more proximal injuries require a longer distance of axonal regeneration and a longer time for the axons to reach the muscle or other end-organ. If there is axonal disruption at the time of the injury, changes start to occur in the nerve and in the denervated muscle, as well as at the neuromuscular junction. Eventually, these changes become irreversible and re-establishing a functional nerve-muscle unit becomes impossible [16, 17]. Thus, the longer distance over which axonal regeneration must occur, the lower the chance of establishing a functional nerve-muscle unit before these irreversible changes set in.

Diagnosis of Sports-Related Nerve Injuries

Accurate diagnosis of SRNIs begins with an understanding of the individual peripheral nerves and their functions, the anatomy of these nerves, particularly the anatomical areas where individual nerves are most susceptible to injury, the common associations of specific sports with specific nerve injuries, and the common associations of specific orthopedic injuries with specific nerve injuries. Ultimately, diagnosis relies on a thorough and skillful history and physical examination, electrodiagnostic testing, and various imaging modalities, most commonly MRI and ultrasound (US). The value of each diagnostic technique varies depending on the potential injury (described in detail below). Importantly, SRNIs often present with symptoms that overlap with those of musculoskeletal injuries. Therefore, electrodiagnostic tests and imaging can provide clarification in cases with nonspecific symptoms.

A thorough history and physical examination is crucial for accurate diagnosis. Mechanism of injury, sensory and motor symptoms, loss of function, pain, numbness, and paresthesias should all be assessed. For acute injuries, it is important to establish care early to allow for early examination. Serial examination done by the same examiner is important for detecting signs of spontaneous improvement, which is ultimately important for treatment recommendations (the topic of the next chapter). Furthermore, establishing a pre-intervention, baseline neurological examination is important for being able to detect any iatrogenic injury that may occur, which may be managed differently, when recognized. A history of decreased performance or difficulty improving performance despite a progressive training regimen is one of the most common early signs of chronic or subacute injury. Physical examination should include standard neurologic exam techniques, including sensory and motor examination and reflex testing. In the cases of chronic injury, the specific mechanism underlying the damage must be determined in order to recommend the appropriate rehabilitation program. This goes beyond characterizing nerve injury as compression versus traction; instead, the clinician's goal should be assessing for muscle imbalance, joint issues, or inappropriate form, positioning, or movements [18].

Electrodiagnostic testing, including electromyography (EMG) and nerve conduction studies (NCS), complements the physical exam. It is important to emphasize that electrodiagnostic testing is not a replacement for a well-conducted history and physical examination. Rather, electrodiagnostic testing is useful in confirming the diagnosis, assisting in localization, assessing severity, and evaluating for signs of improvement. Electrodiagnostic testing is most useful at least 3 weeks after the injury. Wallerian degeneration resulting from axonal disruption takes time to complete, and some of the electrodiagnostic findings will not be present until this process is completed. Thus, electrodiagnostic testing is typically not recommended until at least 3 weeks after the injury. Serial electrodiagnostic testing, as with serial physical examination, is useful in assessing for evidence of spontaneous improvement, which is important in determining treatment.

As with electrodiagnostic testing, imaging has a role in SRNI diagnosis as an adjunct and extension of the history and physical examination. Imaging can be helpful in supporting the localization, helping to clarify the extent/severity of the injury, and evaluating for concomitant injuries to other nearby structures. Ultrasound and MRI are the mainstays of nerve imaging. Ultrasound can be useful in evaluating for nerve continuity, can help identify features of denervation in corresponding muscles, can identify points of primary or secondary nerve compression, and can identify cysts in or around nerves that may have contributed to or resulted from the traumatic injury. In the case of nerve transection, ultrasound can be useful for identifying opposing nerve ends and aids in surgical planning. When done in a delayed fashion, ultrasound can often identify a terminal neuroma at the cut end of the nerve. One of the major advantages of ultrasound is the ability to image dynamically. This allows for the detection of abnormalities that may not be noticed in static images, such as abnormal nerve movement or entrapment that is only found with joint movement [18].

Magnetic resonance imaging, and the specialized version referred to as magnetic resonance neurography (MRN), is useful in assessing peripheral nerves. MRN is useful in assessing both peripheral nerve anatomy and pathology. This technique relies primarily on T1-weighted and T2-weighted fluid-sensitive sequences, such as short tau inversion recovery (STIR). Useful imaging features include signal intensity within the nerve(s) of interest, size and caliber of the nerve(s), fascicular pattern, and any associated lesions, both intrinsic and extrinsic to the nerve [19]. In nonpathologic states, nerves typically are isointense to muscle on T1-weighted sequences and slightly hyperintense to muscle on T2-weighted sequences [20]. Obtaining fat-saturated images is paramount when trying to assess nerves, as is obtaining gadolinium-enhanced images. Owing to the presence of the blood-nerve barrier, healthy peripheral nerves do not normally enhance with contrast administration [21]. Pathologic or injured nerves typically show increased signal intensity on T2-weighted sequences [22].

Similar to Seddon's classification of nerve injuries, a 3-tiered system of injury classification based on MRN findings has been proposed [12]. The most minor form of injury, neurapraxic-type injury, is suggested by T2-hyperintensity within the nerve, without enlargement (or only mild enlargement) relative to nearby nerves.

The middle tier is recognized by T2-hyperintensity plus nerve enlargement and loss of the fascicular architecture, with or without a neuroma-in-continuity. This tier would correlate well with Seddon's axonotmetic injury. Finally, in the most severe neurotmetic injuries, there is complete disruption of the nerve, with an area of discontinuity apparent on imaging, with or without a terminal neuroma.

MRN can also be useful in evaluating entrapment neuropathies associated with sports. Injury to the nerve from entrapment is thought to be related to increased endoneurial fluid pressure, which in turn causes microvascular congestion, infarction, and fibrosis [23]. On MRN, compression or entrapment is suggested by the loss of the fat plane around the affected nerve and/or a change in the structure of the nerve. Potential findings include loss of the fascicular architecture, narrowing of the nerve caliber at the site of entrapment, enlargement of the nerve proximal and distal to the site of entrapment, and T2-hyperintensity within the nerve [21]. When compression is severe, denervation may occur, causing characteristic changes in the corresponding muscles.

Upper Extremity Nerve Injuries

Brachial Plexus

The brachial plexus, comprising the interconnected highway of nerves arising from the C5 to T1 nerve roots, is commonly affected in sports-related injuries. Insult to the brachial plexus can occur from blunt trauma, crush injury, penetrating wounds, or extreme hyperextension or lateral flexion of the neck. Significant traction can be placed on the brachial plexus, particularly when the neck is laterally flexed while the shoulder is pulled, increasing the angle between the neck and shoulder. The severity of symptoms from brachial plexus injuries varies widely and is dependent on the force and mechanism of the initial insult. Complaints range from paresthesias lasting a few minutes to complete arm paralysis [24, 25].

As with all nerve injuries, initial assessment begins with a thorough history and physical examination, in order to identify the affected muscles, reflex circuits, and sensory deficits. This enables the examiner to discern between injury to the brachial plexus, spinal cord, or individual nerve roots. Any patient with upper and lower or bilateral extremity deficits identified on clinical exam must be assessed for possible spinal cord injury. Imaging studies of the cervical spine, including MRI and computed tomography (CT), should be obtained if there is concern for spine or spinal cord injury. If a brachial plexus injury is suspected and symptoms are persistent, an electrodiagnostic study is typically obtained 4–6 weeks after the injury in order to better characterize the injury, support the localization, and establish a baseline so that future studies can be compared and assessed for spontaneous improvement. Serial physical examination should also be performed to assess for evidence of recovery.

Ultimately, through the use of serial physical examination, electrodiagnostic testing, and in some cases, imaging, the goal is to characterize the injury location as pre- versus postganglionic and the injury severity to neurapraxic, axonotmetic, and neurotmetic. Such classification has significant ramifications for prognosis and treatment.

The supraclavicular portion of the brachial plexus is a common site of injury. The upper brachial plexus (C5, C6, +/− C7) receives the most traction when the adducted arm or shoulder is pulled down while the neck is forcefully laterally flexed to the contralateral side. With involvement of the upper brachial plexus, there may be sensory loss or paresthesias along the lateral arm, forearm, and first and second digits plus weakness or paralysis of shoulder abduction and external rotation, elbow flexion, and forearm supination. Isolated injury to the lower brachial plexus (C8, T1) is much rarer in comparison. Stretch of the lower brachial plexus can occur with traction on the fully abducted arm. With involvement of the lower brachial plexus, there may be sensory loss or paresthesias along the medial arm, forearm, and fourth and fifth digits. There may also be weakness or paralysis of the hand intrinsic muscles, finger flexors, and wrist and finger extensors.

Sport-related brachial plexus injuries are usually associated with contact sports. "Stingers" or "burners" are likely the most common form of brachial plexus injury and represent neurapraxic injury to the brachial plexus. Symptoms of a burner or stinger typically include numbness, paresthesias, pain, and less commonly weakness. The symptoms usually last minutes to hours. Sports commonly associated with stingers or burners include football, rugby, and ice hockey [1, 8].

Suprascapular Nerve

The suprascapular nerve is a mixed motor/sensory nerve that derives from the upper trunk of the brachial plexus (C5 and C6 roots). The motor branch innervates the supraspinatus and infraspinatus muscles, while the sensory branch innervates the coracohumeral and coracoacromial ligaments, the subacromial bursa, and the acromioclavicular and glenohumeral joints. While direct trauma can cause suprascapular nerve injury, the most common mechanism is repetitive overhead motion and hyperabduction of the shoulder, such as in baseball (especially pitchers), fencing, volleyball, swimming, or tennis [2, 18, 26, 27].

Suprascapular nerve injury presents with deep-seated shoulder pain, weakness, and sometimes atrophy of the infraspinatus and/or supraspinatus muscles, without involvement of other rotator cuff muscles. Differential diagnosis includes cervical radiculopathy and brachial plexopathy. If the site of compression and injury is at the suprascapular notch, external shoulder rotation and abduction, particularly the first 15 degrees of abduction, will be weak, given involvement of both the infraspinatus and supraspinatus. If the injury is more distal, only the infraspinatus will be affected, limiting the weakness to external rotation. Other C5/upper trunk-innervated muscles should be examined to help differentiate a C5 radiculopathy from an upper trunk brachial plexopathy from a suprascapular neuropathy, including the rhomboids, deltoid, subscapularis, and biceps brachii muscles.

Electrodiagnostic testing can help identify the site of compression by examining both the supraspinatus and infraspinatus for changes, as well as helping to differentiate from a C5 radiculopathy and/or upper trunk brachial plexopathy by examining additional muscles, as suggested above. Imaging, including ultrasound and MRI, may be performed to rule out a structural lesion, such as a ganglion cyst which is a common cause of compression of the suprascapular nerve [2, 18]. For suprascapular neuropathy, it is important to obtain imaging in the diagnostic evaluation, in order to exclude a ganglion cyst [28]. Ganglion cysts may compress the suprascapular nerve at the suprascapular notch or at the spinoglenoid notch. Intraneural ganglion cysts can also occur, using joint branches to the glenohumeral joint as a conduit [29, 30]. Particularly when the primary complaint is pain, a diagnostic nerve block of the suprascapular nerve may be helpful in the evaluation in order to support the diagnosis.

Axillary Nerve

The axillary nerve arises from the posterior cord of the brachial plexus, carrying fibers from the C5 and C6 nerve roots. It innervates the deltoid and teres minor after coursing below the shoulder joint and curving around the proximal humerus. Damage most commonly occurs secondary to direct trauma, humerus fracture, or anterior shoulder dislocation [18]. Due to the circuitous course around the surgical neck of the humerus, the axillary nerve is particularly susceptible to injury with fractures in this location or due to shoulder dislocation. Subacute or chronic injury can also occur, with compression/entrapment of the axillary nerve in the quadrangular space. Common sports causing axillary nerve injuries include skiing, football, rugby, baseball, ice hockey, weightlifting, and wrestling [31].

The most common presentation of acute axillary nerve injury is weakness of arm abduction and shoulder forward flexion, though a thorough examination will often reveal a small area of numbness in the sensory territory supplied by the nerve on the anterolateral aspect of the upper arm. Differential diagnosis includes posterior cord plexopathy. Physical examination and electrodiagnostic assessment of the latissimus dorsi muscle, innervated by the thoracodorsal nerve, which arises just proximal to the axillary nerve takeoff, as well as the radial innervated muscles assist in making the distinction. In the more chronic condition known as quadrilateral space syndrome, the signs and symptoms may be more subtle [32, 33]. Many times there are pain and paresthesias about the shoulder that are difficult to localize. On physical examination, there is often pain with deep palpation in the quadrangular space and there may be subtle weakness of the deltoid and/or sensory changes in the distribution of the axillary nerve. The subjective symptoms are often worsened with resisted shoulder abduction and/or external rotation. Electrodiagnostic studies may be helpful in detecting subtle signs of axillary neuropathy. Imaging can be helpful in detecting denervation changes or atrophy in the teres minor, which is often a prominent feature. Finally, a diagnostic nerve block of the axillary nerve can be helpful in supporting the diagnosis.

Radial Nerve

The radial nerve, one of two terminal branches of the posterior cord of the brachial plexus, courses posterior to the humerus through the triangular interval and then runs in the spiral groove of the humerus. The nerve then runs between the brachialis and brachioradialis. In the proximal forearm, the nerve gives off the superficial radial nerve and a motor branch to the extensor carpi radialis brevis and then continues as the posterior interosseous nerve (PIN). The PIN then runs under the Arcade of Frohse at the supinator inlet. Along the course, the nerve is most susceptible to injury at the spiral groove, either related to bone fractures or compression from the lateral intermuscular septum [34]. The posterior interosseous nerve is prone to compression at the supinator inlet.

Sports-related injuries include proximal humeral fracture, injuring the nerve at the spiral groove. Overall, radial nerve injury is estimated to have 10–15% incidence in association with humeral shaft fractures [35–37]. Chronic injuries are often due to repetitive forceful extension of the elbow [18]. Repetitive pronation and supination, common in racket sports, can cause overuse injury, with compression of the posterior interosseous nerve at the Arcade of Frohse [18]. Compression of the distal radial nerve or posterior interosseous nerve can result in weakness of the posterior interosseous innervated muscles or a pain syndrome that lacks any weakness, often referred to as radial tunnel syndrome [38].

As with all injuries, the history and physical examination serve as the foundation of the evaluation. When possible, a physical examination should be performed at the time of the injury prior to any intervention, particularly since iatrogenic injury to the radial nerve can occur with reduction of humeral fractures. Injury-related radial nerve injuries versus iatrogenic radial nerve injuries may be managed differently. Physical examination should include evaluation of the radial-innervated muscles working from proximal to distal, as this will help localize the injury. The triceps branches come off quite proximally, so involvement of the triceps suggests a very proximal injury. In this case, one should also examine the axillary innervated muscles (e.g., deltoid) to help exclude a posterior cord injury, rather than a radial nerve injury. The brachioradialis should be examined, since sparing (or relative-sparing) of the triceps but involvement of the brachioradialis (and the rest of the distal muscles) localizes to the spiral groove. The nerve branches to the extensor carpi radialis longus and brevis arise proximal to the posterior interosseous nerve, while the branch to the extensor carpi ulnaris arises from the PIN. A PIN palsy is suggested by a finger drop without a wrist drop, with radial deviation on wrist extension. Radial tunnel syndrome is suggested by pain that is exacerbated with resisted extension of the third digit, resisted wrist extension and/or resisted supination [39]. Electrodiagnostic testing may assist in establishing the anatomic site of injury, especially for subacute or chronic presentations [2]. Serial electrodiagnostic studies may be used to examine for evidence of spontaneous recovery. Imaging can be helpful in identifying signal changes within the nerve consistent with nerve injury, for examining the relationship between the radial nerve and fractures, and for evaluating the relationship of the nerve to surgical hardware.

Median Nerve

The median nerve forms from the merging of branches from the lateral and medial cords, with the lateral cord supplying predominantly the sensory fibers and the medial cord supplying predominantly the motor fibers. The median nerve runs between the brachialis and biceps brachii in the arm, passes through the antecubital fossa coursing under the lacertus fibrosus. The nerve continues between the two heads of the pronator teres and eventually passes through the carpal tunnel to enter the hand. The median nerve innervates the pronator teres, flexor carpi radialis, flexor digitorum superficialis, lumbricals 1 and 2, opponens pollicis, abductor pollicis brevis, and flexor pollicis brevis. The median nerve also innervates the flexor pollicis longus, flexor digitorum profundus to the second and third digits, and pronator quadratus through the anterior interosseous nerve, which is a branch of the median nerve arising in the mid-forearm. The sensory innervation of the median nerve includes the radial aspect of the palm to approximately the level of the wrist crease and the palmar aspect of the radial three and a half digits. The median innervation reliably splits the ring finger, with the median nerve innervating the radial side and the ulnar nerve innervating the ulnar side.

Damage to the median nerve in athletes comes from repetitive movements, compression, traction, or direct blunt or penetrating traumatic injuries including elbow fracture or dislocation. The most common median nerve injury manifests as carpal tunnel syndrome, which may be acute after a crush or penetrating injury or bony fracture or chronic secondary to repetitive overuse injury of the wrist. Median nerve injury/entrapment can complicate distal radius fractures, either from the injury or from an ill-fitting cast [40]. Typical symptoms include sensory loss or paresthesias in the median distribution, pain, and median-innervated intrinsic hand weakness.

Repetitive movements of the forearm and elbow can lead to chronic median nerve compression in the forearm. Potential points of compression include the lacertus fibrosus, pronator teres, and sublimis arch. Activities where repeated pronation of the forearm occurs can result in the median nerve being compressed between the two heads of the pronator teres. Patients will complain of pain in the forearm with pronation and numbness in the distribution of the median nerve. On examination, pain can be elicited by compressing the point where the median nerve dives between the heads of the pronator teres muscle [41]. Distal to the antecubital fossa, the median nerve dives inferiorly beneath the fascial extension (lacertus fibrosus) of the biceps brachii tendon that merges with the fascia of the forearm. This tunnel acts as a site for median nerve compression between the lacertus fibrosus and biceps brachii.

EMG/NCS, MRI, and US are useful tools in assessing the severity of nerve dysfunction as well as the location and degree of compression in athletes with median nerve symptoms. For example, EMG and US are commonly used for the diagnosis of carpal tunnel syndrome [42–46]. It is important to remember that median nerve compression in the forearm may be a pure pain syndrome, with few, if any, changes on electrodiagnostic study or imaging.

Ulnar Nerve

The ulnar nerve arises from the medial cord of the brachial plexus. As the nerve descends down the arm, it penetrates the medial intermuscular septum and runs under the arcade of Struthers on the surface of the medial head of the triceps. The nerve then courses posterior to the medial epicondyle, entering the cubital tunnel by passing deep to Osborne's ligament. In addition to muscular branches to the flexor carpi ulnaris and flexor digitorum profundus, in the forearm the nerve gives off the dorsal cutaneous and palmar cutaneous branches. At the wrist, the nerve enters Guyon's canal and bifurcates into the superficial (primarily sensory) and deep (primarily motor) branches.

The ulnar nerve is susceptible to entrapment/compression around the elbow and in some circumstances can be prone to repetitive microtrauma from rubbing against the edge of the medial epicondyle. With ulnar neuropathy at the elbow, patients present with numbness and/or paresthesias in the dorsal and palmar aspect of the ulnar side of the hand and the ulnar 1.5 digits as well as potentially with weakness of the ulnar-innervated hand intrinsic muscles often manifesting as reduced hand dexterity. With injury or compression of the ulnar nerve in the wrist or hand around the area of Guyon's canal, the palmar and dorsal cutaneous distributions will be spared. Compression or injury within Guyon's canal can be divided into three zones: Zone 1 has a combination of sensory and motor symptoms, with compression of the proximal to the bifurcation; Zone 2 has only motor symptoms and occurs with injury to the deep branch around the hook of the hamate; Zone 3 has sensory symptoms and occurs with injury to the superficial branch.

Injury to the ulnar nerve can occur in a variety of sports, but baseball players, especially pitchers, are particularly prone to injury of the ulnar nerve around the elbow. The significant forces generated to throw a baseball pitch generate significant compression of the ulnar nerve within the cubital tunnel. The repetitive nature of throwing then causes repetitive trauma to the ulnar nerve [47, 48]. Injury to the ulnar nerve in the wrist/hand occurs more commonly from repetitive direct pressure on the wrist and hand, with the direct pressure being transmitted to the ulnar nerve. The hook of the hamate is also in close approximation to the ulnar nerve and fractures of the hook of the hamate can result in ulnar nerve injury, as can ganglion cysts that form in the area. Athletes that are prone to ulnar neuropathy around Guyon's canal include wheelchair athletes and cyclists [49, 50].

Evaluation begins with history and physical examination. The examiner should test sensory function in the dorsal cutaneous, palmar cutaneous, and ulnar digital distributions, which can be helpful in differentiating ulnar neuropathy at the elbow versus Guyon's canal. While the flexor carpi ulnaris and flexor digitorum profundus tend to be relatively spared in cubital tunnel syndrome, involvement of these muscles also helps exclude Guyon's canal syndrome, so these muscles should be examined in addition to the ulnar-innervated hand intrinsic muscles. The median-innervated hand intrinsic muscles should be examined to help exclude a C8-T1 radiculopathy or lower trunk plexopathy such as you might see with thoracic outlet syndrome. The median-innervated hand intrinsic muscles should be preserved in an ulnar neuropathy. The ulnar nerve should also be palpated through elbow range of motion to evaluate for subluxation of the ulnar nerve, which may have treatment ramifications. Provocative maneuvers such as the Tinel test or elbow flexion test should also be incorporated into the examination.

US, MRI, and electrodiagnostic studies may confirm physical exam findings and help elucidate the cause of ulnar nerve dysfunction. US is highly effective in visualizing the ulnar nerve throughout its anatomical course. Analysis of the cross-sectional area and ratio of nerve enlargement to normal size allows the examiner to assess the location of nerve damage. Also, US is effective in identifying if abnormal hyper-mobility of the ulnar nerve occurs in the cubital tunnel during movement, for example with subluxation over the medial epicondyle during elbow flexion. MRI is useful for evaluating soft tissue masses or anatomical compression along the length of the ulnar nerve [44, 45, 51, 52].

Lower Extremity Nerve Injuries

Lateral Femoral Cutaneous Nerve

The lateral femoral cutaneous nerve (LFCN) is a pure sensory nerve that arises from L2 and L3 and innervates the anterolateral thigh. Anatomy around the hip is variable, especially the nerve course in relation to the anterior superior iliac spine (ASIS) and inguinal ligament. The most common configuration is for the nerve to pass medial to the ASIS and deep to the inguinal ligament [53]. When the nerve passes over the ASIS and/or through or over the inguinal ligament, the nerve may be more susceptible to injury. Sports-related injuries have been described due to both blunt trauma and entrapment. Two locations along the path of the nerve are most susceptible to direct trauma: at the ASIS and in the distal thigh, where it is most superficial [54, 55]. Unsurprisingly, this mechanism of injury is most common in high-contact sports, such as football and rugby [55]. Entrapment may result from activities that involve repetitive hip flexion and extension, such as in jumping sports, gymnastics, or prolonged skipping, or related to compression from poorly fitting gear, seen most often in SCUBA divers and mountain climbers [2, 3, 55, 56]. In both cases, the nerve injury is generally neurapraxic and avoidable with appropriate technique and equipment [55].

Regardless of mechanism, injury to the LFCN presents with pain, numbness, and/or paresthesias along the anterolateral thigh. There should not be any motor symptoms, since the nerve is a pure sensory nerve. As with other nerves, the history and physical examination are the keys to diagnosis. Consistent with a peripheral nerve injury, the area of sensory symptoms will have a sharply demarcated border. We usually ask the patient to take one finger and trace the area of the sensory symptoms. A well-circumscribed area is consistent with injury to the LFCN, whereas patients that have difficulty doing this may have a more proximal injury (e.g., radiculopathy). The sensory examination should focus on confirming the area of sensory abnormality and the sharply demarcated border. A lower extremity motor examination should be performed to exclude lumbosacral plexopathy or radiculopathy, since the motor exam should be normal with injuries to the LFCN.

Ultrasound can be used effectively to identify this nerve and may have a role in confirming and localizing entrapment; however, it is not commonly used in the literature [57]. Electrodiagnostic testing may be done; however, the utility is questionable, as responses can be absent in normal individuals [58]. In cases where the diagnosis is not clear, electrodiagnostic studies may be useful, primarily to exclude radiculopathy, rather than to confirm lateral femoral cutaneous neuropathy. Ultrasound-guided diagnostic nerve block can also be quite useful in supporting the diagnosis.

Femoral Nerve

The largest branch of the lumbar plexus, the femoral nerve arises from L2, L3, and L4 and provides motor and sensory supply to the anterior compartment of the thigh, as well as sensation to the anteromedial leg. It is most at risk of traumatic injury as it courses through the iliacus compartment, but femoral nerve injury remains rare in sport [18, 22]. When it does occur, it is usually caused by hyperextension of the hip, often following a sudden collision [18, 55]. In most cases, injury to the femoral nerve occurs related to compression as a result of a partial iliopsoas tear and subsequent iliacus hematoma [55, 59, 60]. Sports prone to this injury include football, dancing, basketball, gymnastics, long jump, body-building, and cross-country skiing [18, 55]. Individual muscle branches can also be injured related to direct trauma to the anterior thigh. The saphenous nerve is the terminal branch of the femoral nerve. This nerve, particularly its infrapatellar branch, is susceptible to injury during knee arthroscopy, which is common in athletes [61–63].

Athletes with femoral nerve injury present with some combination of hip flexion weakness, inguinal pain, anterior thigh numbness/paresthesias/pain, quadriceps weakness, and/or anteromedial leg numbness/paresthesias/pain. Physical examination should focus on the sensory and motor distribution of the femoral nerve, including the saphenous nerve distribution. Physical examination may reveal pain with hip extension and/or an absent patellar reflex [2, 18].

As femoral nerve injury is usually secondary to trauma to the surrounding muscle and connective tissue, imaging plays a role in accurate diagnosis. MRI can confirm an iliopsoas tear and hematoma and subsequent mass effect on the nerve [18, 22]. Identification of a compressive hematoma can have significant ramifications for management, so imaging is paramount. Furthermore, when imaging is performed in the subacute to early chronic period, changes in signal intensity of different muscle groups can help identify the specific location of nerve injury. Denervation of the iliopsoas indicates intrapelvic injury, while isolated changes in the signal of the quadriceps group, pectineus, and/or sartorius are more likely following damage to the nerve distal to the inguinal ligament [22].

Sciatic Nerve

The sciatic nerve arises from the L4-S2 roots of the lumbosacral plexus, courses through the gluteal region, runs deep to the piriformis into the posteromedial thigh and divides into two branches, the tibial nerve and the common peroneal nerve, proximal to the popliteal fossa. The proximal sciatic nerve provides motor innervation to the hamstring muscles, while the tibial nerve innervates the ankle plantar flexors, toe flexors, and ankle invertors and the common peroneal nerve innervates the ankle dorsiflexors, toe extensors, and evertors. Finally, the sciatic nerve provides sensory innervation to the anterior, posterior, and lateral leg, as well as the dorsal, plantar, and lateral surfaces of the foot, excluding the medial foot (innervated by the saphenous nerve). Basically, the sciatic nerve through its branches controls all movements distal to the knee and provides all sensation distal to the knee, with the exception of the infrapatellar region and a stripe down the medial leg to the medial foot, which is innervated by the saphenous nerve.

The most common mechanism of injury of the sciatic nerve is due to trauma in contact sports. These traumas generally occur due to a fall, which leads to compression of the nerve against the hip capsule, but can also occur in the presence of a fracture of the hip or proximal tibia [55]. Sciatic nerve injury may also occur in association with proximal hamstring avulsion [64]. Proximal hamstring injuries are common in athletes, especially in sports where rapid acceleration is required or when rapid stretch occurs, such as during a fall related to water skiing [65–67].

Imaging is important in the evaluation of sciatic nerve injuries to evaluate for associated muscle, bone, or tendon injury. Electrodiagnostic testing is useful for both diagnosis and prognosis [68].

Common Peroneal Nerve

The most commonly injured lower extremity peripheral nerve is the common peroneal nerve. This lateral branch of the sciatic nerve runs through the popliteal fossa and then superficially around the fibular head through the fibular tunnel before branching into the superficial peroneal and deep peroneal nerves. The nerve is particularly susceptible to injury as it wraps around the fibular head, either related to stretch, since this is a relative point of fixation, or related to direct trauma to the proximal lateral leg.

Sport-related injury to the nerve can occur via traction, compression, entrapment, and trauma [18, 55, 69]. Repetitive traction at the knee results in irritation along the neck of the fibula, most commonly seen in runners and martial artists [18, 55]. Knee dislocations, especially those associated with ligamentous knee injuries, can cause severe traction injury to the common peroneal nerve and in severe cases, even rupture of the nerve [70–73]. Compression injuries most commonly occur due to exertional compartment syndrome, which is most common in runners and leads to compression and potentially ischemia of the nerve in any or all of the lower leg compartments [18, 69]. Compression of the deep peroneal nerve can occur at the ankle in the setting of improperly fitting equipment (e.g., ski boots or skates) and is often characterized by a self-limited neurapraxia [18]. Injury to the common peroneal nerve from direct trauma is also often neurapraxic and, as with other mechanisms, is most common at the fibular head. This is seen in contact sports such as soccer, hockey, and football [18].

Symptoms vary depending on the mechanism of injury and which branch of the nerve is injured. Classic descriptions of common peroneal nerve injury include impaired foot dorsiflexion (i.e., foot drop) and eversion, along with sensory loss and burning pain in the lateral lower leg and/or dorsal foot [2]. The deep peroneal nerve provides sensation to the dorsal first webspace, while the superficial peroneal nerve provides sensation to the remainder of the dorsum of the foot. The history should be used to tease out the specific distribution of pain, numbness, and paresthesias, focusing on determining whether the distribution matches the superficial peroneal, deep peroneal, or both, in which case a common peroneal neuropathy is more likely. The physical examination should similarly be used to detect sensory changes in these distributions. The major differential diagnosis for a foot drop is an L5 radiculopathy. With a common peroneal neuropathy, the weakness will involve dorsiflexion and eversion. Inversion will not be involved. With an L5 radiculopathy, dorsiflexion may also be weak, but inversion will be involved, rather than eversion, or at least eversion to a lesser degree. Testing of eversion and inversion thus can be used to help differentiate a common peroneal neuropathy from an L5 radiculopathy or sciatic neuropathy. Exacerbating factors should also be sought in the history. Running-related injuries (i.e., repetitive traction at the fibular neck and exertional compartment syndrome) are characterized by lack of symptoms at rest or when walking, with onset of pain, paresthesias, and foot drop when running [18]. However, with repetitive injury, the symptoms may progress to being present at rest.

Imaging—ultrasound and/or MRI—is crucial in the assessment of the common peroneal nerve. Common peroneal nerve injury at the level of the fibular head can be diagnosed by increased signal intensity and size on axial fluid-sensitive images [74]. Imaging (MRI and CT) can also distinguish nerve entrapment from stress fracture or popliteal artery entrapment syndrome in the setting of chronic, diffuse lower leg pain [74]. With severe injuries, it is important to evaluate the integrity of the nerve, as this may change management. The lariat sign on MRI has been described in association with nerve rupture [75, 76]. Extraneural and intraneural ganglion cysts also occur, arising from the superior tibiofibular joint. The intraneural version arises from the superior tibiofibular joint and uses the articular branch of the common peroneal nerve as a conduit for synovial fluid to track into the nerve [77–80]. It is important to recognize these cysts, as their presence changes management. Characteristic MRI findings for peroneal intraneural ganglion cysts, which are the most common form of intraneural ganglion cyst, have been described [81]. Interestingly, ankle injuries that occur in sports can result in ganglion cyst formation at the superior tibiofibular joint due to forces transmitted from the ankle, along the interosseous membrane, and ultimately to the superior tibiofibular joint [82]. In this way, common peroneal neuropathy can occur in association with ankle injuries.

Electrodiagnostic testing is essential in evaluating common peroneal nerve injuries. It helps assess the site, type and extent of injuries, which is crucial for determining recovery and prognosis [2, 83]. Notably, electromyography can help differentiate between an isolated common peroneal nerve injury as opposed to a peroneal-predominant sciatic nerve injury or L5 radiculopathy. EMG abnormalities in the short head of biceps femoris indicate involvement of the peroneal division of the sciatic nerve, since the branch to the short head of the biceps arises proximal to the sciatic bifurcation into the common peroneal and tibial nerves [83]. If the mechanism of injury involves repetitive traction, pre- and post-exercise EMG/NCS can be considered [2]. If exertional compartment syndrome is being considered, needle pressure measurements should be made pre- and post-exercise [18, 69].

Pudendal Nerve

Arising from the S2-S4 roots, the pudendal nerve has a complicated course through the gluteal region and the pelvis, ultimately running through the pudendal (Alcock) canal. It serves a number of roles, include anal and genital region sensation, innervation of rectal and bladder sphincters, sympathetic innervation of erectile tissue, and motor control of the bulbospongiosus and ischiocavernosus muscles [18]. SRNI of the pudendal nerve occurs in the setting of chronic compression, most commonly associated with prolonged bicycle riding without ergonomic seats. Hard, narrow seats predispose to this, as they do not support the ischial tuberosities, which increases pressure on the perineal area overlaying the nerve. Long-term pressure causes thickening of the sacrotuberous and sacrospinous ligaments, leading to nerve compression and potentially ischemia [2, 18].

Athletes present with numbness and/or pain anywhere in the distribution of the pudendal nerve that is exacerbated with sitting and tends to worsen progressively throughout the day [18]. As expected given its end-organs, compression of the pudendal nerve has been associated with sexual, urinary, and bowel dysfunction, including male impotence [18, 84, 85]. Imaging is rarely described in diagnosis of pudendal nerve injury; however, MRI of the pudendal canal can reveal increased signal intensity in the setting of SRNI [86]. Somatosensory evoked potentials may reveal conduction delays and potentially bulbocavernosus reflex abnormalities [2]. Diagnostic nerve block can also be used to support the diagnosis.

Conclusion

Peripheral nerve injuries resulting from sports, exercise, or recreation can cause significant functional impairment and result in lengthy and variable degrees of recovery. There is a wide range of possible mechanisms of injury, including contact-related trauma, acute and chronic stretch, and tissue swelling. Inadequate protective equipment, ill-fitting equipment, overtraining, and use of improper technique or positioning are all factors that increase an athlete's risk for developing a sports-related nerve injury. Diagnosis of sports-related nerve injuries, including physical examination, electrodiagnostics, imaging, and the use of diagnostic nerve blocks, is essential for proper management.

References

1. Olivo R, Tsao B. Peripheral nerve injuries in sport. Neurol Clin. 2017;35(3):559–72. https://doi.org/10.1016/j.ncl.2017.03.010.
2. Lolis AM, Falsone S, Beric A. Common peripheral nerve injuries in sport: diagnosis and management. Elsevier B.V.; 2018. p. 401–19.
3. Hirasawa Y, Sakakida K. Sports and peripheral nerve injury. Am J Sports Med. 1983;11(6):420–6.
4. Li NY, Onor GI, Lemme NJ, Gil JA. Epidemiology of peripheral nerve injuries in sports, exercise, and recreation in the United States, 2009–2018. Phys Sportsmed. 2021;49(3):355–62. https://doi.org/10.1080/00913847.2020.1850151.
5. Charbonneau RME, McVeigh SA, Thompson K. Brachial neuropraxia in Canadian Atlantic University sport football players: what is the incidence of "stingers"? Clin J Sport Med. 2012;22(6):472–7.
6. Krivickas LS, Wilbourn AJ. Peripheral nerve injuries in athletes: a case series of over 200 injuries. Thieme Medical Publishers, Inc; 2000. p. 225–32.
7. Krivickas LS, Wilbourn AJ. Sports and peripheral nerve injuries: report of 190 injuries evaluation in a single electromyography laboratory. Muscle Nerve. 1998;21(8):1092–4. https://doi.org/10.1002/(SICI)1097-4598(199808)21:8<1092::AID-MUS19>3.0.CO;2-W.
8. Feinberg JH. Burners and stingers. W.B. Saunders; 2000. p. 771–84.
9. Zuckerman SL, Kerr ZY, Pierpoint L, Kirby P, Than KD, Wilson TJ. An 11-year analysis of peripheral nerve injuries in high school sports. Phys Sportsmed. 2019;47(2):167–73. https://doi.org/10.1080/00913847.2018.1544453.
10. Seddon HJ. A classification of nerve injuries. Br Med J. 1942;2(4260):237–9.
11. Sunderland S. A classification of peripheral nerve injuries producing loss of function. Brain. 1951;74(4):491–516. https://doi.org/10.1093/brain/74.4.491.
12. Chhabra A, Ahlawat S, Belzberg A, Andreseik G. Peripheral nerve injury grading simplified on MR neurography: as referenced to Seddon and Sunderland classifications. Indian J Radiol Imaging. 2014;24(3):217–24. https://doi.org/10.4103/0971-3026.137025.
13. Chhabra A, Madhuranthakam AJ, Andreisek G. Magnetic resonance neurography: current perspectives and literature review. Eur Radiol. 2018;28(2):698–707. https://doi.org/10.1007/s00330-017-4976-8.
14. Purger DA, Sakamuri S, Hug NF, Biswal S, Wilson TJ. Imaging of damaged nerves. Clin Plast Surg. 2020;47(2):245–59. https://doi.org/10.1016/j.cps.2019.12.003.
15. Robinson LR. How electrodiagnosis predicts clinical outcome of focal peripheral nerve lesions. Muscle Nerve. 2015;52(3):321–33. https://doi.org/10.1002/mus.24709.

16. Borisov AB, Carlson BM. Cell death in denervated skeletal muscle is distinct from classical apoptosis. Anat Rec. 2000;258(3):305–18.
17. Fu SY, Gordon T. Contributing factors to poor functional recovery after delayed nerve repair: prolonged axotomy. J Neurosci. 1995;15(5 Pt 2):3876–85.
18. Hainline BW. Peripheral nerve injury in sports. Continuum (Minneap Minn). 2014;20:1605–28. https://doi.org/10.1212/01.CON.0000458971.86389.9c.
19. Chhabra A, Williams EH, Wang KC, Dellon AL, Carrino JA. MR neurography of neuromas related to nerve injury and entrapment with surgical correlation. AJNR Am J Neuroradiol. 2010;31(8):1363–8. https://doi.org/10.3174/ajnr.A2002.
20. Husarik DB, Saupe N, Pfirrmann CW, Jost B, Hodler J, Zanetti M. Elbow nerves: MR findings in 60 asymptomatic subjects--normal anatomy, variants, and pitfalls. Radiology. 2009;252(1):148–56. https://doi.org/10.1148/radiol.2521081614.
21. Binaghi D, Socolovsky M. Magnetic resonance neurography and peripheral nerve surgery. In: Socolovsky M, Rasulic LG, Midha R, Garozzo D, editors. Manual of peripheral nerve surgery: from the basics to complex procedures. Thieme; 2018. p. 59–64.
22. Petchprapa CN, Rosenberg ZS, Sconfienza LM, Cavalcanti CF, Vieira RL, Zember JS. MR imaging of entrapment neuropathies of the lower extremity. Part 1. The pelvis and hip. Radiographics. 2010;30(4):983–1000. https://doi.org/10.1148/rg.304095135.
23. Garwood ER, Duarte A, Bencardino JT. MR imaging of entrapment neuropathies of the lower extremity. Radiol Clin N Am. 2018;56(6):997–1012. https://doi.org/10.1016/j.rcl.2018.06.012.
24. Sakellariou VI, Badilas NK, Mazis GA, Stavropoulos NA, Kotoulas HK, Kyriakopoulos S, et al. Brachial plexus injuries in adults: evaluation and diagnostic approach. ISRN Orthop. 2014;2014:726103. https://doi.org/10.1155/2014/726103.
25. Gutkowska O, Martynkiewicz J, Urban M, Gosk J. Brachial plexus injury after shoulder dislocation: a literature review. Neurosurg Rev. 2020;43(2):407–23. https://doi.org/10.1007/s10143-018-1001-x.
26. Matzkin E, Suslavich K, Wes D. Swimmer's shoulder: painful shoulder in the competitive swimmer. J Am Acad Orthop Surg. 2016;24(8):527–36. https://doi.org/10.5435/jaaos-d-15-00313.
27. LiBrizzi CL, Rojas JL, Bontrager NC, Srikumaran U, McFarland EG. Suprascapular nerve entrapment in young kayaker: a case report. Phys Sportsmed. 2020;48(2):236–40. https://doi.org/10.1080/00913847.2019.1662273.
28. Antoniadis G, Richter HP, Rath S, Braun V, Moese G. Suprascapular nerve entrapment: experience with 28 cases. J Neurosurg. 1996;85(6):1020–5. https://doi.org/10.3171/jns.1996.85.6.1020.
29. Spinner RJ, Amrami KK. Intraneural ganglion of the suprascapular nerve: case report. J Hand Surg Am. 2006;31(10):1698–9. https://doi.org/10.1016/j.jhsa.2006.09.015.
30. Spinner RJ, Amrami KK, Kliot M, Johnston SP, Casanas J. Suprascapular intraneural ganglia and glenohumeral joint connections. J Neurosurg. 2006;104(4):551–7. https://doi.org/10.3171/jns.2006.104.4.551.
31. Lee S, Saetia K, Saha S, Kline DG, Kim DH. Axillary nerve injury associated with sports. Neurosurg Focus. 2011;31(5):E10. https://doi.org/10.3171/2011.8.focus11183.
32. Cahill BR, Palmer RE. Quadrilateral space syndrome. J Hand Surg Am. 1983;8(1):65–9. https://doi.org/10.1016/s0363-5023(83)80056-2.
33. Flynn LS, Wright TW, King JJ. Quadrilateral space syndrome: a review. J Shoulder Elbow Surg. 2018;27(5):950–6. https://doi.org/10.1016/j.jse.2017.10.024.
34. Latef TJ, Bilal M, Vetter M, Iwanaga J, Oskouian RJ, Tubbs RS. Injury of the radial nerve in the arm: a review. Cureus. 2018;10(2):e2199. https://doi.org/10.7759/cureus.2199.
35. Mahabier KC, Vogels LM, Punt BJ, Roukema GR, Patka P, Van Lieshout EM. Humeral shaft fractures: retrospective results of non-operative and operative treatment of 186 patients. Injury. 2013;44(4):427–30. https://doi.org/10.1016/j.injury.2012.08.003.
36. Bishop J, Ring D. Management of radial nerve palsy associated with humeral shaft fracture: a decision analysis model. J Hand Surg. 2009;34(6):991–6.e1. https://doi.org/10.1016/j.jhsa.2008.12.029.

37. Shao YC, Harwood P, Grotz MR, Limb D, Giannoudis PV. Radial nerve palsy associated with fractures of the shaft of the humerus: a systematic review. J Bone Joint Surg. 2005;87(12):1647–52. https://doi.org/10.1302/0301-620x.87b12.16132.
38. Cha J, York B, Tawfik J. Posterior interosseous nerve compression. Eplasty. 2014;14:ic4.
39. Moradi A, Ebrahimzadeh MH, Jupiter JB. Radial tunnel syndrome, diagnostic and treatment dilemma. Arch Bone Jt Surg. 2015;3(3):156–62.
40. Vaghela KR, Velazquez-Pimentel D, Ahluwalia AK, Choraria A, Hunter A. Distal radius fractures: an evidence-based approach to assessment and management. Br J Hosp Med (Lond). 2020;81(6):1–8. https://doi.org/10.12968/hmed.2020.0006.
41. Adler JA, Wolf JM. Proximal median nerve compression: pronator syndrome. J Hand Surg Am. 2020; https://doi.org/10.1016/j.jhsa.2020.07.006.
42. Soubeyrand M, Melhem R, Protais M, Artuso M, Crézé M. Anatomy of the median nerve and its clinical applications. Hand Surg Rehab. 2020;39(1):2–18. https://doi.org/10.1016/j.hansur.2019.10.197.
43. Cartwright MS, Hobson-Webb LD, Boon AJ, Alter KE, Hunt CH, Flores VH, et al. Evidence-based guideline: neuromuscular ultrasound for the diagnosis of carpal tunnel syndrome. Muscle Nerve. 2012;46(2):287–93. https://doi.org/10.1002/mus.23389.
44. Cartwright MS, Walker FO. Neuromuscular ultrasound in common entrapment neuropathies. Muscle Nerve. 2013;48(5):696–704. https://doi.org/10.1002/mus.23900.
45. Robinson LR. Traumatic injury to peripheral nerves. John Wiley & Sons; 2000. p. 863–73.
46. Robinson LR, Micklesen PJ, Wang L. Optimizing the number of tests for carpal tunnel syndrome. Muscle Nerve. 2000;23(12):1880–2. https://doi.org/10.1002/1097-4598(200012)23:12<1880::aid-mus14>3.0.co;2-a.
47. Post EG, Laudner KG, McLoda TA, Wong R, Meister K. Correlation of shoulder and elbow kinetics with ball velocity in collegiate baseball pitchers. J Athl Train. 2015;50(6):629–33. https://doi.org/10.4085/1062-6040-50.1.06.
48. Treihaft MM. Neurologic injuries in baseball players. Semin Neurol. 2000;20(2):187–93. https://doi.org/10.1055/s-2000-9827.
49. Klenck C, Gebke K. Practical management: common medical problems in disabled athletes. Clin J Sport Med. 2007;17(1):55–60. https://doi.org/10.1097/JSM.0b013e3180302587.
50. Wilbourn AJ. Electrodiagnostic testing of neurologic injuries in athletes. Clin Sports Med. 1990;9(2):229–45.
51. Polatsch DB, Melone CP Jr, Beldner S, Incorvaia A. Ulnar nerve anatomy. Hand Clin. 2007;23(3):283–9, v. https://doi.org/10.1016/j.hcl.2007.05.001.
52. Schickendantz MS, Yalcin S. Conditions and injuries affecting the nerves around the elbow. Clin Sports Med. 2020;39(3):597–621. https://doi.org/10.1016/j.csm.2020.02.006.
53. Tomaszewski KA, Popieluszko P, Henry BM, Roy J, Sanna B, Kijek MR, et al. The surgical anatomy of the lateral femoral cutaneous nerve in the inguinal region: a meta-analysis. Hernia. 2016;20(5):649–57. https://doi.org/10.1007/s10029-016-1493-7.
54. Ecker AD, Woltman HW. Meralgia paraesthetica: a report of one hundred and fifty cases. J Am Med Assoc. 1938;110(20):1650–2. https://doi.org/10.1001/jama.1938.02790200018006.
55. Lorei MP, Hershman EB. Peripheral nerve injuries in athletes: treatment and prevention. Sports Med. 1993;16(2):130–47. https://doi.org/10.2165/00007256-199316020-00005.
56. Toth C. Peripheral nerve injuries attributable to sport and recreation. Phys Med Rehabil Clin N Am. 2009;26:77–100. https://doi.org/10.1016/j.pmr.2008.10.012.
57. Chang K-V, Mezian K, Naňka O, Wu W-T, Lou Y-M, Wang J-C, et al. Ultrasound imaging for the cutaneous nerves of the extremities and RELEVANT entrapment syndromes: from anatomy to clinical implications. J Clin Med. 2018;7(11):457. https://doi.org/10.3390/jcm7110457.
58. Sarala PK, Nishihara T, Oh SJ. Meralgia paresthetica: electrophysiologic study. Arch Phys Med Rehabil. 1979;60(1):30–1.
59. Seijo-Martínez M, Castro Del Río M, Fontoira E, Fontoira M. Acute femoral neuropathy secondary to an iliacus muscle hematoma. J Neurol Sci. 2003;209(1–2):119–22. https://doi.org/10.1016/S0022-510X(03)00005-4.

60. Murray IR, Perks FJ, Beggs I, Moran M. Femoral nerve palsy secondary to traumatic iliacus haematoma - A young athlete's injury. BMJ Case Rep. 2010;2010:bcr0520103045-bcr. https://doi.org/10.1136/bcr.05.2010.3045.
61. Ahn JH, Lee SH, Jung HJ, Koo KH, Kim SH. The relationship of neural structures to arthroscopic posterior portals according to knee positioning. Knee Surg Sports Traumatol Arthrosc. 2011;19(4):646–52. https://doi.org/10.1007/s00167-010-1326-7.
62. Kerver AL, Leliveld MS, den Hartog D, Verhofstad MH, Kleinrensink GJ. The surgical anatomy of the infrapatellar branch of the saphenous nerve in relation to incisions for anteromedial knee surgery. J Bone Joint Surg Am. 2013;95(23):2119–25. https://doi.org/10.2106/jbjs.l.01297.
63. Mochida H, Kikuchi S. Injury to infrapatellar branch of saphenous nerve in arthroscopic knee surgery. Clin Orthop Relat Res. 1995;320:88–94.
64. Wilson TJ, Spinner RJ, Mohan R, Gibbs CM, Krych AJ. Sciatic nerve injury after proximal hamstring avulsion and repair. Orthop J Sports Med. 2017;5(7):2325967117713685. https://doi.org/10.1177/2325967117713685.
65. Ahmad CS, Redler LH, Ciccotti MG, Maffulli N, Longo UG, Bradley J. Evaluation and management of hamstring injuries. Am J Sports Med. 2013;41(12):2933–47. https://doi.org/10.1177/0363546513487063.
66. Ali K, Leland JM. Hamstring strains and tears in the athlete. Clin Sports Med. 2012;31(2):263–72. https://doi.org/10.1016/j.csm.2011.11.001.
67. Cohen S, Bradley J. Acute proximal hamstring rupture. J Am Acad Orthop Surg. 2007;15(6):350–5.
68. Distad BJ, Weiss MD. Clinical and Electrodiagnostic features of sciatic neuropathies. Phys Med Rehabil Clin N Am. 2013;24:107–20. https://doi.org/10.1016/j.pmr.2012.08.023.
69. Rajasekaran S, Kvinlaug K, Finnoff JT. Exertional leg pain in the athlete. PM R. 2012;4(12):985–1000. https://doi.org/10.1016/j.pmrj.2012.10.002.
70. Kahan JB, Li D, Schneble CA, Huang P, Bullock J, Porrino J, et al. The pathoanatomy of posterolateral corner ligamentous disruption in multiligament knee injuries is predictive of Peroneal nerve injury. Am J Sports Med. 2020;48:3541. https://doi.org/10.1177/0363546520962503.
71. Hoit G, Farag J, Whelan DB. Neurologic assessment and management of the multiple ligament injured knee: a review and synthesis of current evidence. J Knee Surg. 2020;33(4):339–45. https://doi.org/10.1055/s-0039-3401828.
72. Mukohara S, Inui A, Mifune Y, Nishimoto H, Kataoka T, Kurosawa T, et al. Isolated nerve grafting for a young patient with a complete common Peroneal nerve palsy following a traumatic knee dislocation: a case report. Kobe J Med Sci. 2020;65(3):E110–e3.
73. Samson D, Ng CY, Power D. An evidence-based algorithm for the management of common peroneal nerve injury associated with traumatic knee dislocation. EFORT Open Rev. 2016;1(10):362–7. https://doi.org/10.1302/2058-5241.160012.
74. Donovan A, Rosenberg ZS, Cavalcanti CF. MR imaging of entrapment neuropathies of the lower extremity: part 2. The knee, leg, ankle, and foot. Radiographics. 2010;30(4):1001–14. https://doi.org/10.1148/rg.304095188.
75. Tran TMA, Lim BG, Sheehy R, Robertson PL. Magnetic resonance imaging for common peroneal nerve injury in trauma patients: are routine knee sequences adequate for prediction of outcome? J Med Imaging Radiat Oncol. 2019;63(1):54–60. https://doi.org/10.1111/1754-9485.12840.
76. Morris BL, Grinde AS, Olson H, Brubacher JW, Schroeppel JP, Everist BM. Lariat sign: an MRI finding associated with common peroneal nerve rupture. Radiol Case Rep. 2018;13(3):743–6. https://doi.org/10.1016/j.radcr.2018.03.015.
77. Spinner RJ, Amrami KK, Wolanskyj AP, Desy NM, Wang H, Benarroch EE, et al. Dynamic phases of peroneal and tibial intraneural ganglia formation: a new dimension added to the unifying articular theory. J Neurosurg. 2007;107(2):296–307. https://doi.org/10.3171/JNS-07/08/0296.
78. Spinner RJ, Atkinson JL, Tiel RL. Peroneal intraneural ganglia: the importance of the articular branch. A unifying theory. J Neurosurg. 2003;99(2):330–43. https://doi.org/10.3171/jns.2003.99.2.0330.

79. Spinner RJ, Hebert-Blouin MN, Skinner JA, Amrami KK. Knee MR arthrographic proof of an articular origin for combined intraneural and adventitial cysts. Acta Neurochir. 2010;152(5):919–23. https://doi.org/10.1007/s00701-009-0574-0.
80. Wilson TJ, Hebert-Blouin MN, Murthy NS, Garcia JJ, Amrami KK, Spinner RJ. The nearly invisible intraneural cyst: a new and emerging part of the spectrum. Neurosurg Focus. 2017;42(3):E10. https://doi.org/10.3171/2016.12.focus16439.
81. Spinner RJ, Luthra G, Desy NM, Anderson ML, Amrami KK. The clock face guide to peroneal intraneural ganglia: critical "times" and sites for accurate diagnosis. Skelet Radiol. 2008;37(12):1091–9. https://doi.org/10.1007/s00256-008-0545-1.
82. Spinner RJ, Ibrahim Elshiekh MA, Tubbs RS, Turner NS 3rd, Amrami KK. Posttraumatic torsional injury as an indirect cause of fibular intraneural ganglion cysts: case illustrations and potential mechanisms. Clin Anat. 2012;25(5):641–6. https://doi.org/10.1002/ca.21290.
83. Marciniak C, Armon C, Wilson J, Miller R. Practice parameter: utility of electrodiagnostic techniques in evaluating patients with suspected peroneal neuropathy: an evidence-based review. Muscle Nerve. 2005;31(4):520–7. https://doi.org/10.1002/mus.20308.
84. Andersen KV, Bovim G. Impotence and nerve entrapment in long distance amateur cyclists. Acta Neurol Scand. 1997;95(4):233–40. https://doi.org/10.1111/j.1600-0404.1997.tb00104.x.
85. Sommer F, König D, Graf C, Schwarzer U, Bertram C, Klotz T, et al. Impotence and genital numbness in cyclists. Int J Sports Med. 2001;22(6):410–3. https://doi.org/10.1055/s-2001-16248.
86. Mitchell CH, Brushart TM, Ahlawat S, Belzberg AJ, Carrino JA, Fayad LM. MRI of sports-related peripheral nerve injuries. Am J Roentgenol. 2014;203(5):1075–84. https://doi.org/10.2214/AJR.13.12183.

Chapter 9
Nonoperative and Operative Management of Sports-Related Peripheral Nerve Injury

Brandon W. Smith, Megan M. Jack, and Robert J. Spinner

Introduction

As discussed in the previous chapter on the diagnostic evaluation of sports-related nerve injuries, these injuries, although rare, do occur and can affect almost every major peripheral nerve in the body and in every sport [1–4]. The preceding chapter 8 focused on the recognition, workup, and diagnosis of peripheral nerve injury. This chapter will now discuss management, both nonoperative and operative, of these injuries. The same principles and tools that you became familiar with in the preceding text will be reutilized in the management.

The physical examination, imaging, and electro-diagnostic testing are key to understanding which nerve(s) have been affected, but the critical information that directs the initial management is in the history (Fig. 9.1). You will learn in this chapter that the management of nerve injury in sports is not dictated by the location of the specific nerve injury, but rather the timing, mechanism, severity, and overall trajectory of nerve function and recovery. When urgent treatment is not recommended based on the initial history and presentation, the exam and electrodiagnostic testing will again come to the forefront.

Understanding the underlying physiology of nerve injury and recovery will dictate the principles and treatment options. The severity of nerve injury needs to be met with realistic expectations for recovery. In severe nerve injury, whether treated medically or surgically, the goal is for functional improvement, not high-performance. This can often be life-altering for the high-performance athlete; thus, providing realistic expectations is essential [5].

B. W. Smith · M. M. Jack · R. J. Spinner (✉)
Neurological Surgery, Mayo Clinic, Rochester, MI, USA
e-mail: Spinner.Robert@Mayo.edu

M. E. Oppenlander (ed.), *Neurosurgical Care of Athletes*,
https://doi.org/10.1007/978-3-030-88227-3_9

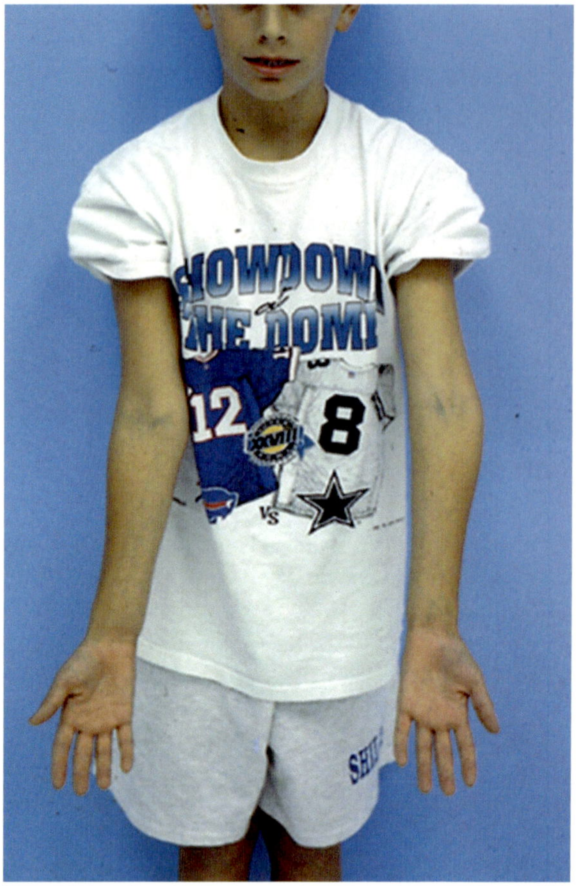

Fig. 9.1 This teenager presented with symptoms and signs of ulnar neuropathy at the left elbow. He had a previous supracondylar humeral fracture treated years earlier which went onto malunion. He developed a cubitus varus deformity and ulnar neuropathy

Foundational Principles

To understand the treatment of peripheral nerve injuries, it is important to think about the microanatomy of the nerve. The layers of the nerve, including epineurium that surrounds the nerve, perineurium which surrounds the fascicles, and endoneurium which surrounds the axons, can all be injured. Myelin is an insulating layer of cholesterol and glycolipids that speeds conduction along select axons. This layered anatomy is the basis for nerve injury classification; the severity of injury based on this classification predicts the potential for recovery dictating our treatment.

Seddon and Sunderland classifications are the most widely utilized injury classifications [6, 7]. The injury subtypes range from demyelinating injuries with generally good recovery prognosis to complete nerve disruptions which necessitate surgical repair. There are multiple levels of injury between these two major classifications, but the key point for determining surgical intervention is whether the underlying injury has retained the potential for regeneration [6, 7].

When an axon is injured, it undergoes Wallerian degeneration at the point of injury and begins the repair process. The distal axon undergoes complete degeneration leaving behind the structural scaffolding, and the proximal nerve dies back a small distance from the point of injury. After this process, axonal regrowth can commence if the structural scaffolding is present across the injury [8]. Denervation changes can begin to occur within the end organ following nerve injury [9, 10].

Although regeneration is advantageous for patients, the rate of nerve growth is slow, averaging just 1 inch per month. In a race against time, the hope is that the nerve re-grows and reaches its target before irreversible damage within the end organ, in this case muscle, occurs [9, 10]. The classic teaching is that the motor endplate can remain viable for up to a year; however, many believe that any small amount of remaining innervation will protect the endplate during regrowth. This slow repair process is the basis why many nerve injuries are treated with a "watchful waiting" period.

The Rule of 3's Plus 1

In nerve surgery, there is an often referred to "rule of 3's" [11]; for a more comprehensive multidisciplinary approach, we have modified this to be a "rule of 3's plus 1" to accommodate patients who would benefit from additional function after either delayed presentations or insufficient recovery (from nonoperative or operative interventions). The rule of 3's defines timing of surgical intervention based on the type of nerve injury: acute surgery within 3 days following sharp clean injuries with laceration of a nerve, subacute surgery within 3 weeks for ragged injuries, and delayed surgery within 3 months for blunt or contusion injuries. The "plus 1" highlights the option for soft tissue (such as tendon or free muscle transfers) or bony procedures (such as fusions) 1 year or several years following the initial injury (and surgery, if performed). This will be discussed in the following text, but the pathologic and regenerative process just described is crucial to understanding the principle.

Nonoperative Management Strategies

The most common clinical scenario for the treating physician is serial observation following peripheral nerve injury. Once an emergent or acute situation has been ruled out, the patient's mechanism and clinical trajectory will dictate management. It is important to document clear detailed exams as part of your ongoing care of a patient with a peripheral nerve injury. The basic motor exam we use in the care of spine patients is not sufficient for the care of a patient with a peripheral nerve injury. Most nerve injuries will recover from proximal to distal, and this can usually be seen clinically on a detailed peripheral nerve exam [9, 10]. The specific grading score or metric used can be debated; however, consistency is key. We find that written description of active motion (with or without gravity, and with or without resistance) can be helpful for patients with complicated exams. Recording the presence and location of a Tinel's sign can also be helpful in following recovery, as this will migrate distally as the nerve grows down the limb [12]. Nerve regeneration is slow and, following monthly exams in the beginning of care, is long enough to see changes, but short enough that the patient does not slip outside of an interventional window if needed.

Initial workup should include imaging which helps assess the continuity of the nerve and to rule out any acute compression. Electrodiagnostic exams are quite useful in follow up. Remember that the role of electrodiagnostic testing, especially EMG, is typically limited for the first few weeks after initial injury. Nerve and muscle injuries will follow a predictable electrodiagnostic pattern [13]. Follow-up EMG can show which muscles are being denervated and, more importantly which muscles, if any, are showing evidence of reinnervation. After the first few weeks, EMG will demonstrate denervation changes as noted by fibrillations or sharp waves. If there is recovery, eventually polyphasic motor units will appear [13]. Generally, indications for surgical exploration would include no motor recovery on examination, and no motor recovery on EMG, which would represent an injury with little or no spontaneous recovery potential. The electrodiagnostic testing in this case can be used as an extension of your history and physical exam [13]. The role of imaging (i.e., high resolution MRI or US) is evolving and is being included into the armamentarium of many peripheral nerve surgeons' evaluations. It may localize the injury and define its extent (either focal or diffuse). It can also be utilized to evaluate for sites of distal compression that could hinder or plateau nerve recovery [14].

The focus of observation is to see if the recovery is happening in a predictable fashion. You can expect approximately 1 inch per month of nerve recovery once it has started. We tell our patients that they will reach their maximum recovery two or more years from surgery or injury, but a majority of their gains will happen in the first year. If the nerve recovery never begins, stalls, or it does not appear that the patient will regain antigravity function, then surgery can be considered. Again, the "rules of 3's plus 1" can be quite helpful in determining the surgical management; all surgical intervention on nerves should be accomplished within 6–12 months to achieve the best surgical outcomes.

During the serial appointments, it is important to monitor for and prevent secondary issues from arising [15–17]. One of the most detrimental complications following peripheral nerve injury is contracture formation. This is particularly problematic in the patient that is recovering neurologic function, as a contracture will limit range of motion despite functional power or strength recovery. The role for careful documentation of passive range of motion is of importance in the serial exams; physical therapy and rehabilitation efforts cannot be overstated in importance. A recovered nerve does no good at powering an immovable joint. Contractures are largely preventable, and it is important to educate the patient on these so that they continue range of motion and strengthening exercises to keep joints supple.

Management of Acute Nerve Injuries

Clean Open Injuries

Open injuries are rare occurrences in sports but can result from laceration from equipment such as a hockey skate or sharp material from the arena such as glass. The management of laceration injuries to the nerve can be either in the acute phase for clean transections without much contamination or delayed with ragged transections with contamination, which will be discussed later. Clean transection injuries require repair as there is no potential for spontaneous regeneration in these injuries. There are no proven methods for immediate repair with instant restoration of nerve function. Since the distal nerve continues to undergo Wallerian degeneration despite surgical repair and the proximal nerve will have to grow to the motor end plate, an emergent repair is not required. In the rule of 3's plus 1, the clean transection falls under the 3-day rule. A repair within the first 3 days of injury is the current gold standard; the reasoning behind this is that nerves tend to retract when not under some longitudinal tension. A delay of more than 3 days may hinder the ability to perform direct tension-free end to end nerve repair, which will be described later in this chapter.

Acute Compression

Acute ongoing compression is one of the few emergent treatment indications in peripheral nerve surgery. Decompression, either direct or indirect, in a timely fashion is the gold standard of treatment. Given that the acute indications for intervention result from pathologies either of orthopedic or vascular origin, a multidisciplinary approach will likely be required. Neurosurgeons will often be consulted for these issues and assist other surgical specialists in these cases as the nerve injury and loss of function is secondary to other similarly acute issues.

Fractures/Dislocations

The management of bony/joint injuries in the acute setting remains somewhat controversial. Most orthopedic surgeons would consider early exploration for open fractures in patients with associated nerve injury, or those patients with a new neurologic deficit or severe neuropathic pain after reduction. The rare occurrence of an entrapped nerve within a reduced fracture or joint would require direct intervention. In contrast, most nerve injuries associated with closed fractures or dislocations undergo closed reduction which indirectly decompresses the nerve, but the nerve injury is observed for spontaneous recovery for several months.

Vascular Causes

Acute compressive neuropathies may be encountered in athletes, particularly in the case of an expanding masses such as pseudoaneurysms or hematomas [18–20]. The general rule is that nerve injuries are maximal at onset of injury. Any patient with active worsening likely has ongoing compression. Hematomas and pseudoaneurysms continue to grow and can cause ongoing compression requiring evacuation and decompression.

Acute Compartment Syndrome

Acute compartment syndrome is a medical emergency that requires immediate intervention to spare the limb from ongoing neurovascular damage [21]. Any severe sports injury that causes trauma and swelling, such as fractures or blunt trauma, could lead to elevated compartment pressures. In athletes, the leg is the most common area to develop acute compartment syndrome. Prompt evaluation is necessary to first identify the potential for compartment syndrome, followed by accurate measurement of compartment pressures. Urgent surgical fasciotomy is necessary to minimize peripheral nerve injury in the setting of compartment syndrome [21].

Management of Subacute Nerve Injuries

Though controversial, a delayed intervention for a known ragged laceration nerve injury will often be performed at the 3-week mark. As mentioned earlier, this will give enough time for the wound to be cleared of infection, and for the extent of injury to the nerve ends to be apparent. A primary repair can sometimes be done at this point with the techniques mentioned below, but it is more likely that a nerve graft will be utilized.

Management of Chronic Nerve Injuries

Closed Nerve Injuries

There are two main types of closed nerve injuries that may be encountered in sporting events. The first is blunt nerve trauma resulting from contact with another player, piece of equipment, or part of the playing arena. The skin remains intact in these injuries, but the underlying injury can range from a demyelinating neuropraxic injury with great recovery potential to severe neurotmetic injuries that will require surgical intervention for any chance of recovery. In the aforementioned "rule of 3's," the closed blunt type (contusive) nerve injuries fall into the 3-month category. Thus, the decision for operative exploration would be reached by 3 months after injury, making early referral to a nerve surgeon critical. A blunt injury with initial complete loss of function has the potential for recovery based on the continuity of the nerve. Three months gives both an adequate time for spontaneous recovery and highlights the importance of serial examinations and EMG. If the patient has no recovery or the recovery stalls, surgical exploration can be done. Electrodiagnostic testing is used serially to monitor for signs of recovery.

The other type of closed injury would be a stretch injury. This can happen in many scenarios, but the most common is a brachial plexus injury from downward pressure on the shoulder. Commonly seen in football and other contact sports, the "stinger" is a type of transient neuropraxic injury. Given its transient nature, it is rare to see this in referral. However, when the injury is more severe, even potentially leading to rupture or avulsion, more long-standing weakness, numbness, and/or pain can occur [22]. Patients with these symptoms will be evaluated with imaging and electrodiagnostic studies. Despite the severity of these injuries, it is again commonplace to follow serial examinations and electrodiagnostic testing to see if there is any evidence of spontaneous recovery. If there is none, then again at 3–6 months, operative exploration may be pursued (Fig. 9.2). The general principles of this type of surgery will be detailed later in the chapter. If there is some recovery, continued serial examinations will be performed to monitor for improvement.

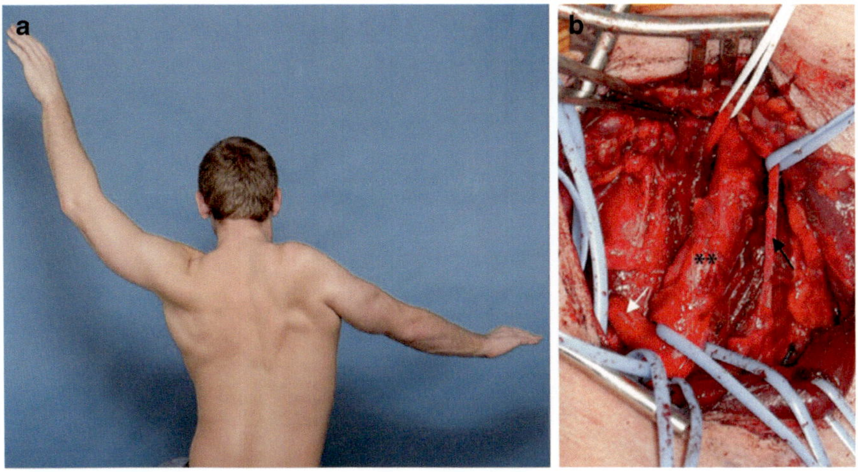

Fig. 9.2 Traumatic right upper trunk brachial plexus injury in a football player sustained while making a tackle. (**a**) The right upper extremity demonstrates wasting of the deltoids and spinati, and inability to fully abduct the shoulder. (**b**) Intraoperative photograph demonstrated the upper trunk neuroma (**) exiting between the anterior scalene and middle scalene muscles. The phrenic nerve is coursing inferomedially (black arrow). In this case, a graft from C5 to the suprascapular nerve (white arrow) was performed in addition to an ulnar fascicular nerve transfer to the biceps motor branch (not pictured)

Overuse Injuries

Given the repetitive mechanical nature of sports, some nerve issues can develop prematurely due to chronic use. Carpal tunnel and cubital tunnel syndrome can present or be exacerbated in athletes from overuse. Some impingement syndromes, like suprascapular nerve palsies (Fig. 9.3), have been observed in athletes who participate in sports with overhead movements like swimming and throwing sports, although there is some speculation that a majority of these rare palsies are inflammatory in nature. The general management of overuse injuries is to discontinue the offending movement. This is an easier suggestion in the standard population than that of high performing athletes who depend on these movements for their sport and/or livelihood. Should the symptoms persist, most of these would be managed the same way as if they were caused by degenerative changes in older patients. Begin first with conservative measures such as limiting the provocative movements, bracing, and, in some cases, steroid injections.

There is some description of compartment syndrome in young athletes causing peripheral nerve palsies [23]. Chronic exertional compartment syndrome is a condition characterized by high compartment pressures that may result in compression of peripheral nerves [23]. Typically, the symptoms are brought on with exercise and improve with rest. Initial workup includes a thorough history followed by measuring intra-compartmental pressures following activity. If the patient has elevated compartment pressures indicative of compartment syndrome and has failed conservative treatment, referral can be made for fasciotomies. In

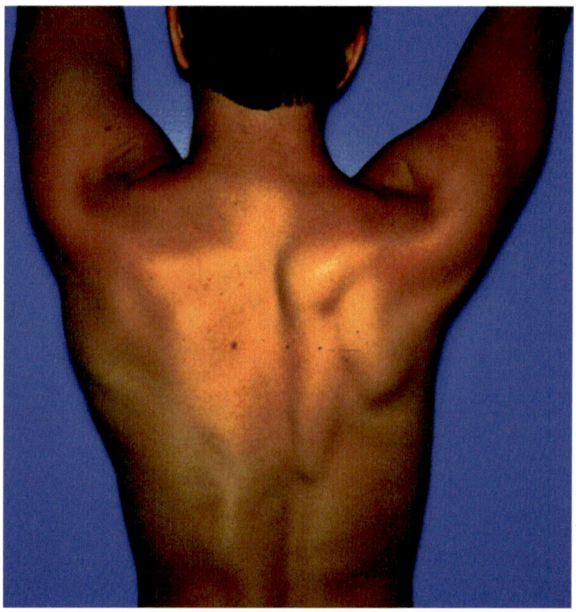

Fig. 9.3 This athlete sustained a right suprascapular nerve lesion. Note atrophy of the supraspinatus and infraspinatus muscles and the incomplete right shoulder abduction

exertional compartment syndrome involving the leg, nerve decompression can also be performed at characteristic compression zones such as the common peroneal nerve at the fibular neck (underneath the fascia of the peroneus longus), the deep peroneal nerve at the anterior intermuscular septum, or the superficial peroneal nerve in the distal leg. Determining chronic or exertional compartment syndrome from compression syndromes can be difficult; new imaging modalities are being introduced [24–26].

Post-traumatic Inflammatory Neuropathies

Post-traumatic inflammatory neuropathies such as Parsonage Turner syndrome are rare conditions; however, they can also affect athletes [27]. The underlying pathology is not well understood, but is thought to be immune-mediated [27]. Inflammatory neuropathies may or may not have an associated inciting event. Typically, inflammatory neuropathies are characterized by an acute onset of severe pain followed by weakness that often occurs 1–2 weeks later. Certain nerves may be affected, including suprascapular, axillary, long thoracic, anterior interosseous, and posterior interosseous nerves. Athletes may associate a sports injury or overuse condition with weakness or pain that is actually the result of an inflammatory neuropathy (Fig. 9.4). Recovery often (but not always) occurs over 1–2 years. Pain management and physical therapy are important to maximize recovery.

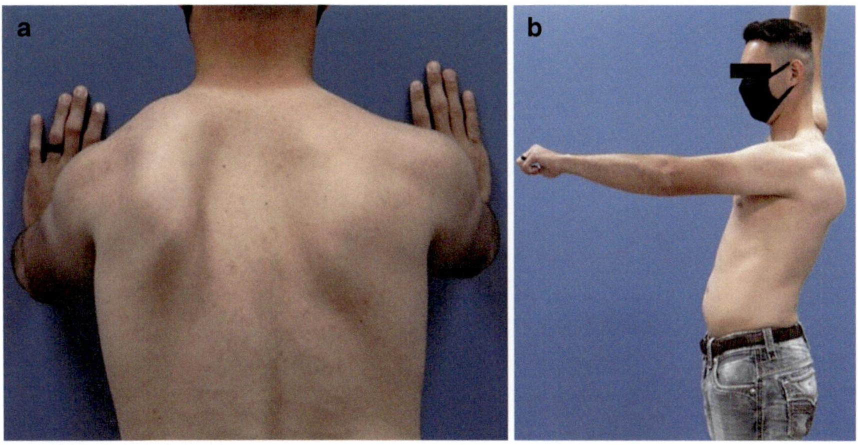

Fig. 9.4 This patient presented with left shoulder dysfunction and a winging scapula from a long thoracic nerve lesion and serratus anterior paralysis which was attributed to overuse from his recreational athletics. It remains important to remember athletes are also at risk for other processes that may be temporally linked to sports, but may not be pathophysiologically associated, such as with an inflammatory mononeuropathy. Note the medial winging of the left scapula (**a**) and the decreased forward flexion from the scapular instability (**b**)

Operative Management Strategies

Primary Nerve Repair

The goal of primary nerve repair is to bring the two ends of the injured nerve together in a tension-free fashion. There are detailed texts describing operative exposures for nerve surgery; however, in open trauma settings for which you would be doing a primary nerve repair, wound exploration will be your approach. Normal anatomy will be obscured due to the local trauma, but the general advice is to find normal nerve both proximally and distally. If you are unable to find the injured nerve ends in the exposed field, finding the nerve proximally and distally in their normal locations and tracing them to the free end is advised. Once found, distal and proximal neurolysis and exploration can ensure the trauma to the nerve is focal. A circumferential nerve dissection is also helpful in gaining extra length and mobility to ensure a tension-free repair.

Nerve coaptation can be achieved with epineurial sutures; 8–0 or 9–0 nylon sutures are our preferred suture for most nerve repairs. The data support that primary repairs are best when done without tension.

Although it seems counter-intuitive, less tension and even a small gap would be preferred over an overambitious repair with the ends effectively strangulated together. A small gap can be covered with fibrin glue. There are some proponents of using collagen tubes to guide the growing axons to the distal end. Entubulation, as this is referred to, is a growing area of investigation in peripheral nerve surgery, proposed by some, to bridge small gaps.

Nerve Grafting

It is imperative to expose a portion of nerve both proximal and distal to the visible neuroma-in-continuity. A neuroma in continuity cannot be accurately assessed without intraoperative testing. Nerve action potentials across the area of injury for blunt nerve injuries are key for decision making [28]. Nerve action potentials should be used to define if there is evidence of recovery occurring across the nerve lesion. If a nerve action potential is present across the neuroma, then neurolysis alone is indicated and no nerve resection/reconstruction is performed. If a neuroma is found that does not conduct a nerve action potential, then excision of the neuroma to the point of healthy nerve is performed. The reconstruction will utilize either a direct repair or, more commonly, an interposition graft.

The most common, and most studied, technique to traverse a gap between the proximal and distal ends of a nerve would be an autologous nerve graft. This in our opinion, represents the current gold standard. The nerves that are harvested are most commonly sensory nerves, and in our practice the most common is the sural nerve. The role of nerve tubes as sole conduits is reported, but again most of the data are focused on autologous nerve grafting. If necessary, multiple nerve grafts can be glued together to form a cable graft for a better size match in the repair. Various methods of securing the grafts are used, we utilize suture fixation with 8–0 nylon and fibrin glue, whereas some surgeons use fibrin glue or sutures alone. It is important to consider the donor site morbidity for nerve grafting in specific relation to the athlete's sport, although the classic nerve grafting sites show limited functional morbidity. The donor sites will have permanent sensation loss either to the dorsum of the hand from a superficial radial or the dorsal-lateral foot from a sural nerve harvest, two of the more common donors. Reduced outcomes are associated with the use of long grafts, especially those over considerable distance (e.g., 12 cm) [29–31].

Nerve Transfer Reconstruction

Entire texts are focused on nerve transfers for functional restoration, and the individual nuances are beyond the scope of this chapter. However, nerve transfers deserve mention as they are potentially important procedures to help patients with sports nerve injuries. To date, there are successful nerve transfer strategies to restore critical motion of the upper extremity [32–36]. In the case of sports injury, these are more likely to be utilized as reconstructive options later in a patient's care. For familiarity, nerve transfers take expendable nerves, branches, or fascicles from functioning muscle groups and bypass the area of injury to reinnervate targeted muscles closer to their motor end plates. The proponents of nerve transfers in brachial plexus surgery cite the shorter distance to reinnervation and single site of coaptation as the major advantages [35, 36]. The detractors of nerve transfers are that they require some motor relearning and they do not offer sensory recovery in the same way that a primary or graft repair does.

Secondary Reconstruction

Secondary reconstruction techniques are often utilized following peripheral nerve injury in two key instances: those outside the 12-month operative window for primary nerve procedures and those that do not achieve good functional recovery following surgical intervention. Tendon or muscle transfer surgery moves a working but expendable muscle/tendon to replace the function that is lost. For example, the tibialis posterior tendon can be used to aid with dorsiflexion in cases of foot drop from a common peroneal nerve (division) injury [37]. Other reconstructive techniques such as joint fusions can also be used typically in severe injuries where the patient has difficulty with controlling the placement of a limb in space. Thus, athletes with ongoing functional deficits should be referred to specialists to be evaluated for other procedures to ensure that all surgical options have been considered.

Adaptive Sports

While nonoperative and operative management of sports injuries to peripheral nerves can lead to good functional outcomes, this may not be achieved in the case of devastating injuries and the athlete may not return to their former high baseline performance. Thus, adaptive sports provide an opportunity with those with a disability to participate either on a competitive or recreational level. Specific equipment is used based on the specific need of the athlete. Adaptive sports may be an option for athletes who can no longer participate in conventional competitive sports.

Conclusion

Athletic peripheral nerve injuries can occur in almost every major peripheral nerve and from all sports. Acute or emergent surgery is indicated for those rare injuries with clean transection or ongoing compression. Otherwise, serial examinations and EMG/NCS are crucial to determine if the injuries are demonstrating recovery or not. If the athlete is demonstrating motor recovery on electrodiagnostic and muscle group testing, nonoperative management along with physical therapy can be continued. If there is limited or no functional recovery, "the rule of 3's plus 1" will help guide surgical intervention based on the injury classification. Primary repair, nerve grafts, and nerve transfers are all operative techniques that, in the right setting, can be used to help repair peripheral nerves following athletic injuries.

References

1. Krivickas LS, Wilbourn AJ. Peripheral nerve injuries in athletes: a case series of over 200 injuries. Semin Neurol. Published online 2000. https://doi.org/10.1055/s-2000-9832.
2. Toth C. Peripheral nerve injuries attributable to sport and recreation. Phys Med Rehabil Clin N Am. Published online 2009. https://doi.org/10.1016/j.pmr.2008.10.012.
3. Feinberg JH, Nadler SF, Krivickas LS. Peripheral nerve injuries in the athlete. Sport Med. Published online 1997. https://doi.org/10.2165/00007256-199724060-00004.
4. Daly CA, Payne SH, Seiler JG. Severe brachial plexus injuries in American football. Orthopedics. Published online 2016. https://doi.org/10.3928/01477447-20160721-03.
5. Kirsch M, Brown S, Smith BW, Chang KWC, Koduri S, Yang LJS. The presence and persistence of unrealistic expectations in patients undergoing nerve surgery. Neurosurgery. Published online 2020. https://doi.org/10.1093/neuros/nyz335.
6. Seddon HJ, Medawar PB, Smith H. Rate of regeneration of peripheral nerves in man. J Physiol. 1943;102(2):191–215.
7. Sunderland S. A classification of peripheral nerve injuries producing loss of function. Brain. 1951;74(4):491–516.
8. Stoll G, Jander S, Myers RR. Degeneration and regeneration of the peripheral nervous system: from Augustus Waller's observations to neuroinflammation. J Peripher Nerv Syste. 2002; https://doi.org/10.1046/j.1529-8027.2002.02002.x.

9. Gordon T. Nerve regeneration. Understanding biology and its influence on return of function after nerve transfers. Hand Clin. 2016;32(2):103–17. https://doi.org/10.1016/j.hcl.2015.12.001.
10. Gupta R, Chan JP, Uong J, et al. Human motor endplate remodeling after traumatic nerve injury. J Neurosurg. Published online 2020. https://doi.org/10.3171/2020.8.jns201461.
11. Kline DG. Surgical repair of peripheral nerve injury. Muscle Nerve. Published online 1990. https://doi.org/10.1002/mus.880130911.
12. Meadows JR, Finnoff JT. Lower extremity nerve entrapments in athletes. Curr Sports Med Rep. Published online 2014. https://doi.org/10.1249/JSR.0000000000000083.
13. Quan D, Bird S. Nerve conduction studies and electromyography in the evaluation of peripheral nerve injuries. Univ Pa Orthop J. Published online 1999.
14. Wilson TJ, Kleiber GM, Nunley RM, Mackinnon SE, Spinner RJ. Distal peroneal nerve decompression after sciatic nerve injury secondary to total hip arthroplasty. J Neurosurg. Published online 2019. https://doi.org/10.3171/2017.8.JNS171260.
15. Safran MR. Nerve injury about the shoulder in athletes, part 1: suprascapular nerve and axillary nerve. Am J Sports Med. Published online 2004. https://doi.org/10.1177/0363546504264582.
16. Safran MR. Nerve injury about the shoulder in athletes, part 2: long thoracic nerve, spinal accessory nerve, burners/stingers, thoracic outlet syndrome. Am J Sports Med. Published online 2004. https://doi.org/10.1177/0363546504265193.
17. Perlmutter GS, Apruzzese W. Axillary nerve injuries in contact sports. Recommendations for treatment and rehabilitation. Sport Med. Published online 1998. https://doi.org/10.2165/00007256-199826050-00005.
18. Steinman S, Bastrom TP, Newton PO, Mubarak SJ. Beware of ulnar nerve entrapment in flexion-type supracondylar humerus fractures. J Child Orthop. Published online 2007. https://doi.org/10.1007/s11832-007-0034-4.
19. Bevoni R. Common peroneal nerve palsy due to hematoma at the fibular neck. J Knee Surg. Published online 2013. https://doi.org/10.1055/s-0032-1330055.
20. Smith BW, Sakamuri S, Spain DA, Joseph JR, Yang LJS, Wilson TJ. An update on the management of adult traumatic nerve injuries – replacing old paradigms: a review. J Trauma Acute Care Surg. Published online 2019. https://doi.org/10.1097/TA.0000000000002081.
21. Von Keudell AG, Weaver MJ, Appelton PT, et al. Diagnosis and treatment of acute extremity compartment syndrome. Lancet. Published online 2015. https://doi.org/10.1016/S0140-6736(15)00277-9.
22. Saliba S, Saliba EN, Pugh KF, Chhabra A, Diduch D. Rehabilitation considerations of a brachial plexus injury with complete avulsion of C5 and C6 nerve roots in a college football player: a case study. Sports Health. Published online 2009. https://doi.org/10.1177/1941738109343544.
23. Rajasekaran S, Kvinlaug K, Finnoff JT. Exertional leg pain in the athlete. PM R. Published online 2012. https://doi.org/10.1016/j.pmrj.2012.10.002.
24. Litwiller D V., Amrami KK, Dahm DL, et al. Chronic exertional compartment syndrome of the lower extremities: improved screening using a novel dual birdcage coil and in-scanner exercise protocol. Skeletal Radiol. Published online 2007. https://doi.org/10.1007/s00256-007-0360-0.
25. Lauder TD, Stuart MJ, Amrami KK, Felmlee JP. Exertional compartment syndrome and the role of magnetic resonance imaging. Am J Phys Med Rehabil. Published online 2002. https://doi.org/10.1097/00002060-200204000-00016.
26. Ringler MD, Litwiller D V., Felmlee JP, et al. MRI accurately detects chronic exertional compartment syndrome: a validation study. Skeletal Radiol. Published online 2013. https://doi.org/10.1007/s00256-012-1487-1.
27. Feinberg JH, Radecki J. Parsonage-turner syndrome. HSS J. Published online 2010. https://doi.org/10.1007/s11420-010-9176-x.
28. Tiel RL, Happel LT, Kline DG. Nerve action potential recording method and equipment. Neurosurgery. Published online 1996. https://doi.org/10.1097/00006123-199607000-00019.
29. Kim DH, Kam AC, Chandika P, Tiel RL, Kline DG. Surgical management and outcome in patients with radial nerve lesions. J Neurosurg. Published online 2001. https://doi.org/10.3171/jns.2001.95.4.0573.

30. Kline DG, Kim DH. Axillary nerve repair in 99 patients with 101 stretch injuries. J Neurosurg. Published online 2003. https://doi.org/10.3171/jns.2003.99.4.0630.
31. Kim DH, Han K, Tiel RL, Murovic JA, Kline DG. Surgical outcomes of 654 ulnar nerve lesions. J Neurosurg. Published online 2003. https://doi.org/10.3171/jns.2003.98.5.0993.
32. Oberlin C, Beal D, Leechavengvongs S, Salon A, Dauge MC, Sarcy JJ. Nerve transfer to biceps muscle using a part of ulnar nerve for C5-C6 avulsion of the brachial plexus: anatomical study and report of four cases. J Hand Surg Am. 1994;19(2):232–7. https://doi.org/10.1016/0363-5023(94)90011-6.
33. Witoonchart K, Leechavengvongs S, Uerpairojkit C, Thuvasethakul P, Wongnopsuwan V. Nerve transfer to deltoid muscle using the nerve to the long head of the triceps, part I: an anatomic feasibility study. J Hand Surg Am. Published online 2003. https://doi.org/10.1016/S0363-5023(03)00200-4.
34. Tse R, Marcus JR, Curtis CG, Dupuis A, Clarke HM. Suprascapular nerve reconstruction in obstetrical brachial plexus palsy: spinal accessory nerve transfer versus C5 root grafting. Plast Reconstr Surg. 2011;127(6):2391–6. https://doi.org/10.1097/PRS.0b013e3182131c7c.
35. Mackinnon SE, Novak CB. Nerve transfers. New options for reconstruction following nerve injury. Hand Clin. 1999;15(4):643–66. ix
36. Ray WZ, Chang J, Hawasli A, Wilson TJ, Yang L. Motor nerve transfers: a comprehensive review. Neurosurgery. 2015;78(1):1–25. https://doi.org/10.1227/NEU.0000000000001029.
37. Schweitzer KM, Jones CP. Tendon transfers for the drop foot. Foot Ankle Clin. Published online 2014. https://doi.org/10.1016/j.fcl.2013.12.002.

Chapter 10
Concussion in Sports: What Is It and How Is It Managed?

Arjang Ahmadpour, Valentina Vasenina, Vimal Patel, and Julian E. Bailes

Introduction: Defining Sports-Related Concussion

Sports-related concussion (SRC) is broadly defined as the immediate and transient symptoms of traumatic brain injury (TBI) [1]. The underlying issue with this definition is that it does not provide insight into the underlying processes causing brain impairment. This definition also does not distinguish between different grades of severity. The term mild traumatic brain injury (mTBI) is often used interchangeably with concussion. This term is also vague and lacks validated criteria in this context. Therefore, the term concussion with this usage is imprecise.

The most commonly recognized definition of concussion stems from the consensus statement from the 5th International Conference on Concussion in Sport, which states that sports-related concussion (SRC) is a traumatic brain injury (TBI) induced by biomechanical forces [1].

Several common features that may be utilized in clinically defining the nature of a concussive head injury include:

- SRC may be caused either by a direct blow to the head, face, neck, or elsewhere on the body with an impulsive force transmitted to the head.
- SRC typically results in the rapid onset of short-lived impairment of neurological function that resolves spontaneously. However, in some cases, signs and symptoms evolve over a number of minutes to hours.

A. Ahmadpour · V. Vasenina
Department of Neurosurgery, University of Chicago Medical Center, Chicago, IL, USA
e-mail: Arjang.Ahmadpour@uchospitals.edu; Valentina.Vasenina@uchospitals.edu

V. Patel · J. E. Bailes (✉)
Department of Neurosurgery, North Shore Hospital, Evanston, IL, USA
e-mail: VPatel2@northshore.org; JBailes@northshore.org

M. E. Oppenlander (ed.), *Neurosurgical Care of Athletes*,
https://doi.org/10.1007/978-3-030-88227-3_10

- SRC may result in neuropathological changes, but the acute clinical signs and symptoms largely reflect a functional disturbance rather than a structural injury and, as such, no abnormality is seen on standard structural neuroimaging studies.
- SRC results in a range of clinical signs and symptoms that may or may not involve loss of consciousness. Resolution of the clinical and cognitive features typically follows a sequential course. However, in some cases, symptoms may be prolonged.
- The clinical signs and symptoms cannot be explained by drug, alcohol, or medication use, other injuries (such as cervical injuries, peripheral vestibular dysfunction, etc.) or other comorbidities (e.g., psychological factors or coexisting medical conditions).

Several definitions of mild traumatic brain injury (mTBI) have been used over the past decades [2]. Traumatic brain injury (TBI) is typically graded from mild to severe, with use of the clinical assessment of the Glasgow Coma Scale (GCS). The GCS has a composite score ranging from 3 to 15. A numerical assignment is awarded according to the patient's eye opening, motor responses to verbal and physical stimuli, and verbal responses to questions and commands. Based on this scale, mTBI refers to patients with a GCS score of 13 to 15. The World Health Organization (WHO) Collaborating Centre for Neurotrauma Prevention, Management and Rehabilitation Task Force on Mild Traumatic Brain Injury proposed the following mTBI definition [3]:

> MTBI is an acute brain injury resulting from mechanical energy to the head from external physical forces. Operational criteria for clinical identification include: (i) 1 or more of the following: confusion or disorientation, loss of consciousness for 30 minutes or less, post-traumatic amnesia for less than 24 hours, and/or other transient neurological abnormalities such as focal signs, seizure, and intracranial lesion not requiring surgery; (ii) Glasgow Coma Scale score of 13–15 after 30 minutes post-injury or later upon presentation for health care. These manifestations of MTBI must not be due to drugs, alcohol, medications, caused by other injuries or treatment for other injuries (e.g. systemic injuries, facial injuries or intubation), caused by other problems (e.g. psychological trauma, language barrier or coexisting medical conditions) or caused by penetrating craniocerebral injury.

This definition set forth by the WHO was created as an attempt to standardize an operational definition of mTBI for research purposes.

MTBI may also apply to patients in whom structural lesions are found on standard neuroimaging, or those with focal neurological deficits. This is not consistent with the most commonly accepted definition of concussion. Such imaging findings may include epidural or subdural hematoma, subarachnoid hemorrhage, parenchymal contusion, skull fractures, etc. [4]. The focus of this chapter is traumatic brain injury as it relates to functional brain abnormalities, without the structural changes seen on standard neuroimaging. Please refer to Table 10.1, which provides descriptions of various levels of TBI severity according to GCS score.

Table 10.1 Classification of head injury severity

Classification	Glasgow Coma Scale Score
Mild TBI	13–15
Moderate TBI	9–12
Severe TBI	3–8

TBI traumatic brain injury

Epidemiology

TBI is a global healthcare-related problem of paramount importance [5]. An estimated 1.7 million TBIs occur annually in the United States. A majority of these TBIs are mild [6]. TBI incidence in military personnel, commonly overshadowed by the focus on sports-related injuries, has gained increased attention in recent years. Mild TBI occurred in 20% of deployed personnel, and accounted for the majority of military-associated head injuries during the conflicts in Iraq and Afghanistan [7]. Blast injury caused by improvised explosive devices (IEDs) is an especially common cause of mTBI and concussion, contributing to as much as 79% of these injuries [8–13].

The number of American patients seeking care for traumatic brain injuries, most of which are mild in nature, has been on the rise. Marin and colleagues [14] estimated that there were 2,544,087 visits to emergency departments (EDs) for TBI in 2010. This represents a 29.1% increase when compared to the number of ED visits in 2006. This rate of increase is nearly eight times greater than the rate of increase of total ED visits over the same time frame; it is most likely attributed to a combination of factors such as increases in TBI awareness, exposure, and diagnoses. Children <3 years old, and adults >60 years old had the highest rates of ED visits, with falls serving as the leading mechanisms of injury [14].

The annual incidence of sports-related concussion in the United States is estimated to be approximately 3.8 million. This number likely underestimates the true incidence given that many concussions might go unreported or affected athletes might have no gateway to formal medical follow-up [15]. Clay and associates [16] performed a systematic review of the epidemiology of concussion in sport, and reported that the highest reported incidences of concussion, in descending order, are related to football, female and male soccer, wrestling, and female basketball. Between 2% and 15% of athletes participating in organized sports will suffer a concussion during one season (Table 10.2) [17–35].

Football accounts for the highest proportion of sports-related concussion overall [16]. The incidence ranges from 0.48 to 1.03 per 1000 athletic exposures (AEs) at the high school level, 0.52 to 0.81 per 1000 AEs at the college level, and 4.56 per 1000 game AEs in the National Football League (NFL). This NFL data does not include concussions sustained during practice [16, 36–40] Linebackers are the most commonly concussed players in football in all levels of play overall. Quarterbacks are the

Table 10.2 Seasonal risk of concussion in sports

Author	Type of athletes	Years of study	Seasons (n)	Athletes (n)	Concussed	Concussed per player/season (%)
Football						
Barr and McCrea [19]	High school and college football	1997–1999	2	1313	50	1.9
McCrea [18]	High school and college football	1998–1999	2	1325	63	2.4
McCrea et al. [17]	High school and college football	1999–2001	3	2385	91	3.8
McCrea et al. [19]	College football	1999–2001	2		94	3.9
Barr et al. [16]	High school and college football	2008–2009	2	823	59	7.2
Seidman et al. [24]	High school football	2013	1	343	9	2.6
Dompier et al. [25]	Football	2012–2013	2	20,479	1178	5.8
	Youth football	2012–2013	2	4092	136	3.3
	High school football	2012–2013	2	11,957	767	6.4
	College football	2012–2013	2	4430	275	6.7
	College football	2011–2014	4	9718	518	5.3
Houck et al. [26]	College football	2006–2015	9	945[a]	118	12.5
Bretzin et al. [14]	High school football	2015–2016	1	39,520	1530	3.9
Total football				**67,133**	**3192**	**4.8**
All sports						
Galetta et al. [27]	Football, sprint football, men's and women's soccer and basketball	2010–2011	1	219	10	4.6
Marinides et al. [20]	College athletes	2011–2012	1	217	30	13.8
Galetta et al. [21]	Ice hockey/lacrosse youth and college		1	332	12	3.6
Leong et al. [28]	Football, men's and women's basketball	2012–2013	1	127	11	8.7
Putukian et al. [22]	College athletes	2011–2012	1	263	32	12.2

Table 10.2 (continued)

Author	Type of athletes	Years of study	Seasons (n)	Athletes (n)	Concussed	Concussed per player/season (%)
Chin et al. [23]	High school and college athletes	2012–2014	3	2018	166	2.7
Kerr et al. [12]	NCAA athletes	2011–2014	4	32,156	1410	4.4
	Men's baseball	2011–2014	4	1757	13	0.7
	Men's basketball	2011–2014	4	1889	74	3.9
	College football	2011–2014	4	9718	518	5.3
	Men's ice hockey	2011–2014	4	3689	253	6.9
	Men's lacrosse	2011–2014	4	1768	44	2.5
	Men's soccer	2011–2014	4	1810	29	1.6
	Men's wrestling	2011–2014	4	821	65	7.9
	Women's basketball	2011–2014	4	1690	90	5.3
	Women's ice hockey	2011–2014	4	1301	94	7.2
	Women's lacrosse	2011–2014	4	1522	49	3.2
	Women's softball	2011–2014	4	1569	38	2.4
	Women's soccer	2011–2014	4	2831	93	3.3
	Women's volleyball	2011–2014	4	1791	50	2.8
Dhawan et al. [29]	Youth hockey		1	141	20	14.2
Tsushima et al. [13]	Athletes grades 8–12	2013–2014	1	10,334	1250	12.1
Bretzin et al. [14]	High school athletes in 15 sports	2015–2016	1	193,757	3352	1.7
Total				**239,564**	**6293**	**2.6**

Table reproduced from Harmon et al. [17]

[a]Total number of athletes estimated using 105 athletes per year on football roster. NCAA, National Collegiate Athletic Association

most frequently concussed players in the NFL [16]. The majority of concussions are sustained during competition rather than practices, with high-speed player-to-player impact serving as the most common mechanism for concussive injury [41–43].

The majority of concussions are sustained during competition rather than practices, with high-speed player-to-player impact serving as the most common mechanism for concussive injury. This correlates with helmet accelerometer data collected in a study of a college football team. Data from this study demonstrated that impacts during football games are nearly three times higher than those during practice [44].

It is unclear why high school athletes report a higher incidence of concussion when compared to college and professional athletes. These findings are unexpected, given that increased high impact exposure and increased cumulative concussions are established risk factors for sustaining concussions in the future [16, 45]. Proposed explanations, which are not well established, have included the immature anatomy of younger athletes, style of play differences (more running plays vs. passing plays in high school football), injury reporting differences, and greater force per hit due to lack of experience [46]. In most sex-comparable sports (excluding lacrosse), concussion incidence is consistently higher in females than in males [17–23]. A study of the National College Athletic Association ice hockey found that in women's hockey, which prohibits body checking, player contact was the source of 41% of concussions, compared with 72% in men's hockey [47]. Additionally, women suffer fewer impacts and experience lower head acceleration than men. This suggests that these factors are not the direct cause of an overall higher incidence of concussion in female athletes [48]. Various studies have proposed that differences in incidence may relate to differences in reporting, as well as the differences in the size and strength of head and neck musculature between males and females [49].

Concussion Diagnosis

The diagnosis of concussion is based on assessment of a range of domains, which includes physical signs, cognitive impairment, clinical symptoms, neurobehavioral features, and sleep disturbance [1]. If even one of these signs is present, concussion should be suspected, and the proper management strategy should be implemented [1]. Diagnosis requires awareness of multiple symptoms that may be present with concussive injury paired with a focused clinical examination. On-site assessment tools may aid the provider in the diagnosis of concussion. Adjuncts to the clinical assessment, such as advanced neuropsychological testing, neuroimaging techniques, and blood-based biomarkers of injury, can also be used to aid in identifying injury and secure the diagnosis of concussion. Although these new technologies are not required or recommended for routine clinical care, they show promise as investigative tools to advance our understanding of the pathophysiology of concussion and recovery. Through advanced imaging techniques and analysis of biomarkers that are released following injury, research has conceded that considering concussion as only a functional entity is an inappropriate underestimate.

There is a wide range of variability in the quality of training and experience of health care professionals diagnosing and caring for concussed athletes. This contributes to uncertainty and inconsistency in the various aspects of concussion diagnosis, prognostication, and treatment in affected athletes. In 2013, The Guideline Development Subcommittee of the American Academy of Neurology (AAN) published the "Evidence-based Guideline Update: Evaluation and Management of Concussion in Sports." [50] This comprehensive publication reviews evidence in children, adolescents, and adults from 1955 through 2012 in an attempt to bring consistency to this clinical entity.

Concussion: Signs and Symptoms

The clinical manifestations of concussion affect one or more of the domains of somatic, cognitive, behavioral, emotional, vestibular, cervical, autonomic, and sleep/wake symptoms. Common signs and symptoms of concussion are headache, fatigue, dizziness, amnesia, irritability, anxiety, poor concentration, photophobia/phonophobia, disorientation, and postural instability. See Table 10.3 for a summary of commonly reported signs and symptoms of injury.

Table 10.3 Common signs and symptoms of mild traumatic brain injury

Signs of injury
Loss of consciousness
Retrograde amnesia (forgetting events that happened before the concussion)
Anterograde or post-traumatic amnesia (forgetting events that happen after the concussion)
"Dazed" look
Confusion about injury events or details
Disorientation to person, place, or time
Emotional lability
Inappropriate emotions
Behavior or personality changes
Symptoms of injury
Headache
Dizziness
Balance problems
Fatigue
Visual changes (double or blurry vision most common)
Insomnia
Hypersomnia
Drowsiness
Attentional dysfunction
Short-term memory and learning problems
Difficulty multitasking
Phonophobia
Photophobia
Bradyphrenia
Feeling mentally "foggy"
Emotional changes

These signs and symptoms are sometimes associated with other conditions in athletes, including dehydration, exertional migraines, heat-related illness, and sleep disorders. Thus, it is important to establish a relationship between mechanism of injury and the onset or worsening of symptoms [51–55]. Physicians and others caring for athletes must remember that although symptoms typically begin immediately following the inciting trauma, some patients may not experience symptoms for several hours after the injury [56].

Headache is the most common reported symptom of concussion, present in 83–86% of patients with concussion [57, 58]. The headache characteristics experienced after concussion or mTBI may include tension-type, cluster-like, migraine-type, and mixed. The mechanism for headache following head injury is not well understood. Both migraine and mTBI have common pathophysiologic effects, including increases in intracellular sodium, calcium, chloride, and extracellular potassium. Both conditions have been linked to increased release of excitatory amino acids, such as glutamate [59].

Post-concussion headache may be associated with slowed reaction time, memory impairment, on-field anterograde amnesia, and increased overall symptoms [60]. Patients with migrainous headache after concussion scored lower on several neurocognitive measures (processing speed, verbal and visual memory, and reaction time) than those with nonmigrainous headaches or no headache after concussion [61]. Patients with migrainous headache also reported more or worse symptoms relative to the other two groups [61].

Mental status changes and subtle neurocognitive deficits are also quite common with concussion. Confusion has been a longstanding hallmark of concussion [62]. Confusion may also include a disturbance of vigilance with heightened distractibility, inability to maintain a coherent stream of thought, or the inability to carry out a sequence of goal-directed movements. Although disorientation may be present during a concussion, more subtle changes, as described previously, are more common and should be sought during examination of the patient or athlete [63]. One study highlighted that concussed athletes exhibiting "fogginess" have demonstrated poor performance on memory, reaction time, and processing speed measures, and an overall higher total symptom score [64].

Loss of consciousness (LOC) was previously viewed as a requisite for concussion, whereas the literature shows that more than 90% of concussions occur without LOC. Concussions of higher severity with corresponding signs and symptoms may occur with no LOC [65]. LOC occurs in 8–19% of sports-related concussions, with most LOC lasting less than one minute [66, 67]. The duration of LOC is not correlated to injury severity in concussion studies [68, 69]. This is contrary to what is reported in moderate and severe TBI studies [68, 69].

Posttraumatic amnesia can occur immediately, or several minutes after concussive injury in athletes [70–72]. Both retrograde and anterograde amnesia may be associated with neurocognitive deficits, and more reported symptoms in the days immediately following concussion [73]. The presence or absence of post-concussive amnesia as a predictor of long-term outcome is not currently established in the literature [1].

Decreased postural control after concussion is well established [74]. Assessing for this may be carried out by having the patient stand upright with the eyes closed.

Eliminating visual referencing with eye closure accentuates postural control deficit that is associated with an inability to process altered sensory information [74]. Decreased postural stability symptoms typically persist up to 3 days following injury [75].

It is important to recognize that a variety of immediate post-concussive motor phenomena, such as convulsive movements and tonic posturing, may accompany a concussion [1]. These clinical features are typically benign and do not require specific management [1].

Acute Concussion: On-Field Assessment and Sideline Assessment Tools

The Consensus Statement on Concussion in Sport from the International Conference on Concussion in Sport states [1]:

When a player shows any symptoms or signs of an SRC:

(a) The player should be evaluated by a physician or other licensed healthcare provider on site using standard emergency management principles, and particular attention should be given to excluding a cervical spine injury.
(b) The appropriate disposition of the player must be determined by the treating healthcare provider in a timely manner. If no healthcare provider is available, the player should be safely removed from practice or play and urgent referral to a physician arranged.
(c) Once the first aid issues are addressed, an assessment of the concussive injury should be made using the SCAT5 or other sideline assessment tools.
(d) The player should not be left alone after the injury, and serial monitoring for deterioration is essential over the initial few hours after injury.
(e) A player with diagnosed SRC should not be allowed to return to play on the day of injury.

Signs and symptoms which are of particular concern include severe or progressively worsening headaches, positive findings on neurological examination, emesis, or rapid decline in mental status that may indicate a more life-threatening injury (e.g., epidural or subdural hematoma, intraparenchymal hemorrhage) and necessitates immediate transfer to the emergency department.

There are a variety of sideline assessment tools that gauge concussion-related symptoms, neuropsychologic function, and balance [1, 76–79]. The most commonly used sideline assessment tool is the Sports Concussion Assessment Tool, fifth edition (SCAT5). This assessment includes a standardized evaluation of signs and symptoms, neurologic function, cognition, and balance [1]. The original SCAT was developed by the second International Conference on Concussion in Sport [1]. The SCAT5 is designed for use in athletes age 13 years or older, and combines aspects of several previously published concussion tools into multiple components (Fig. 10.1) [1]. In order to eliminate the possible confounding effects of fatigue from competitive play when testing for concussive symptoms, the athlete should be

BJSM Online First, published on April 26, 2017 as 10.1136/bjsports-2017-097506SCAT5

To download a clean version of the SCAT tools please visit the journal online (http://dx.doi.org/10.1136/bjsports-2017-097506SCAT5)

SCAT5©

SPORT CONCUSSION ASSESSMENT TOOL – 5TH EDITION

DEVELOPED BY THE CONCUSSION IN SPORT GROUP
FOR USE BY MEDICAL PROFESSIONALS ONLY

supported by

FIFA®

FEI

Patient details

Name: ____________________

DOB: ____________________

Address: ____________________

ID number: ____________________

Examiner: ____________________

Date of Injury: ____________________ Time: ____________________

WHAT IS THE SCAT5?

The SCAT5 is a standardized tool for evaluating concussions designed for use by physicians and licensed healthcare professionals[1]. The SCAT5 cannot be performed correctly in less than 10 minutes.

If you are not a physician or licensed healthcare professional, please use the Concussion Recognition Tool 5 (CRT5). The SCAT5 is to be used for evaluating athletes aged 13 years and older. For children aged 12 years or younger, please use the Child SCAT5.

Preseason SCAT5 baseline testing can be useful for interpreting post-injury test scores, but is not required for that purpose.Detailed instructions for use of the SCAT5 are provided on page 7. Please read through these instructions carefully before testing the athlete. Brief verbal instructions for each test are given in italics. The only equipment required for the tester is a watch or timer.

This tool may be freely copied in its current form for distribution to individuals, teams, groups and organizations. It should not be altered in any way, re-branded or sold for commercial gain. Any revision, translation or reproduction in a digital form requires specific approval by the Concussion in Sport Group.

Recognise and Remove

A head impact by either a direct blow or indirect transmission of force can be associated with a serious and potentially fatal brain injury. If there are significant concerns, including any of the red flags listed in Box 1, then activation of emergency procedures and urgent transport to the nearest hospital should be arranged.

Key points

- Any athlete with suspected concussion should be REMOVED FROM PLAY, medically assessed and monitored for deterioration. No athlete diagnosed with concussion should be returned to play on the day of injury.
- If an athlete is suspected of having a concussion and medical personnel are not immediately available, the athlete should be referred to a medical facility for urgent assessment.
- Athletes with suspected concussion should not drink alcohol, use recreational drugs and should not drive a motor vehicle until cleared to do so by a medical professional.
- Concussion signs and symptoms evolve over time and it is important to consider repeat evaluation in the assessment of concussion.
- The diagnosis of a concussion is a clinical judgment, made by a medical professional. The SCAT5 should NOT be used by itself to make, or exclude, the diagnosis of concussion. An athlete may have a concussion even if their SCAT5 is "normal".

Remember:

- The basic principles of first aid (danger, response, airway, breathing, circulation) should be followed.
- Do not attempt to move the athlete (other than that required for airway management) unless trained to do so.
- Assessment for a spinal cord injury is a critical part of the initial on-field assessment.
- Do not remove a helmet or any other equipment unless trained to do so safely.

Davis GA, *et al. Br J Sports Med* 2017;**0**:1–8. doi:10.1136/bjsports-2017-097506SCAT5

Fig. 10.1 Developed by the concussion in sport group, SCAT5 is a standardized tool used by Medical professionals and qualified health care professionals to aid in evaluation of athletes suspected of having sustained a concussion [1]. SCAT 5 can also be used to obtain baseline data among health athletes for future reference

1

Name: ______________________

DOB: ______________________

Address: ______________________

ID number: ______________________

Examiner: ______________________

Date: ______________________

IMMEDIATE OR ON-FIELD ASSESSMENT

The following elements should be assessed for all athletes who are suspected of having a concussion prior to proceeding to the neurocognitive assessment and ideally should be done on-field after the first first aid / emergency care priorities are completed.

If any of the "Red Flags" or observable signs are noted after a direct or indirect blow to the head, the athlete should be immediately and safely removed from participation and evaluated by a physician or licensed healthcare professional.

Consideration of transportation to a medical facility should be at the discretion of the physician or licensed healthcare professional.

The GCS is important as a standard measure for all patients and can be done serially if necessary in the event of deterioration in conscious state. The Maddocks questions and cervical spine exam are critical steps of the immediate assessment; however, these do not need to be done serially.

STEP 1: RED FLAGS

RED FLAGS:

- Neck pain or tenderness
- Double vision
- Weakness or tingling/ burning in arms or legs
- Severe or increasing headache
- Seizure or convulsion
- Loss of consciousness
- Deteriorating conscious state
- Vomiting
- Increasingly restless, agitated or combative

STEP 2: OBSERVABLE SIGNS

Witnessed ☐ Observed on Video ☐

Lying motionless on the playing surface	Y	N
Balance / gait difficulties / motor incoordination: stumbling, slow / laboured movements	Y	N
Disorientation or confusion, or an inability to respond appropriately to questions	Y	N
Blank or vacant look	Y	N
Facial injury after head trauma	Y	N

STEP 3: MEMORY ASSESSMENT MADDOCKS QUESTIONS[2]

"I am going to ask you a few questions, please listen carefully and give your best effort. First, tell me what happened?"

____

____

Mark Y for correct answer / N for incorrect

What venue are we at today?	Y	N
Which half is it now?	Y	N
Who scored last in this match?	Y	N
What team did you play last week / game?	Y	N
Did your team win the last game?	Y	N

Note: Appropriate sport-specific questions may be substituted.

STEP 4: EXAMINATION GLASGOW COMA SCALE (GCS)[3]

Time of assessment			
Date of assessment			
Best eye response (E)			
No eye opening	1	1	1
Eye opening in response to pain	2	2	2
Eye opening to speech	3	3	3
Eyes opening spontaneously	4	4	4
Best verbal response (V)			
No verbal response	1	1	1
Incomprehensible sounds	2	2	2
Inappropriate words	3	3	3
Confused	4	4	4
Oriented	5	5	5
Best motor response (M)			
No motor response	1	1	1
Extension to pain	2	2	2
Abnormal flexion to pain	3	3	3
Flexion / Withdrawal to pain	4	4	4
Localizes to pain	5	5	5
Obeys commands	6	6	6
Glasgow Coma score (E + V + M)			

CERVICAL SPINE ASSESSMENT

Does the athlete report that their neck is pain free at rest?	Y	N
If there is NO neck pain at rest, does the athlete have a full range of ACTIVE pain free movement?	Y	N
Is the limb strength and sensation normal?	Y	N

In a patient who is not lucid or fully conscious, a cervical spine injury should be assumed until proven otherwise.

Davis GA, *et al. Br J Sports Med* 2017;**0**:1–8. doi:10.1136/bjsports-2017-097506SCAT5

Fig. 10.1 (continued)

OFFICE OR OFF-FIELD ASSESSMENT

Please note that the neurocognitive assessment should be done in a distraction-free environment with the athlete in a resting state.

STEP 1: ATHLETE BACKGROUND

Sport / team / school: ______

Date / time of injury: ______

Years of education completed: ______

Age: ______

Gender: M / F / Other

Dominant hand: left / neither / right

How many diagnosed concussions has the athlete had in the past?: ______

When was the most recent concussion?: ______

How long was the recovery (time to being cleared to play) from the most recent concussion?: ______ (days)

Has the athlete ever been:

Hospitalized for a head injury?	Yes	No
Diagnosed / treated for headache disorder or migraines?	Yes	No
Diagnosed with a learning disability / dyslexia?	Yes	No
Diagnosed with ADD / ADHD?	Yes	No
Diagnosed with depression, anxiety or other psychiatric disorder?	Yes	No

Current medications? If yes, please list:

______

______

______

______

______

______

Name: ______

DOB: ______

Address: ______

ID number: ______

Examiner: ______

Date: ______

2

STEP 2: SYMPTOM EVALUATION

The athlete should be given the symptom form and asked to read this instruction paragraph out loud then complete the symptom scale. For the baseline assessment, the athlete should rate his/her symptoms based on how he/she typically feels and for the post injury assessment the athlete should rate their symptoms at this point in time.

Please Check: ☐ **Baseline** ☐ **Post-Injury**

Please hand the form to the athlete

	none	mild		moderate		severe	
Headache	0	1	2	3	4	5	6
"Pressure in head"	0	1	2	3	4	5	6
Neck Pain	0	1	2	3	4	5	6
Nausea or vomiting	0	1	2	3	4	5	6
Dizziness	0	1	2	3	4	5	6
Blurred vision	0	1	2	3	4	5	6
Balance problems	0	1	2	3	4	5	6
Sensitivity to light	0	1	2	3	4	5	6
Sensitivity to noise	0	1	2	3	4	5	6
Feeling slowed down	0	1	2	3	4	5	6
Feeling like "in a fog"	0	1	2	3	4	5	6
"Don't feel right"	0	1	2	3	4	5	6
Difficulty concentrating	0	1	2	3	4	5	6
Difficulty remembering	0	1	2	3	4	5	6
Fatigue or low energy	0	1	2	3	4	5	6
Confusion	0	1	2	3	4	5	6
Drowsiness	0	1	2	3	4	5	6
More emotional	0	1	2	3	4	5	6
Irritability	0	1	2	3	4	5	6
Sadness	0	1	2	3	4	5	6
Nervous or Anxious	0	1	2	3	4	5	6
Trouble falling asleep (if applicable)	0	1	2	3	4	5	6

Total number of symptoms:	of 22
Symptom severity score:	of 132
Do your symptoms get worse with physical activity?	Y N
Do your symptoms get worse with mental activity?	Y N
If 100% is feeling perfectly normal, what percent of normal do you feel?	

If not 100%, why?

______

______

______

Please hand form back to examiner

Davis GA, *et al. Br J Sports Med* 2017;**0**:1–8. doi:10.1136/bjsports-2017-097506SCAT5

Fig. 10.1 (continued)

3

STEP 3: COGNITIVE SCREENING

Standardised Assessment of Concussion (SAC)[4]

ORIENTATION

What month is it?	0	1
What is the date today?	0	1
What is the day of the week?	0	1
What year is it?	0	1
What time is it right now? (within 1 hour)	0	1
Orientation score		of 5

IMMEDIATE MEMORY

The Immediate Memory component can be completed using the traditional 5-word per trial list or optionally using 10-words per trial to minimise any ceiling effect. All 3 trials must be administered irrespective of the number correct on the first trial. Administer at the rate of one word per second.

Please choose EITHER the 5 or 10 word list groups and circle the specific word list chosen for this test.

I am going to test your memory. I will read you a list of words and when I am done, repeat back as many words as you can remember, in any order. For Trials 2 & 3: I am going to repeat the same list again. Repeat back as many words as you can remember in any order, even if you said the word before.

List	Alternate 5 word lists					Score (of 5)		
						Trial 1	Trial 2	Trial 3
A	Finger	Penny	Blanket	Lemon	Insect			
B	Candle	Paper	Sugar	Sandwich	Wagon			
C	Baby	Monkey	Perfume	Sunset	Iron			
D	Elbow	Apple	Carpet	Saddle	Bubble			
E	Jacket	Arrow	Pepper	Cotton	Movie			
F	Dollar	Honey	Mirror	Saddle	Anchor			
					Immediate Memory Score			of 15
					Time that last trial was completed			

List	Alternate 10 word lists					Score (of 10)		
						Trial 1	Trial 2	Trial 3
G	Finger	Penny	Blanket	Lemon	Insect			
	Candle	Paper	Sugar	Sandwich	Wagon			
H	Baby	Monkey	Perfume	Sunset	Iron			
	Elbow	Apple	Carpet	Saddle	Bubble			
I	Jacket	Arrow	Pepper	Cotton	Movie			
	Dollar	Honey	Mirror	Saddle	Anchor			
					Immediate Memory Score			of 30
					Time that last trial was completed			

Name: __________

DOB: __________

Address: __________

ID number: __________

Examiner: __________

Date: __________

CONCENTRATION

DIGITS BACKWARDS

Please circle the Digit list chosen (A, B, C, D, E, F). Administer at the rate of one digit per second reading DOWN the selected column.

I am going to read a string of numbers and when I am done, you repeat them back to me in reverse order of how I read them to you. For example, if I say 7-1-9, you would say 9-1-7.

Concentration Number Lists (circle one)					
List A	List B	List C			
4-9-3	5-2-6	1-4-2	Y	N	0
6-2-9	4-1-5	6-5-8	Y	N	1
3-8-1-4	1-7-9-5	6-8-3-1	Y	N	0
3-2-7-9	4-9-6-8	3-4-8-1	Y	N	1
6-2-9-7-1	4-8-5-2-7	4-9-1-5-3	Y	N	0
1-5-2-8-6	6-1-8-4-3	6-8-2-5-1	Y	N	1
7-1-8-4-6-2	8-3-1-9-6-4	3-7-6-5-1-9	Y	N	0
5-3-9-1-4-8	7-2-4-8-5-6	9-2-6-5-1-4	Y	N	1
List D	List E	List F			
7-8-2	3-8-2	2-7-1	Y	N	0
9-2-6	5-1-8	4-7-9	Y	N	1
4-1-8-3	2-7-9-3	1-6-8-3	Y	N	0
9-7-2-3	2-1-6-9	3-9-2-4	Y	N	1
1-7-9-2-6	4-1-8-6-9	2-4-7-5-8	Y	N	0
4-1-7-5-2	9-4-1-7-5	8-3-9-6-4	Y	N	1
2-6-4-8-1-7	6-9-7-3-8-2	5-8-6-2-4-9	Y	N	0
8-4-1-9-3-5	4-2-7-9-3-8	3-1-7-8-2-6	Y	N	1
		Digits Score:			of 4

MONTHS IN REVERSE ORDER

Now tell me the months of the year in reverse order. Start with the last month and go backward. So you'll say December, November. Go ahead.

Dec - Nov - Oct - Sept - Aug - Jul - Jun - May - Apr - Mar - Feb - Jan	0 1
Months Score	of 1
Concentration Total Score (Digits + Months)	of 5

Davis GA, *et al. Br J Sports Med* 2017;**0**:1–8. doi:10.1136/bjsports-2017-097506SCAT5

Fig. 10.1 (continued)

4

STEP 4: NEUROLOGICAL SCREEN

See the instruction sheet (page 7) for details of test administration and scoring of the tests.

Can the patient read aloud (e.g. symptom check-list) and follow instructions without difficulty?	Y	N
Does the patient have a full range of pain-free PASSIVE cervical spine movement?	Y	N
Without moving their head or neck, can the patient look side-to-side and up-and-down without double vision?	Y	N
Can the patient perform the finger nose coordination test normally?	Y	N
Can the patient perform tandem gait normally?	Y	N

BALANCE EXAMINATION

Modified Balance Error Scoring System (mBESS) testing[5]

Which foot was tested (i.e. which is the non-dominant foot) ☐ Left ☐ Right

Testing surface (hard floor, field, etc.) ____________

Footwear (shoes, barefoot, braces, tape, etc.) ____________

Condition	Errors
Double leg stance	of 10
Single leg stance (non-dominant foot)	of 10
Tandem stance (non-dominant foot at the back)	of 10
Total Errors	of 30

Name: ____________

DOB: ____________

Address: ____________

ID number: ____________

Examiner: ____________

Date: ____________

5

STEP 5: DELAYED RECALL:

The delayed recall should be performed after 5 minutes have elapsed since the end of the Immediate Recall section. Score 1 pt. for each correct response.

Do you remember that list of words I read a few times earlier? Tell me as many words from the list as you can remember in any order.

Time Started ____

Please record each word correctly recalled. Total score equals number of words recalled.

____

____

____

Total number of words recalled accurately: of 5 or of 10

6

STEP 6: DECISION

Domain	Date & time of assessment:		
Symptom number (of 22)			
Symptom severity score (of 132)			
Orientation (of 5)			
Immediate memory	of 15 of 30	of 15 of 30	of 15 of 30
Concentration (of 5)			
Neuro exam	Normal Abnormal	Normal Abnormal	Normal Abnormal
Balance errors (of 30)			
Delayed Recall	of 5 of 10	of 5 of 10	of 5 of 10

Date and time of injury: ____________

If the athlete is known to you prior to their injury, are they different from their usual self?
☐ **Yes** ☐ **No** ☐ **Unsure** ☐ **Not Applicable**
(If different, describe why in the clinical notes section)

Concussion Diagnosed?
☐ **Yes** ☐ **No** ☐ **Unsure** ☐ **Not Applicable**

If re-testing, has the athlete improved?
☐ **Yes** ☐ **No** ☐ **Unsure** ☐ **Not Applicable**

I am a physician or licensed healthcare professional and I have personally administered or supervised the administration of this SCAT5.

Signature: ____________

Name: ____________

Title: ____________

Registration number (if applicable): ____________

Date: ____________

SCORING ON THE SCAT5 SHOULD NOT BE USED AS A STAND-ALONE METHOD TO DIAGNOSE CONCUSSION, MEASURE RECOVERY OR MAKE DECISIONS ABOUT AN ATHLETE'S READINESS TO RETURN TO COMPETITION AFTER CONCUSSION.

Davis GA, *et al. Br J Sports Med* 2017;**0**:1–8. doi:10.1136/bjsports-2017-097506SCAT5

Fig. 10.1 (continued)

CLINICAL NOTES:

Name: ____________________

DOB: ____________________

Address: ____________________

ID number: ____________________

Examiner: ____________________

Date: ____________________

CONCUSSION INJURY ADVICE

(To be given to the person monitoring the concussed athlete)

This patient has received an injury to the head. A careful medical examination has been carried out and no sign of any serious complications has been found. Recovery time is variable across individuals and the patient will need monitoring for a further period by a responsible adult. Your treating physician will provide guidance as to this timeframe.

If you notice any change in behaviour, vomiting, worsening headache, double vision or excessive drowsiness, please telephone your doctor or the nearest hospital emergency department immediately.

Other important points:

Initial rest: Limit physical activity to routine daily activities (avoid exercise, training, sports) and limit activities such as school, work, and screen time to a level that does not worsen symptoms.

1) Avoid alcohol
2) Avoid prescription or non-prescription drugs without medical supervision. Specifically:
   a) Avoid sleeping tablets
   b) Do not use aspirin, anti-inflammatory medication or stronger pain medications such as narcotics
3) Do not drive until cleared by a healthcare professional.
4) Return to play/sport requires clearance by a healthcare professional.

Clinic phone number: ____________________

Patient's name: ____________________

Date / time of injury: ____________________

Date / time of medical review: ____________________

Healthcare Provider: ____________________

Contact details or stamp

Davis GA, *et al. Br J Sports Med* 2017;**0**:1–8. doi:10.1136/bjsports-2017-097506SCAT5

Fig. 10.1 (continued)

INSTRUCTIONS

Words in *Italics* throughout the SCAT5 are the instructions given to the athlete by the clinician

Symptom Scale

The time frame for symptoms should be based on the type of test being administered. At baseline it is advantageous to assess how an athlete "typically" feels whereas during the acute/post-acute stage it is best to ask how the athlete feels at the time of testing.

The symptom scale should be completed by the athlete, not by the examiner. In situations where the symptom scale is being completed after exercise, it should be done in a resting state, generally by approximating his/her resting heart rate.

For total number of symptoms, maximum possible is 22 except immediately post injury, if sleep item is omitted, which then creates a maximum of 21.

For Symptom severity score, add all scores in table, maximum possible is 22 x 6 = 132, except immediately post injury if sleep item is omitted, which then creates a maximum of 21x6=126.

Immediate Memory

The Immediate Memory component can be completed using the traditional 5-word per trial list or, optionally, using 10-words per trial. The literature suggests that the Immediate Memory has a notable ceiling effect when a 5-word list is used. In settings where this ceiling is prominent, the examiner may wish to make the task more difficult by incorporating two 5–word groups for a total of 10 words per trial. In this case, the maximum score per trial is 10 with a total trial maximum of 30.

Choose one of the word lists (either 5 or 10). Then perform 3 trials of immediate memory using this list.

Complete all 3 trials regardless of score on previous trials.

"I am going to test your memory. I will read you a list of words and when I am done, repeat back as many words as you can remember, in any order." The words must be read at a rate of one word per second.

Trials 2 & 3 MUST be completed regardless of score on trial 1 & 2.

Trials 2 & 3:

"I am going to repeat the same list again. Repeat back as many words as you can remember in any order, even if you said the word before."

Score 1 pt. for each correct response. Total score equals sum across all 3 trials. Do NOT inform the athlete that delayed recall will be tested.

Concentration

Digits backward

Choose one column of digits from lists A, B, C, D, E or F and administer those digits as follows:

Say: *"I am going to read a string of numbers and when I am done, you repeat them back to me in reverse order of how I read them to you. For example, if I say 7-1-9, you would say 9-1-7."*

Begin with first 3 digit string.

If correct, circle "Y" for correct and go to next string length. If incorrect, circle "N" for the first string length and read trial 2 in the same string length. One point possible for each string length. Stop after incorrect on both trials (2 N's) in a string length. The digits should be read at the rate of one per second.

Months in reverse order

"Now tell me the months of the year in reverse order. Start with the last month and go backward. So you'll say December, November ... Go ahead"

1 pt. for entire sequence correct

Delayed Recall

The delayed recall should be performed after 5 minutes have elapsed since the end of the Immediate Recall section.

"Do you remember that list of words I read a few times earlier? Tell me as many words from the list as you can remember in any order."

Score 1 pt. for each correct response

Modified Balance Error Scoring System (mBESS)[5] testing

This balance testing is based on a modified version of the Balance Error Scoring System (BESS)[5]. A timing device is required for this testing.

Each of 20-second trial/stance is scored by counting the number of errors. The examiner will begin counting errors only after the athlete has assumed the proper start position. The modified BESS is calculated by adding one error point for each error during the three 20-second tests. The maximum number of errors for any single condition is 10. If the athlete commits multiple errors simultaneously, only one error is recorded but the athlete should quickly return to the testing position, and counting should resume once the athlete is set. Athletes that are unable to maintain the testing procedure for a minimum of five seconds at the start are assigned the highest possible score, ten, for that testing condition.

OPTION: For further assessment, the same 3 stances can be performed on a surface of medium density foam (e.g., approximately 50cm x 40cm x 6cm).

Balance testing – types of errors

1. Hands lifted off iliac crest
2. Opening eyes
3. Step, stumble, or fall
4. Moving hip into > 30 degrees abduction
5. Lifting forefoot or heel
6. Remaining out of test position > 5 sec

"I am now going to test your balance. Please take your shoes off (if applicable), roll up your pant legs above ankle (if applicable), and remove any ankle taping (if applicable). This test will consist of three twenty second tests with different stances."

(a) Double leg stance:

"The first stance is standing with your feet together with your hands on your hips and with your eyes closed. You should try to maintain stability in that position for 20 seconds. I will be counting the number of times you move out of this position. I will start timing when you are set and have closed your eyes."

(b) Single leg stance:

"If you were to kick a ball, which foot would you use? [This will be the dominant foot] *Now stand on your non-dominant foot. The dominant leg should be held in approximately 30 degrees of hip flexion and 45 degrees of knee flexion. Again, you should try to maintain stability for 20 seconds with your hands on your hips and your eyes closed. I will be counting the number of times you move out of this position. If you stumble out of this position, open your eyes and return to the start position and continue balancing. I will start timing when you are set and have closed your eyes."*

(c) Tandem stance:

"Now stand heel-to-toe with your non-dominant foot in back. Your weight should be evenly distributed across both feet. Again, you should try to maintain stability for 20 seconds with your hands on your hips and your eyes closed. I will be counting the number of times you move out of this position. If you stumble out of this position, open your eyes and return to the start position and continue balancing. I will start timing when you are set and have closed your eyes."

Tandem Gait

Participants are instructed to stand with their feet together behind a starting line (the test is best done with footwear removed). Then, they walk in a forward direction as quickly and as accurately as possible along a 38mm wide (sports tape), 3 metre line with an alternate foot heel-to-toe gait ensuring that they approximate their heel and toe on each step. Once they cross the end of the 3m line, they turn 180 degrees and return to the starting point using the same gait. Athletes fail the test if they step off the line, have a separation between their heel and toe, or if they touch or grab the examiner or an object.

Finger to Nose

"I am going to test your coordination now. Please sit comfortably on the chair with your eyes open and your arm (either right or left) outstretched (shoulder flexed to 90 degrees and elbow and fingers extended), pointing in front of you. When I give a start signal, I would like you to perform five successive finger to nose repetitions using your index finger to touch the tip of the nose, and then return to the starting position, as quickly and as accurately as possible."

References

1. McCrory et al. Consensus Statement On Concussion In Sport – The 5th International Conference On Concussion In Sport Held In Berlin, October 2016. British Journal of Sports Medicine 2017 (available at www.bjsm.bmj.com)
2. Maddocks, DL; Dicker, GD; Saling, MM. The assessment of orientation following concussion in athletes. Clinical Journal of Sport Medicine 1995; 5: 32-33
3. Jennett, B., Bond, M. Assessment of outcome after severe brain damage: a practical scale. Lancet 1975; i: 480-484
4. McCrea M. Standardized mental status testing of acute concussion. Clinical Journal of Sport Medicine. 2001; 11: 176-181
5. Guskiewicz KM. Assessment of postural stability following sport-related concussion. Current Sports Medicine Reports. 2003; 2: 24-30

Davis GA, *et al. Br J Sports Med* 2017;**0**:1–8. doi:10.1136/bjsports-2017-097506SCAT5

Fig. 10.1 (continued)

CONCUSSION INFORMATION

Any athlete suspected of having a concussion should be removed from play and seek medical evaluation.

Signs to watch for

Problems could arise over the first 24-48 hours. The athlete should not be left alone and must go to a hospital at once if they experience:

- Worsening headache
- Drowsiness or inability to be awakened
- Inability to recognize people or places
- Repeated vomiting
- Unusual behaviour or confusion or irritable
- Seizures (arms and legs jerk uncontrollably)
- Weakness or numbness in arms or legs
- Unsteadiness on their feet.
- Slurred speech

Consult your physician or licensed healthcare professional after a suspected concussion. Remember, it is better to be safe.

Rest & Rehabilitation

After a concussion, the athlete should have physical rest and relative cognitive rest for a few days to allow their symptoms to improve. In most cases, after no more than a few days of rest, the athlete should gradually increase their daily activity level as long as their symptoms do not worsen. Once the athlete is able to complete their usual daily activities without concussion-related symptoms, the second step of the return to play/sport progression can be started. The athlete should not return to play/sport until their concussion-related symptoms have resolved and the athlete has successfully returned to full school/learning activities.

When returning to play/sport, the athlete should follow a stepwise, **medically managed exercise progression, with increasing amounts of exercise.** For example:

Graduated Return to Sport Strategy

Exercise step	Functional exercise at each step	Goal of each step
1. Symptom-limited activity	Daily activities that do not provoke symptoms.	Gradual reintroduction of work/school activities.
2. Light aerobic exercise	Walking or stationary cycling at slow to medium pace. No resistance training.	Increase heart rate.
3. Sport-specific exercise	Running or skating drills. No head impact activities.	Add movement.
4. Non-contact training drills	Harder training drills, e.g., passing drills. May start progressive resistance training.	Exercise, coordination, and increased thinking.
5. Full contact practice	Following medical clearance, participate in normal training activities.	Restore confidence and assess functional skills by coaching staff.
6. Return to play/sport	Normal game play.	

In this example, it would be typical to have 24 hours (or longer) for each step of the progression. If any symptoms worsen while exercising, the athlete should go back to the previous step. Resistance training should be added only in the later stages (Stage 3 or 4 at the earliest).

Written clearance should be provided by a healthcare professional before return to play/sport as directed by local laws and regulations.

Graduated Return to School Strategy

Concussion may affect the ability to learn at school. The athlete may need to miss a few days of school after a concussion. When going back to school, some athletes may need to go back gradually and may need to have some changes made to their schedule so that concussion symptoms do not get worse. If a particular activity makes symptoms worse, then the athlete should stop that activity and rest until symptoms get better. To make sure that the athlete can get back to school without problems, it is important that the healthcare provider, parents, caregivers and teachers talk to each other so that everyone knows what the plan is for the athlete to go back to school.

Note: If mental activity does not cause any symptoms, the athlete may be able to skip step 2 and return to school part-time before doing school activities at home first.

Mental Activity	Activity at each step	Goal of each step
1. Daily activities that do not give the athlete symptoms	Typical activities that the athlete does during the day as long as they do not increase symptoms (e.g. reading, texting, screen time). Start with 5-15 minutes at a time and gradually build up.	Gradual return to typical activities.
2. School activities	Homework, reading or other cognitive activities outside of the classroom.	Increase tolerance to cognitive work.
3. Return to school part-time	Gradual introduction of schoolwork. May need to start with a partial school day or with increased breaks during the day.	Increase academic activities.
4. Return to school full-time	Gradually progress school activities until a full day can be tolerated.	Return to full academic activities and catch up on missed work.

If the athlete continues to have symptoms with mental activity, some other accomodations that can help with return to school may include:

- Starting school later, only going for half days, or going only to certain classes
- More time to finish assignments/tests
- Quiet room to finish assignments/tests
- Not going to noisy areas like the cafeteria, assembly halls, sporting events, music class, shop class, etc.
- Taking lots of breaks during class, homework, tests
- No more than one exam/day
- Shorter assignments
- Repetition/memory cues
- Use of a student helper/tutor
- Reassurance from teachers that the child will be supported while getting better

The athlete should not go back to sports until they are back to school/learning, without symptoms getting significantly worse and no longer needing any changes to their schedule.

Davis GA, *et al. Br J Sports Med* 2017;**0**:1–8. doi:10.1136/bjsports-2017-097506SCAT5

Fig. 10.1 (continued)

removed from play and be "in a resting state" before testing is performed [1]. This usually requires at least ten minutes or more, which gives time for the athlete's heart rate to return to the resting state. Therefore, it is important to recognize that the SCAT5 cannot be performed correctly if less than 10 minutes have passed since time of suspected concussion. A preseason baseline evaluation can provide tremendous benefit. Possession of a baseline "scorecard" for reference facilitates serial tracking of a concussion over time, should injury occur during competitive regular season events. This may be helpful given reports regarding the variability in baseline testing, as well as test reliability for earlier SCAT versions. One study reported baseline values for 260 collegiate athletes utilizing the original SCAT [80]. This study demonstrated gender differences in baseline values. A history of previous concussion in athletes also accounted for differences in baseline scores. Another study investigating representative baseline values on the SCAT2 reported differences in scores associated with age, gender, and self-reported concussion. This further highlights the benefit of baseline testing of athletes before initiation of competitive events during the regular season [81]. It should be noted that scores for the SCAT5 are not "pass/fail" scores, but rather, the tool is used by the healthcare professional to assist in the diagnosis of concussion, to determine overall injury severity, and management of concussion.

For children aged 5–12 years, the Child SCAT5 was developed, and contains modifications from the SCAT5 that are more appropriate to children [82]. Some of the differences between the Child SCAT5 and the SCAT5 include a child-specific symptoms list, which includes both child and parent reported symptoms, simpler concentration questions for children, removal of orientation questions for children, and simplified balance testing for younger children. A large body of evidence supports balance testing (which includes balance assessed with tandem gait.), particularly in the first few days, as a sensitive component of the diagnosis of concussion [83–85]. This influenced the inclusion of the Balance Error Scoring System (BESS) that was included in the SCAT5.

The examiner should follow this with a more detailed evaluation of cervical range of motion (ROM). Range of motion testing should assess flexion, extension, and rotation in all directions, both passively and actively [86]. This should be followed with formal assessment of motor strength testing in all muscle groups. The athlete should be withheld from participation (even in the absence of deficits on previous portions of the concussion assessment) for further evaluation, because limitations in these areas may place the athlete at risk for further injury by restricting the athlete's ability to protect the head and anticipate impacts from oncoming opponents [87]. For athletes who have performed at or above baseline for all other aspects of the assessment, functional testing marks the final step in the concussion evaluation.

The goal of functional testing is to elicit symptoms that may be exhibited with the physical and cognitive demands the athlete may experience upon return to play [87]. Simple tasks such as push-ups, and sit-ups, and Valsalva maneuver should be performed first [87].

Next, physical activity may be advanced by having the athlete jog. This may be followed by more strenuous aerobic activity such as interval sprinting exercises. Successful completion of the progression culminates with sport-specific activities (e.g., dribbling/shooting a basketball, passing drills with a soccer ball, throwing/catching a football, shooting a hockey puck, etc.) performed at a similar intensity level necessary for safe return to play [86]. With each step, the practitioner should ask the athlete whether any concussion-related symptoms have been elicited before moving on to an increase in activity level. If at any time, an athlete reports symptoms that result from the exertion, the player should not be permitted to return to play (or progressed to the next step). If no symptoms are elicited through these functional tests and all other assessments demonstrate normal findings, the athlete has not likely sustained a concussion and may be considered for return to play.

Although standardized sideline assessment tools may be useful in the evaluation of concussion, several points must be kept in mind. These tools are designed for rapid screening of concussion by the wider spectrum of practitioner types and should not be used to replace comprehensive neuropsychologic testing by a trained neuropsychologist [1]. Furthermore, no sideline assessment tool should be used for the ongoing management of sports-related concussions [1]. A standardized clinical evaluation of concussion is useful, but should not substitute for clinician's judgment [87].

Adjuncts to the Clinical Assessment for Concussion

Neuropsychologic Testing

Neuropsychologists have contributed greatly to our knowledge of the effects of concussion on cognition and emotional functioning. The application of neuropsychologic testing has been long recognized in the evaluation and treatment of individuals with concussive injuries [88] Well-known sequelae of concussion include deficits in attention, processing speed, reaction time, and learning [89–91]. If a neuropsychological assessment is deemed necessary by the treating physician, it should be performed by a trained neuropsychologist [1]. Neuropsychological assessment can be especially helpful in the cognitive assessment of athletes when distinction between true cognitive impairment secondary to a concussion versus other factors are difficult to determine.

Multiple studies have demonstrated the usefulness of neuropsychologic assessment with concussed patients and in return-to-play (RTP) protocols [1, 92–98]. Neuropsychologists employ computerized measures to examine cognitive functions such as attention, memory, language, visual abilities, and executive functioning as well as affective functioning. Computerized tests offer the advantage of decreased administration time, availability of multiple alternative forms for serial testing, and more precise measurements [99, 100]. Perhaps the most widely-used computerized test is the Immediate Post-Concussion Assessment and Cognitive Testing (ImPACT) program [101]. This is a 20-minute assessment that contains a symptom checklist, and measures visual and verbal memory, reaction time, and information processing time [102, 103]. Validity measures with computerized tests such as the ImPACT program reduce the risk of intentionally poor performance reporting on baseline testing without reaching threshold on the test validity indicators, which alert the administrator to an invalid test [104]. These validity measures may be used with or without baseline data, in which case normative data may be applied.

Various studies have demonstrated the utility of the ImPACT program in concussion [95, 103, 105–111]. Although the use of computerized instruments in concussion has become widely accepted, there are still legitimate concerns regarding this assessment method. Among some of the concerns raised are: privacy and data security, test reliability and validity, cultural, experiential, and disability effects, and checks on effort validity [112].

One study reported low reliability scores with ImPACT and other tests [113]. This study demonstrated that, even with alternative forms, practice effects can be seen on ImPACT, particularly with processing speed scores. Broglio and colleagues reported lack of test-retest reliability of three computerized tests (ImPACT, CogSport, and Headminders) in an often-cited study as argument against the validity of computerized testing [114].

Advanced Neuroimaging

Conventional neuroimaging findings seen in computed tomography (CT) and magnetic resonance imaging (MRI) are typically normal in concussion. CT and MRI of the brain are utilized when there is concern for intracerebral hemorrhage or a structural lesion is suspected in the setting of focal neurological deficit, prolonged loss of consciousness, or progressive worsening of symptoms. Several advanced neuroimaging techniques, such as diffusion tensor imaging (DTI), functional MRI (fMRI), magnetic resonance spectroscopy (MRS), and high-definition fiber tracking (HDFT), and positron emission tomography (PET), might possibly increase the sensitivity of neuroimaging to detect both structural and functional abnormalities associated with concussion—both in the acute setting and subsequently in the subacute and chronic phases of recovery.

Several studies have used advanced MRI techniques to assess for acute concussion. These studies demonstrate acute changes in brain function and structure following concussion. These acute changes were shown to gradually revert back to a normal pre-concussive state, which is comparable to non-concussed control patients. These acute MRI findings include changes in white matter integrity on diffusion imaging, changes in cerebral blood flow on arterial spin labeling (ASL), altered functional connectivity on resting state functional MRI (rs-fMRI), and appearance of microhemmorhage on perfusion imaging.

Several studies have evaluated and discussed fMRI findings in sports-related concussion [84, 115–123]. One study examined performance of memory and sensory tasks in a group of college football players, some of whom had suffered concussion. Brain activation was found to be more widespread following concussion than before injury (baseline fMRI used for comparison). This cohort was compared to un-injured control subjects [124]. The mid-dorsolateral prefrontal cortex (DLPC) is an area associated with working memory. Less task-related activation in the DLPC was observed in subjects with persistent post-concussion symptoms 1–14 months following concussion. These findings were present in the absence of abnormalities seen on structural MRI. Of particular interest was one subject who demonstrated resolution of symptoms with associated normalization of the observed widespread activation pattern. Some studies have also demonstrated a correlation between fMRI abnormalities and cognitive test results. Athletes with post-injury fMRI findings that demonstrated hyperactivation experienced a longer clinical recovery when compared to those without hyperactivation [125].

PET measures certain components of cerebral metabolism, including blood flow and the cerebral metabolic oxygen consumption. Some limitations of PET include expense, exposure to radiolabeled tracers, and the time required to complete the study. Despite these limitations, studies have demonstrated interesting findings when PET is performed after mTBI. Umile et al. observed adults after mTBI who exhibited persistent post-concussion symptoms. This study found the subjects to have significantly reduced metabolism in the medial temporal lobe [126]. Chen et al. demonstrated differences in cerebral metabolism during a visual-spatial working memory task in adult subjects with persistent symptoms following mTBI [127].

MRS measures concentrations of compounds in the brain within a sampled region. It is a useful tool that is commonly used in the evaluation of brain lesions [119]. TBI is associated with specific metabolites, which may include choline, a marker of membrane damage and turnover; lactate, an indirect marker for ischemia and hypoxia; *N*-acetyl aspartate (NAA), a marker of neuronal integrity; creatine (Cr), a cellular energy marker for adenosine triphosphate (ATP) resynthesis; and myoinositol, a glial marker [117, 128].

In a study of 14 patients with sports-related concussion, reduced NAA:Cr ratios were observed 3 days after concussion, with normalization of the NAA:Cr ratio 30 days post injury [129]. This reduced ratio persisted despite resolution of symptoms which occurred, on average, after 3 days. This suggests that metabolic normalization may be different than symptom recovery. Reduction in NAA and other metabolic derangements in post-concussion patients is supported by various studies comparing athletes with and without concussion [130, 131].

HDFT and DTI, both techniques that are capable of providing information regarding fiber tract integrity and white matter microstructure, have been increasingly utilized following mTBI and concussion. Many DTI studies have shown correlation between mTBI and widespread structural changes in cortical white matter tracts [132–146].

These studies report abnormalities in various regions of the brain. These areas include the corona radiate, corpus callosum, uncinate fasciculus, inferior and superior longitudinal fasciculus, cingulum bundle, inferior fronto-occipital fasciculus, internal capsule, as well as the acoustic and posterior thalamic radiations [135]. Studies have demonstrated a correlation between DTI and injury severity with symptoms [145] as well as functional deficits measured by neuropsychologic testing and other behavioral measures [138, 141, 147, 148].

HDFT provides high-resolution details of axonal pathways and projection fields that allow detection of the specific location and degree of damage [149, 150]. HDFT was used in one study to identify a specific lesion of the corona radiata corticospinal pathway that was associated with left-sided weakness in a patient 4 months after injury [149].

HDFT may overcome some of the shortcomings of DTI, but routine use of either modality for concussion is premature [149]. The results of initial studies using HDFT are preliminary and must be validated in larger studies, but emerging data is encouraging.

Cerebrospinal Fluid and Serum-Based Biomarkers of Injury

There has been a drastic increase in research in both cerebrospinal fluid (CSF) and serum biomarkers of neuronal, axonal, and astroglial injury with a goal of improving diagnosis and helping predict the clinical course after concussion and mTBI. Despite these efforts, there remains a lack of sufficient evidence to justify their routine clinical use [1, 151].

Recent studies have demonstrated changes in common TBI biomarkers after SRC, suggesting evidence of neuronal cell body damage, axonal injury, and neuroinflammatory response to injury. Serum may seem to be an attractive biofluid for analysis given its lower cost and lower associated risk of acquisition, but extensive studies with sampling of both biofluids suggest otherwise. Trauma to areas outside of the brain, as well as non-trauma-related athletic exertion, is associated with increased levels of certain biomarkers that may give a false representation of levels in the brain. For example, S100 calcium-binding protein (S100B) and glial fibrillary acidic protein (GFAP), both markers of astroglial injury, have been shown to be elevated in the serum of mTBI patients [152–154].

Other biomarkers, such as myelin basic protein (MBP), tau protein, and neuron-specific enolase (NSE) are being actively studied. Immunoassay technique sensitivity, validity, clinical assays for quantification, and the amount of longitudinal data in concussion need to improve before these biomarkers can be routinely used [151].

Concussion Management

The mainstays in concussion management have previously been both physical and cognitive rest. The Berlin consensus statement states [1]:

> There is currently insufficient evidence that prescribing complete rest achieves these objectives. After a brief period of rest during the acute phase (24–48 hours) after injury, patients can be encouraged to become gradually and progressively more active while staying below

their cognitive and physical symptom-exacerbation thresholds (ie, activity level should not bring on or worsen their symptoms). It is reasonable for athletes to avoid vigorous exertion while they are recovering. The exact amount and duration of rest is not yet well defined in the literature and requires further study.

Fortunately, most symptoms resolve relatively shortly over the course of several days following injury, thus allowing the patient to gradually return to social and academic activities.

A stepwise program is generally accepted with regard to return to athletic play [1]. This program begins with a period of no activity. This is followed by light aerobic exercise, followed by sport-specific exercise, noncontact training drills, full-contact practice, and finally return to play. Each of these levels is performed over a 24-hour period. The program may be initiated when the athlete is asymptomatic at rest. If the athlete exhibits any post-concussion symptoms at any of these steps, another 24-hour period of rest is completed, and the athlete reverts back to the previous step in the program. Same-day RTP should not be permitted on the day of injury. This is due to evidence that RTP on the day of injury may be associated with prolonged neuropsychological deficits with delayed onset.

It is uncommon for post-concussion symptoms to persist beyond 10 days, but it is possible in a subset of patients. This may prompt clinicians to consider pharmacologic treatments for management of symptoms. If this option is to be employed, the patient and clinician should come to a mutual agreement that that benefit of treatment outweighs any possible adverse effect of a medication under consideration [155, 156]. There are no clinically validated treatments that have demonstrated benefit with regards to expedited recovery or amelioration of deficits attributed to TBI [157]. However, athletes with post-concussion syndrome or prolonged post-concussion syndrome may experience some benefit from symptomatic medical treatment during the recovery phase [157–160].

Several factors must be considered by a physician considering use of medication for the treatment of post-concussion symptoms. Medications that lower seizure threshold, or those that contribute to fatigue, cognitive slowing, or daytime drowsiness should be avoided. Medical therapies should be initiated at the lowest effective dose, with a slow dose titration according to patient tolerability, clinical response, and side effects. In order to prevent adverse interactions, special care should be taken to review all medications and over-the counter supplements the patient is currently using [155, 156, 161].

The treatment of concussion should be specific to patient symptoms, which are grouped into the following four categories: cognitive, emotional, somatic complaints, and sleep disturbance [155, 160]. However, it should be noted that alleviating one symptom may improve upon others. A concise review of selected agents studied in mTBI or concussion for the management of various symptoms is provided below.

The most common symptom reported after concussion is post-traumatic headache, which occurs in more than 90% of patients [162–164]. Patients with persistent post-concussion headaches most commonly develop migraine-like or tension-type headaches [165–167]. Aspirin and other nonsteroidal anti-inflammatory drugs

(NSAIDs) are typically avoided in the acute period following concussion. Therefore, acetaminophen is a reasonable choice for post-concussion headache treatment in the acute period. A majority of patients experience spontaneous resolution of the headache; patients with persistent headaches may require further treatment. Amitriptyline (an antidepressant) has shown efficacy in the treatment of post-concussion headaches [161, 168, 169]. Data is currently limited regarding other treatments, such as triptans, dihydroergotamine (DHE), anticonvulsants (valproic acid, gabapentin, and topiramate), calcium channel blockers, and beta clockers [155, 166, 167, 170].

Neurostimulants are often used for moderate or severe TBI with associated fatigue, but data on their usage in mTBI is sparse. Methylphenidate (a norepinephrine–dopamine reuptake inhibitor), modafinil (an atypical, selective, and weak dopamine reuptake inhibitor), and amantadine (a weak antagonist of the NMDA-type glutamate receptor) are pharmacologic agents that have been studied in randomized trials for use in mTBI, and shown variable success [155, 171, 172].

Acutely following a concussion, difficulty falling asleep is a common source of significant morbidity. This is especially true for student athletes [155, 164]. Trazodone is an antidepressant which antagonizes serotonin 2A (5-HT_{2A}) receptors and inhibits serotonin reuptake, and is commonly used to treat sleep disturbance in post-concussion patients [155, 173]. Prazosin, zolpidem, and melatonin are other agents that have shown varied results for treatment of mTBI and concussion [173–181].

Antidepressants have been generally used for most emotional symptoms following concussion [155, 156]. Most evidence for use of selective serotonin reuptake inhibitors (SSRIs) in concussion comes from small, uncontrolled studies and case reports, thus efficacy is not well validated at this time. Despite this, SSRIs have become the primary treatment for TBI-associated depression due to their perceived clinical efficacy and relatively few side effects. A subset of patients may continue to experience cognitive deficits, as evidenced by neuropsychologic testing for a prolonged period following mTBI or concussion. Amantadine acts through several pharmacologic mechanisms and is a weak antagonist of the NMDA-type glutamate receptor, increases dopamine and norepinephrine release from free nerve endings, and blocks dopamine reuptake; it has been used to improve post-concussion neurocognitive recovery with varied success [182–185].

Recommendations for Concussion Management

The AAN makes several recommendations for health care providers regarding management of suspected concussion [50]. All athletes with suspected concussion should be removed from play immediately to avoid further injury. This should be followed by an evaluation by a provider experienced in diagnosis of concussion, and more severe TBI. Any athlete with concussion should be restricted from return to contact sports play until he or she is asymptomatic without medication use, and the concussion is resolved.

Licensed providers may use neurocognitive testing or other tools to determine concussion resolution.

The development of graded plans for return to cognitive and physical activity, in a monitored clinical setting, may help providers minimize exacerbation of early post-concussion impairments. Cognitive restructuring is a form of psychologic counseling focused on reassurance, education, and reattribution of symptoms that may help decrease the likelihood of the development of chronic post-concussion syndrome.

Post-concussion Syndrome

Symptoms associated with concussion typically resolve several days following injury. Symptoms that persist beyond 10 days occur in up to 10–15% of patients [1].

Post-concussion complications include acute symptoms, post-concussion syndrome (PCS), persistent or prolonged PCS (PPCS), mild cognitive impairment, chronic traumatic encephalopathy (CTE), and dementia pugilistica. The WHO's *International Statistical Classification of Diseases and Related Health Problems,* tenth revision (ICD-10) defines diagnosis of PCS requiring the presence of three or more of the following symptoms: headache, dizziness, fatigue, irritability, insomnia, concentration difficulty, and memory difficulty. There is no universally agreed upon time frame for symptom duration that constitutes the aforementioned syndromes; however, the persistence of symptoms for between 6 weeks and 3 months is generally consistent with PCS, and the presence of any symptom for longer than 3 months is consistent with PPCS [156–186].

There is also some controversy regarding the pathophysiology of these phenomena, with some authorities suggesting that the symptoms associated with PCS are a direct consequence of brain injury, while others propose that the symptoms are functional and represent the emotional or psychologic sequelae of the brain injury [187–189].

It is important to note that symptoms associated with concussion may also be associated with various other conditions. Differentiating among etiologies can prove to be difficult. For example, comparison of the diagnostic criteria for post-traumatic stress disorder (PTSD), major depressive disorder, acute stress disorder, anxiety disorders, and PCS shows considerable overlap [190]. The differential diagnosis also can include vestibular dysfunction, visual dysfunction, cervical injury, somatization, chronic fatigue and pain, or a combination of these in some form [191, 192]. When clinical recovery extends outside the expected window, management by a multidisciplinary team with experience in concussion management should be undertaken [1].

It is unclear which patients will continue to experience PCS spectrum symptoms far beyond their injury, but certain variables may increase the risk. These clinical variables may include prior concussions, female sex, a history of cognitive dysfunction, and the presence of affective disorders, such as depression and anxiety

[192–198]. The average time to normalization to pre-concussion baseline on neurocognitive testing has been reported as 10–14 days in high school students, 5–7 days in collegiate athletes, and 2–5 days in professional athletes [199–201].

Children may experience more severe, prolonged, and more widespread cerebral edema after brain injury [202–204]. The reasons for this are unclear, but may be due to differences in glutamate receptor expression and/or sensitivity, or weakened neck musculature that may result in greater rotational acceleration on impact when compared to that seen in adults [205–208].

There is no widely accepted explanation for the higher risk of PCS and PPCS in patients with underlying cognitive dysfunction. Patients with lower IQ scores have been found to be more likely to experience persistent post-concussion symptoms and to be diagnosed with PCS after brain injury [197, 209]. Several studies suggest that specific premorbid emotional and personality characteristics potentially put some people at increased risk for poor outcome following concussion [198, 210]. Post-concussion symptoms may be mediated by an interaction of psychologic and neurological factors after TBI. Psychiatric disease preceding or following brain injury, including PTSD, anxiety, depression, acute stress disorder, has been associated with increased risk of poor outcome following concussion [197, 209, 211].

Repetitive Mild Traumatic Brain Injury: Cumulative Effects

The short- and long-term sequela of repetitive concussion has gained increased focus in the media and medical community over the last several years. The biggest short-term fear regarding repetitive head injury is that of "second impact syndrome." This is defined as the quick deterioration and death of an athlete who experiences a second mild head injury following return to play subsequent to the first injury. Most case reports pertaining to this syndrome are not associated with space occupying lesions. Death was associated with severe and rapid cerebral edema [212]. This condition has been reported primarily in adolescent and young adult athletes. Proponents of this syndrome believe that following initial mild TBI in younger patients, there exists an increased underlying risk for development of autoregulation and catecholamine release that may result in diffuse cerebral edema and possibly death after even a mild secondary impact [213–215]. The pathophysiology leading to the severe edema and small hematomas that are often encountered is not fully understood. Furthermore, it remains unclear whether the edema or hematomas are the result of one of the individual blows to the head rather than the proposed pathophysiologic mechanisms leading to severe disability or death [215–217].

Suffering multiple concussions has been associated with increased risk for future concussion, cognitive deficit, delayed mild cognitive deficit, and sleep disruption. The association with CTE and suffering multiple concussions has gained increased attention in the media, and the mainstream public [218, 219]. First defined by Omalu et al. in 2005, CTE is defined as a progressive neurodegenerative syndrome caused by repetitive and episodic blunt force impact to the head that cause acceleration-deceleration forces to the brain [220]. A systematic review by Manley et al. examined potential long-term sequelae of concussion by examining cognitive, mental health, neuroimaging, and neuropathological features of CTE. This review demonstrated that despite reports with a small number of retired athletes who exhibited some mental health and cognitive problems, the majority of studies demonstrated these changes to be similar to the incidence in the general population [221]. These authors concluded that while multiple concussions appear to be a risk factor for mental health problems and cognitive impairment in some individuals, more research is needed to better understand the prevalence of CTE and other neurological conditions, and the degree to which they are related to concussions and sports-related repetitive neurotrauma.

A systematic review examining potential long term sequelae of concussion studied the neuroimaging, cognitive, mental health, and neuropathological features of CTE, and identified that whilst a very small number of retired athletes have some mental health and cognitive problems, the majority of studies demonstrate these changes to be similar to the incidence in the general population and the Berlin consensus paper stated that: [1, 221]

> However, there is much more to learn about the potential cause-and-effect relationships of repetitive head-impact exposure and concussions. The potential for developing chronic traumatic encephalopathy (CTE) must be a consideration, as this condition appears to represent a distinct tauopathy with an unknown incidence in athletic populations.
>
> A cause-and-effect relationship has not yet been demonstrated between CTE and SRCs or exposure to contact sports. As such, the notion that repeated concussion or sub-concussive impacts cause CTE remains unknown.

There is significant debate regarding both the clinical and pathological diagnostic criteria for CTE. There is also debate over the theory around a causal and exclusive link between exposure to repetitive head impact and risk for CTE. While case studies have received a great deal of attention, several studies have failed to find a link [222]. Tauopathy changes in the brain that meet the pathological criteria of CTE have been identified in multiple cases with a notable absence of history of head trauma [223, 224]. Therefore, the causal association between the pathological findings of CTE and the clinical condition requires continuing study.

The clinical features of CTE involve a prolonged latency period prior to a composite syndrome of neuropsychiatric disturbance, mood disorder, and cognitive impairment [225, 226]. Insidious onset of poor attention, loss of recent memory, frequent headaches, and bouts of confusion and disorientation are common early in the syndrome [226]. There is often a progression of effects referable to poor prefrontal cortex executive function and limbic system dysfunction, including worsening disorientation and confusion, poor insight and judgment, and the onset of antisocial behaviors [226]. The pathophysiologic mechanisms responsible for the clinical sequelae associated with repetitive brain injury are not entirely understood, but microvascular changes, blood-brain barrier (BBB) breakdown, diffuse axonal injury (DAI), and immunoexcitotoxicity have been implicated [227]. Currently, the diagnosis of CTE relies on autopsy and subsequent neuropathologic examination, with the defining feature of CTE being that of tauopathy, which may be seen in the form of neuropil threads (NT), glial tangles (GTs), or neurofibrillary tangles (NFTs), in an irregular, superficial cortical distribution [226, 228]. The development of tau-binding radiolabeled ligands will likely enhance the ability to diagnose CTE in living patients [218, 229]. Limited cases have demonstrated the ability to identify an increased tau burden within the brains of retired professional football players subjected to repetitive neurotrauma [229]. This work represents the first effort to clearly show the potential of premortem CTE diagnosis [219, 229].

Conclusion

The definition of concussion continues to evolve. Concussion epidemiology, signs and symptoms, and on-field assessment are important for the sports neurosurgeon. Concussion clinical assessment can be supported by neuropsychological testing, advanced neuroimaging, and cerebrospinal fluid and serum-based biomarkers. The American Academy of Neurology Guideline Recommendations for Concussion Management should be heeded by the sports neurosurgeon.

References

1. McCrory P, Meeuwisse W, Dvorak J, et al. Consensus statement on concussion in sport—the 5th international conference on concussion in sport held in Berlin, October 2016. Br J Sports Med. 2017;51:838–47.
2. Kristman VL, Borg J, Godbolt AK, et al. Methodological issues and research recommendations for prognosis after mild traumatic brain injury: results of the International Collaboration on Mild Traumatic Brain Injury Prognosis. Arch Phys Med Rehabil. 2014;95(suppl):S265–77.
3. Carroll LJ, Cassidy JD, Holm L, et al. Injury WHOCCTFoMTB. Methodological issues and research recommendations for mild traumatic brain injury: the WHO Collaborating Centre Task Force on Mild Traumatic Brain Injury. J Rehabil Med. 2004;36(suppl 43):113–25.
4. Tator CH. Let's standardize the definition of concussion and get reliable incidence data. Can J Neurol Sci. 2009;36(4):405–6.
5. Lopez AD, Murray CC. The global burden of disease, 1990–2020. Nat Med. 1998;4(11):1241–3.
6. Thurman DJ, Alverson C, Dunn KA, et al. Traumatic brain injury in the United States: a public health perspective. J Head Trauma Rehabil. 1999;14(6):602–15.
7. Bryan CJ, Clemans TA. Repetitive traumatic brain injury, psychological symptoms, and suicide risk in a clinical sample of deployed military personnel. JAMA Psychiat. 2013;70(7):686–91.
8. Erickson JC. Treatment outcomes of chronic post-traumatic headaches after mild head trauma in US soldiers: an observational study. Headache. 2011;51(6):932–44.
9. Hoge CW, McGurk D, Thomas JL, et al. Mild traumatic brain injury in U.S. Soldiers returning from Iraq. N Engl J Med. 2008;358(5):453–63.

10. Okie S. Traumatic brain injury in the war zone. N Engl J Med. 2005;352(20):2043–7.
11. Schwab KA, Ivins B, Cramer G, et al. Screening for traumatic brain injury in troops returning from deployment in Afghanistan and Iraq: initial investigation of the usefulness of a short screening tool for traumatic brain injury. J Head Trauma Rehabil. 2007;22(6):377–89.
12. Terrio H, Brenner LA, Ivins BJ, et al. Traumatic brain injury screening: preliminary findings in a US Army Brigade Combat Team. J Head Trauma Rehabil. 2009;24(1):14–23.
13. Felber ES. Combat-related posttraumatic headache: diagnosis, mechanisms of injury, and challenges to treatment. J Am Osteopath Assoc. 2010;110(12):737–8.
14. Marin JR, Weaver MD, Yealy DM, et al. Trends in visits for traumatic brain injury to emergency departments in the United States. JAMA. 2014;311(18):1917–9.
15. Langlois JA, Rutland-Brown W, Wald MM. The epidemiology and impact of traumatic brain injury: a brief overview. J Head Trauma Rehabil. 2006;21(5):375–8.
16. Clay MB, Glover KL, Lowe DT. Epidemiology of concussion in sport: a literature review. J Chiropr Med. 2013;12(4):230–51.
17. Harmon KG, Drezner JA, Gammons M Endorsed by the National Trainers' Athletic Association and the American College of Sports Medicine, et al. American Medical Society for Sports Medicine position statement: concussion in sport. Br J Sports Med. 2013;47:15–26.
18. Kerr ZY, Roos KG, Djoko A, et al. Epidemiologic measures for quantifying the incidence of concussion in national collegiate athletic association sports. J Athl Train. 2017;52:167–74. https://doi.org/10.4085/1062-6050-51.6.05.
19. Tsushima WT, Siu AM, Ahn HJ, et al. Incidence and risk of concussions in youth athletes: comparisons of age, sex, concussion history, sport, and football position. Arch Clin Neuropsychol. 2018;126 https://doi.org/10.1093/arclin/acy019.
20. Bretzin AC, Covassin T, Fox ME, et al. Sex differences in the clinical incidence of concussions, missed school days, and time loss in high school student-athletes: part 1. Am J Sports Med. 2018;46:2263–9. https://doi.org/10.1177/0363546518778251.
21. Barr WB, McCrea M. Sensitivity and specificity of standardized neurocognitive testing immediately following sports concussion. J Int Neuropsychol Soc. 2001;7:693–702. https://doi.org/10.1017/S1355617701766052.
22. Barr WB, Prichep LS, Chabot R, et al. Measuring brain electrical activity to track recovery from sport-related concussion. Brain Inj. 2012;26:58–66. https://doi.org/10.3109/02699052.2011.608216.
23. McCrea M, Kelly JP, Randolph C, et al. Immediate neurocognitive effects of concussion. Neurosurgery. 2002;50:1032–40.
24. McCrea M. Standardized mental status assessment of sports concussion. Clin J Sport Med. 2001;11:176–81. https://doi.org/10.1097/00042752-200107000-00008.
25. McCrea M, Barr WB, Guskiewicz K, et al. Standard regression-based methods for measuring recovery after sport-related concussion. J Int Neuropsychol Soc. 2005;11:58–69. https://doi.org/10.1017/S1355617705050083.
26. Marinides Z, Galetta KM, Andrews CN, et al. Vision testing is additive to the sideline assessment of sports-related concussion. Neurol Clin Pract. 2015;5:25–34. https://doi.org/10.1212/CPJ.0000000000000060.
27. Galetta KM, Morganroth J, Moehringer N, et al. Adding vision to concussion testing: a prospective study of sideline testing in youth and collegiate athletes. J Neuroophthalmol. 2015;35:235–41. https://doi.org/10.1097/WNO.0000000000000226.
28. Putukian M, Echemendia R, Dettwiler-Danspeckgruber A, et al. Prospective clinical assessment using Sideline Concussion Assessment Tool-2 testing in the evaluation of sport-related concussion in college athletes. Clin J Sport Med. 2015;25:36–42. https://doi.org/10.1097/JSM.0000000000000102.
29. Chin EY, Nelson LD, Barr WB, et al. Reliability and validity of the sport concussion assessment tool-3 (SCAT3) in high school and collegiate athletes. Am J Sports Med. 2016;44:2276–85. https://doi.org/10.1177/0363546516648141.

30. Seidman DH, Burlingame J, Yousif LR, et al. Evaluation of the King-devick test as a concussion screening tool in high school football players. J Neurol Sci. 2015;356:97–101. https://doi.org/10.1016/j.jns.2015.06.021.
31. Dompier TP, Kerr ZY, Marshall SW, et al. Incidence of concussion during practice and games in youth, high school, and collegiate american football players. JAMA Pediatr. 2015;169:659–65. https://doi.org/10.1001/jamapediatrics.2015.0210.
32. Houck Z, Asken B, Bauer R, et al. Epidemiology of sport-related concussion in an ncaa division i football bowl subdivision sample. Am J Sports Med. 2016;44:2269–75. https://doi.org/10.1177/0363546516645070.
33. Galetta KM, Brandes LE, Maki K, et al. The King-Devick test and sports-related concussion: study of a rapid visual screening tool in a collegiate cohort. J Neurol Sci. 2011;309(1–2):34–9. https://doi.org/10.1016/j.jns.2011.07.039.
34. Leong DF, Balcer LJ, Galetta SL, et al. The King-Devick test for sideline concussion screening in collegiate football. J Optom. 2015;8:131–9. https://doi.org/10.1016/j.optom.2014.12.005.
35. Dhawan PS, Leong D, Tapsell L, et al. King-devick test identifies real-time concussion and asymptomatic concussion in youth athletes. Neurol Clin Pract. 2017;7:1–73. https://doi.org/10.1212/CPJ.0000000000000381.
36. Shankar PR, Fields SK, Collins CL, et al. Epidemiology of high school and collegiate football injuries in the United States, 2005–2006. Am J Sports Med. 2007;35(8):1295–303.
37. Guskiewicz KM, Weaver NL, Padua DA, et al. Epidemiology of concussion in collegiate and high school football players. Am J Sports Med. 2000;28(5):643–50.
38. Yard EE, Comstock RD. Effects of field location, time in competition, and phase of play on injury severity in high school football. Res Sports Med. 2009;17(1):35–49.
39. Guskiewicz KM, McCrea M, Marshall SW, et al. Cumulative effects associated with recurrent concussion in collegiate football players: the NCAA Concussion Study. JAMA. 2003;290(19):2549–55.
40. Pellman EJ, Powell JW, Viano DC, et al. Concussion in professional football: epidemiological features of game injuries and review of the literature—part 3. Neurosurgery. 2004;54(1):81–94; discussion 94–86.
41. Rechel JA, Yard EE, Comstock RD. An epidemiologic comparison of high school sports injuries sustained in practice and competition. J Athl Train. 2008;43(2):197–204.
42. Wisniewski JF, Guskiewicz K, Trope M, et al. Incidence of cerebral concussions associated with type of mouthguard used in college football. Dent Traumatol. 2004;20(3):143–9.
43. Meehan WP 3rd, d'Hemecourt P, Comstock RD. High school concussions in the 2008–2009 academic year: mechanism, symptoms, and management. Am J Sports Med. 2010;38(12):2405–9.
44. Crisco JJ, Fiore R, Beckwith JG, et al. Frequency and location of head impact exposures in individual collegiate football players. J Athl Train. 2010;45(6):549–59.
45. Gessel LM, Fields SK, Collins CL, et al. Concussions among United States high school and collegiate athletes. J Athl Train. 2007;42(4):495–503.
46. Kimbler DE, Murphy M, Dhandapani KM. Concussion and the adolescent athlete. J Neurosci Nurs. 2011;43(6):286–90.
47. Agel J, Harvey EJ. A 7-year review of men's and women's ice hockey injuries in the NCAA. Can J Surg. 2010;53(5):319–23.
48. Brainard LL, Beckwith JG, Chu JJ, et al. Gender differences in head impacts sustained by collegiate ice hockey players. Med Sci Sports Exerc. 2012;44(2):297–304.
49. Niedfeldt MW. Head injuries, heading, and the use of headgear in soccer. Curr Sports Med Rep. 2011;10(6):324–9.
50. Giza CC, Kutcher JS, Ashwal S, et al. Summary of evidence-based guideline update: evaluation and management of concussion in sports: report of the Guideline Development Subcommittee of the American Academy of Neurology. Neurology. 2013;80(24):2250–7.
51. Ellemberg D, Henry LC, Macciocchi SN, et al. Advances in sport concussion assessment: from behavioral to brain imaging measures. J Neurotrauma. 2009;26(12):2365–82.
52. Meehan WP 3rd, Bachur RG. Sport-related concussion. Pediatrics. 2009;123(1):114–23.

53. Patel AV, Mihalik JP, Notebaert AJ, et al. Neuropsychological performance, postural stability, and symptoms after dehydration. J Athl Train. 2007;42(1):66–75.
54. Patel DR, Reddy V. Sport-related concussion in adolescents. Pediatr Clin N Am. 2010;57(3):649–70.
55. Scorza KA, Raleigh MF, O'Connor FG. Current concepts in concussion: evaluation and management. Am Fam Physician. 2012;85(2):123–32.
56. McCrea M, Guskiewicz KM, Marshall SW, et al. Acute effects and recovery time following concussion in collegiate football players: the NCAA Concussion Study. JAMA. 2003;290(19):2556–63.
57. McCrory PR, Ariens T, Berkovic SF. The nature and duration of acute concussive symptoms in Australian football. Clin J Sport Med. 2000;10(4):235–8.
58. Pardini J, Bailes JE, Maroon JC. Mild traumatic brain injury in adults and concussion in sports. In: Winn HR, editor. Youmans neurological surgery, vol. 4. 6th ed. Philadelphia, PA: Saunders; 2011. p. 3380–9.
59. Packard RC. Epidemiology and pathogenesis of posttraumatic headache. J Head Trauma Rehabil. 1999;14(1):9–21.
60. Collins MW, Field M, Lovell MR, et al. Relationship between postconcussion headache and neuropsychological test performance in high school athletes. Am J Sports Med. 2003;31(2):168–73.
61. Mihalik JP, Stump JE, Collins MW, et al. Posttraumatic migraine characteristics in athletes following sports-related concussion. J Neurosurg. 2005;102(5):850–5.
62. McCrea M. Sideline assessment of concussion. In: Bailes JE, Day AL, editors. Neurological sports medicine: a guide for physicians and trainers. Rolling Meadows, IL: American Association of Neurological Surgeons; 2001. p. 109–22.
63. McCrea M, Kelly JP, Randolph C, et al. Standardized assessment of concussion (SAC): on-site mental status evaluation of the athlete. J Head Trauma Rehabil. 1998;13(2):27–35.
64. Iverson GL, Gaetz M, Lovell MR, et al. Relation between subjective fogginess and neuropsychological testing following concussion. J Int Neuropsychol Soc. 2004;10(6):904–6.
65. Cantu RC. Return to play guidelines after a head injury. Clin Sports Med. 1998;17:46–60.
66. Maddocks DL, Dicker GD, Saling MM. The assessment of orientation following concussion in athletes. Clin J Sport Med. 1995;5:32–5.
67. Halstead ME, Walter KD, Council on Sports Medicine and Fitness. American Academy of Pediatrics. Clinical report—sport-related concussion in children and adolescents. Pediatrics. 2010;126(3):597–615.
68. Leininger BE, Gramling SE, Farrell AD, et al. Neuropsychological deficits in symptomatic minor head injury patients after concussion and mild concussion. J Neurol Neurosurg Psychiatry. 1990;53(4):293–6.
69. Lovell MR, Iverson GL, Collins MW, et al. Does loss of consciousness predict neuropsychological decrements after concussion? Clin J Sport Med. 1999;9(4):193–8.
70. Fisher CM. Concussion amnesia. Neurology. 1966;16:826–30.
71. Yarnell PR, Lynch S. Retrograde memory immediately after concussion. Lancet. 1970;1(7652):863–4.
72. Yarnell PR, Lynch S. Progressive retrograde amnesia in concussed football players: observation shortly postimpact. Neurology. 1970;20(4):416–7.
73. McCrea M, Kelly JP, Kluge J, et al. Standardized assessment of concussion in football players. Neurology. 1997;48(3):586–8.
74. Peterson CL, Ferrara MS, Mrazik M, et al. Evaluation of neuropsychological domain scores and postural stability following cerebral concussion in sports. Clin J Sport Med. 2003;13(4):230–7.
75. Riemann BL, Guskiewicz KM. Effects of mild head injury on postural stability as measured through clinical balance testing. J Athl Train. 2000;35(1):19–25.
76. Guskiewicz KM, Bruce SL, Cantu RC, et al. National Athletic Trainers' Association position statement: management of sport-related concussion. J Athl Train. 2004;39(3):280–97.

77. Maddocks DL, Dicker GD, Saling MM. The assessment of orientation following concussion in athletes. Clin J Sport Med. 1995;5(1):32–5.
78. McCrea M. Standardized mental status assessment of sports concussion. Clin J Sport Med. 2001;11(3):176–81.
79. Guskiewicz KM. Assessment of postural stability following sport-related concussion. Curr Sports Med Rep. 2003;2(1):24–30.
80. Shehata N, Wiley JP, Richea S, et al. Sport concussion assessment tool: baseline values for varsity collision sport athletes. Br J Sports Med. 2009;43(10):730–4.
81. Valovich McLeod TC, Bay RC, Lam KC, et al. Representative baseline values on the Sport Concussion Assessment Tool 2 (SCAT2) in adolescent athletes vary by gender, grade, and concussion history. Am J Sports Med. 2012;40(4):927–33.
82. Davis GA, Purcell L, Schneider KJ, et al. The child sport concussion assessment tool 5th edition (child SCAT5): background and rationale. Br J Sports Med. 2017;51:859–61.
83. Cavanaugh JT, Guskiewicz KM, Giuliani C, et al. Detecting altered postural control after cerebral concussion in athletes with normal postural stability. Br J Sports Med. 2005;39(11):805–11.
84. Guskiewicz KM, Ross SE, Marshall SW. Postural stability and neuropsychological deficits after concussion in collegiate athletes. J Athl Train. 2001;36(3):263–73.
85. Davis GA, Iverson GL, Guskiewicz KM, et al. Contributions of neuroimaging, balance testing, electrophysiology and blood markers to the assessment of sport-related concussion. Br J Sports Med. 2009;43(suppl 1):i36–45.
86. Arfanakis K, Haughton VM, Carew JD, et al. Diffusion tensor MR imaging in diffuse axonal injury. AJNR Am J Neuroradiol. 2002;23(5):794–802.
87. Putukian M, Raftery M, Guskiewicz K, et al. Onfield assessment of concussion in the adult athlete. Br J Sports Med. 2013;47(5):285–8.
88. Echemendia RJ, Herring S, Bailes J. Who should conduct and interpret the neuropsychological assessment in sports-related concussion? Br J Sports Med. 2009;43:i32–5.
89. Belanger HG, Curtis G, Demery JA, et al. Factors moderating neuropsychological outcomes following mild traumatic brain injury: a meta-analysis. J Int Neuropsychol Soc. 2005;11(3):215–7.
90. Iverson GL, Brooks BL, Collins MW, et al. Tracking neuropsychological recovery following concussion in sport. Brain Inj. 2006;20(3):245–52.
91. Iverson GL, Zasler NF, Lange RT. Post-concussion disorder. New York: Demos Medical Publishing; 2006.
92. Belanger HG, Vanderploeg RD. The neuropsychological impact of sports-related concussion: a meta-analysis. J Int Neuropsychol Soc. 2005;11(4):345–7.
93. Broglio SP, Sosnoff JJ, Ferrara MS. The relationship of athlete-reported concussion symptoms and objective measures of neurocognitive function and postural control. Clin J Sport Med. 2009;19(5):377–82.
94. Collie A, Makdissi M, Maruff P, et al. Cognition in the days following concussion: comparison of symptomatic versus asymptomatic athletes. J Neurol Neurosurg Psychiatry. 2006;77(2):241–5.
95. Fazio VC, Lovell MR, Pardini JE, et al. The relation between post concussion symptoms and neurocognitive performance in concussed athletes. NeuroRehabilitation. 2007;22(3):207–16.
96. Iverson GL, Lovell MR, Collins MW. Validity of ImPACT for measuring processing speed following sports-related concussion. J Clin Exp Neuropsychol. 2005;27(6):683–9.
97. Van Kampen DA, Lovell MR, Pardini JE, et al. The "value added" of neurocognitive testing after sports-related concussion. Am J Sports Med. 2006;34(10):1630–5.
98. Echemendia RJ, Iverson GL, McCrea M, et al. Role of neuropsychologists in the evaluation and management of sport-related concussion: an inter-organization position statement. Arch Clin Neuropsychol. 2012;27:119–22.
99. McCrory P, Johnston P, Meeuwisse W, et al. Summary and agreement statement of the 2nd International Conference on Concussion in Sport, Prague 2004. Br J Sports Med. 2005;43(suppl 1):i76–84.

100. McCrory P, Makdissi M, Davis G, et al. Value of neuropsychological testing after head injuries in football. Br J Sports Med. 2005;39:i58–63.
101. Meehan WP, d'Hemecourt P, Collins CL, et al. Computerized neurocognitive testing for the management of sport-related concussions. Pediatrics. 2012;129(1):38–44.
102. ImPACT 6.0 [computer program]. Pittsburgh, PA; NeuroHealth Systems; 2007.
103. ImPACT: Immediate post-concussion assessment and cognitive testing. [computer program]. Pittsburgh, PA: NeuroHealth Systems; 2000.
104. Erdal K. Neuropsychological testing for sports-related concussion: how athletes can sandbag their baseline testing without detection. Arch Clin Neuropsychol. 2012;27:473–9.
105. Elbin RJ, Schatz P, Covassin T. One-year test-retest reliability of the online version of ImPACT in high school athletes. Am J Sports Med. 2011;39(11):2319–24.
106. Gl I, Lange RT. Examination of "post-concussion-like" symptoms in a healthy sample. Appl Neuropsychol. 2003;21:303–10.
107. Lau BC, Collins MW, Lovell MR. Sensitivity and specificity of subacute computerized neurocognitive testing and symptom evaluation in predicting outcomes after sport-related concussion. Am J Sports Med. 2011;39(6):1209–16.
108. Schatz P. Long-term test-retest reliability of baseline cognitive assessments using ImPACT. Am J Sports Med. 2010;38(1):47–53.
109. Schatz P, Pardini JE, Lovell MR, et al. Sensitivity and specificity of the ImPACT test battery for concussion in athletes. Arch Clin Neuropsychol. 2006;21:91–9.
110. Schatz P, Putz BO. Cross-validation of measures used for computer-based assessment of concussion. Appl Neuropsychol. 2006;13(3):151–9.
111. Schatz P, Sandel N. Sensitivity and specificity of the online version of ImPACT in high school and collegiate athletes. Am J Sports Med. 2013;41:321–6.
112. Bauer RM, Iverson GL, Cernich AN, et al. Computerized neuropsychological assessment devices: joint position paper of the American Academy of Clinical Neuropsychology and the National Academy of Neuropsychology. Clin Neuropsychol. 2012;26(2):177–96.
113. Register-Mihalik JK, Kontos DL, Guskiewicz KM, et al. Age-related differences and reliability on computerized and paper-pencil neurocognitive assessment batteries. J Athl Train. 2012;47(3):297–305.
114. Broglio SP, Ferrara MS, Macciocchi SN, et al. Test-retest reliability of computerized concussion assessment programs. J Athl Train. 2007;42(4):509–14.
115. Gosselin N, Saluja RS, Chen JK, et al. Brain functions after sports-related concussion: insights from event-related potentials and functional MRI. Phys Sportsmed. 2010;38(3):27–37.
116. Johnston KM, Ptito A, Chankowsky J, et al. New frontiers in diagnostic imaging in concussive head injury. Clin J Sport Med. 2001;11(3):166–75.
117. Khurana VG, Kaye AH. An overview of concussion in sport. J Clin Neurosci. 2012;19(1):1–11.
118. Mendez CV, Hurley RA, Lassonde M, et al. Mild traumatic brain injury: neuroimaging of sports-related concussion. J Neuropsychiatry Clin Neurosci. 2005;17(3):297–303.
119. Prabhu SP. The role of neuroimaging in sport-related concussion. Clin Sports Med. 2011;30(1):103–14, ix.
120. Pulsipher DT, Campbell RA, Thoma R, et al. A critical review of neuroimaging applications in sports concussion. Curr Sports Med Rep. 2011;10(1):14–20.
121. Chen JK, Johnston KM, Collie A, et al. A validation of the post concussion symptom scale in the assessment of complex concussion using cognitive testing and functional MRI. J Neurol Neurosurg Psychiatry. 2007;78(11):1231–8.
122. Chen JK, Johnston KM, Frey S, et al. Functional abnormalities in symptomatic concussed athletes: an fMRI study. NeuroImage. 2004;22(1):68–82.
123. Ptito A, Chen JK, Johnston KM. Contributions of functional magnetic resonance imaging (fMRI) to sport concussion evaluation. NeuroRehabilitation. 2007;22(3):217–27.
124. Jantzen KJ, Anderson B, Steinberg FL, et al. A prospective functional MR imaging study of mild traumatic brain injury in college football players. AJNR Am J Neuroradiol. 2004;25(5):738–45.

125. Lovell MR, Pardini JE, Welling J, et al. Functional brain abnormalities are related to clinical recovery and time to return-to-play in athletes. Neurosurgery. 2007;61(2):352–9; discussion 359–360.
126. Umile EM, Sandel ME, Alavi A, et al. Dynamic imaging in mild traumatic brain injury: support for the theory of medial temporal vulnerability. Arch Phys Med Rehabil. 2002;83(11):1506–13.
127. Chen SH, Kareken DA, Fastenau PS, et al. A study of persistent post-concussion symptoms in mild head trauma using positron emission tomography. J Neurol Neurosurg Psychiatry. 2003;74(3):326–32.
128. DiFiori JP, Giza CC. New techniques in concussion imaging. Curr Sports Med Rep. 2010;9(1):35–9.
129. Vagnozzi R, Signoretti S, Tavazzi B, et al. Temporal window of metabolic brain vulnerability to concussion: a pilot 1H-magnetic resonance spectroscopic study in concussed athletes—part III. Neurosurgery. 2008;62(6):1286–95; discussion 1295–1286.
130. Cimatti M. Assessment of metabolic cerebral damage using proton magnetic resonance spectroscopy in mild traumatic brain injury. J Neurosurg Sci. 2006;50(4):83–8.
131. Henry LC, Tremblay S, Boulanger Y, et al. Neurometabolic changes in the acute phase after sports concussions correlate with symptom severity. J Neurotrauma. 2010;27(1):65–76.
132. Krishna R, Grinn M, Giordano N, et al. Diagnostic confirmation of mild traumatic brain injury by diffusion tensor imaging: a case report. J Med Case Rep. 2012;6(1):66.
133. Bazarian JJ, Zhong J, Blyth B, et al. Diffusion tensor imaging detects clinically important axonal damage after mild traumatic brain injury: a pilot study. J Neurotrauma. 2007;24(9):1447–59.
134. Bazarian JJ, Zhu T, Blyth B, et al. Subject-specific changes in brain white matter on diffusion tensor imaging after sports-related concussion. Magn Reson Imaging. 2012;30(2):171–80.
135. Cubon VA, Putukian M, Boyer C, et al. A diffusion tensor imaging study on the white matter skeleton in individuals with sports-related concussion. J Neurotrauma. 2011;28(2):189–201.
136. Henry LC, Tremblay J, Tremblay S, et al. Acute and chronic changes in diffusivity measures after sports concussion. J Neurotrauma. 2011;28(10):2049–59.
137. Huisman TA, Schwamm LH, Schaefer PW, et al. Diffusion tensor imaging as potential biomarker of white matter injury in diffuse axonal injury. AJNR Am J Neuroradiol. 2004;25(3):370–6.
138. Lipton ML, Gellella E, Lo C, et al. Multifocal white matter ultrastructural abnormalities in mild traumatic brain injury with cognitive disability: a voxel-wise analysis of diffusion tensor imaging. J Neurotrauma. 2008;25(11):1335–42.
139. Mayer AR, Ling J, Mannell MV, et al. A prospective diffusion tensor imaging study in mild traumatic brain injury. Neurology. 2010;74(8):643–50.
140. Messe A, Caplain S, Paradot G, et al. Diffusion tensor imaging and white matter lesions at the subacute stage in mild traumatic brain injury with persistent neurobehavioral impairment. Hum Brain Mapp. 2011;32(6):999–1011.
141. Niogi SN, Mukherjee P, Ghajar J, et al. Extent of microstructural white matter injury in postconcussive syndrome correlates with impaired cognitive reaction time: a 3T diffusion tensor imaging study of mild traumatic brain injury. AJNR Am J Neuroradiol. 2008;29(5):967–73.
142. Niogi SN, Mukherjee P, McCandliss BD. Diffusion tensor imaging segmentation of white matter structures using a Reproducible Objective Quantification Scheme (ROQS). NeuroImage. 2007;35(1):166–74.
143. Rutgers DR, Fillard P, Paradot G, et al. Diffusion tensor imaging characteristics of the corpus callosum in mild, moderate, and severe traumatic brain injury. AJNR Am J Neuroradiol. 2008;29(9):1730–5.
144. Rutgers DR, Toulgoat F, Cazejust J, et al. White matter abnormalities in mild traumatic brain injury: a diffusion tensor imaging study. AJNR Am J Neuroradiol. 2008;29(3):514–9.
145. Smits M, Houston GC, Dippel DW, et al. Microstructural brain injury in post-concussion syndrome after minor head injury. Neuroradiology. 2011;53(8):553–63.

146. Wilde EA, McCauley SR, Hunter JV, et al. Diffusion tensor imaging of acute mild traumatic brain injury in adolescents. Neurology. 2008;70(12):948–55.
147. Kraus MF, Susmaras T, Caughlin BP, et al. White matter integrity and cognition in chronic traumatic brain injury: a diffusion tensor imaging study. Brain. 2007;130(Pt 10):2508–19.
148. Niogi SN, Mukherjee P, Ghajar J, et al. Structural dissociation of attentional control and memory in adults with and without mild traumatic brain injury. Brain. 2008;131(Pt 12):3209–21.
149. Shin SS, Verstynen T, Pathak S, et al. High-definition fiber tracking for assessment of neurological deficit in a case of traumatic brain injury: finding, visualizing, and interpreting small sites of damage. J Neurosurg. 2012;116(5):1062–9.
150. Fernandez-Miranda JC, Pathak S, Engh J, et al. High-definition fiber tractography of the human brain: neuroanatomical validation and neurosurgical applications. Neurosurgery. 2012;71(2):430–53.
151. Zetterberg H, Smith DH, Blennow K. Biomarkers of mild traumatic brain injury in cerebrospinal fluid and blood. Nat Rev Neurol. 2013;9(4):201–10.
152. Mussack T, Kirchhoff C, Buhmann S, et al. Significance of Elecsys S100 immunoassay for real-time assessment of traumatic brain damage in multiple trauma patients. Clin Chem Lab Med. 2006;44(9):1140–5.
153. Stalnacke BM, Ohlsson A, Tegner Y, et al. Serum concentrations of two biochemical markers of brain tissue damage S-100B and neurone specific enolase are increased in elite female soccer players after a competitive game. Br J Sports Med. 2006;40(4):313–6.
154. Metting Z, Wilczak N, Rodiger LA, et al. GFAP and S100B in the acute phase of mild traumatic brain injury. Neurology. 2012;78(18):1428–33.
155. Meehan WP 3rd. Medical therapies for concussion. Clin Sports Med. 2011;30(1):115–24, ix.
156. Petraglia AL, Maroon JC, Bailes JE. From the field of play to the field of combat: a review of the pharmacological management of concussion. Neurosurgery. 2012;70(6):1520–33; discussion 1533.
157. Beauchamp K, Mutlak H, Smith WR, et al. Pharmacology of traumatic brain injury: where is the "golden bullet"? Mol Med. 2008;14(11–12):731–40.
158. Mittenberg W, Burton DB. A survey of treatments for post-concussion syndrome. Brain Inj. 1994;8(5):429–37.
159. Mittenberg W, Canyock EM, Condit D, et al. Treatment of post-concussion syndrome following mild head injury. J Clin Exp Neuropsychol. 2001;23(6):829–36.
160. Reddy C. A treatment paradigm for sports concussion. Brain Inj Professional. 2004;4:24–5.
161. Comper P, Bisschop SM, Carnide N, et al. A systematic review of treatments for mild traumatic brain injury. Brain Inj. 2005;19(11):863–80.
162. Arciniegas DB, Anderson CA, Topkoff J, et al. Mild traumatic brain injury: a neuropsychiatric approach to diagnosis, evaluation, and treatment. Neuropsychiatr Dis Treat. 2005;1(4):311–27.
163. Faux S, Sheedy J. A prospective controlled study in the prevalence of posttraumatic headache following mild traumatic brain injury. Pain Med. 2008;9(8):1001–11.
164. Paniak C, Reynolds S, Phillips K, et al. Patient complaints within 1 month of mild traumatic brain injury: a controlled study. Arch Clin Neuropsychol. 2002;17(4):319–34.
165. Haas DC. Chronic post-traumatic headaches classified and compared with natural headaches. Cephalalgia. 1996;16(7):486–93.
166. Lenaerts ME, Couch JR. Posttraumatic headache. Curr Treat Options Neurol. 2004;6(6):507–17.
167. Lew HL, Lin PH, Fuh JL, et al. Characteristics and treatment of headache after traumatic brain injury: a focused review. Am J Phys Med Rehabil. 2006;85(7):619–27.
168. Tyler GS, McNeely HE, Dick ML. Treatment of post-traumatic headache with amitriptyline. Headache. 1980;20(4):213–6.
169. Weiss HD, Stern BJ, Goldberg J. Post-traumatic migraine: chronic migraine precipitated by minor head or neck trauma. Headache. 1991;31(7):451–6.

170. Lane JC, Arciniegas DB. Post-traumatic headache. Curr Treat Options Neurol. 2002;4(1):89–104.
171. Jha A, Weintraub A, Allshouse A, et al. A randomized trial of modafinil for the treatment of fatigue and excessive daytime sleepiness in individuals with chronic traumatic brain injury. J Head Trauma Rehabil. 2008;23(1):52–63.
172. Kaiser PR, Valko PO, Werth E, et al. Modafinil ameliorates excessive daytime sleepiness after traumatic brain injury. Neurology. 2010;75(20):1780–5.
173. Flanagan SR, Greenwald B, Wieber S. Pharmacological treatment of insomnia for individuals with brain injury. J Head Trauma Rehabil. 2007;22(1):67–70.
174. Rao V, Rollings P. Sleep disturbances following traumatic brain injury. Curr Treat Options Neurol. 2002;4(1):77–87.
175. Nutritional support after spinal cord injury. Neurosurgery. 2002;50(suppl 3):S81–S84.
176. Ruff RL, Ruff SS, Wang XF. Improving sleep: initial headache treatment in OIF/OEF veterans with blast-induced mild traumatic brain injury. J Rehabil Res Dev. 2009;46(9):1071–84.
177. Samantaray S, Das A, Thakore NP, et al. Therapeutic potential of melatonin in traumatic central nervous system injury. J Pineal Res. 2009;47(2):134–42.
178. Orff HJ, Ayalon L, Drummond SP. Traumatic brain injury and sleep disturbance: a review of current research. J Head Trauma Rehabil. 2009;24(3):155–65.
179. Maldonado MD, Murillo-Cabezas F, Terron MP, et al. The potential of melatonin in reducing morbidity-mortality after craniocerebral trauma. J Pineal Res. 2007;42(1):1–11.
180. Kemp S, Biswas R, Neumann V, et al. The value of melatonin for sleep disorders occurring post-head injury: a pilot RCT. Brain Inj. 2004;18(9):911–9.
181. Buscemi N, Vandermeer B, Pandya R, et al. Melatonin for treatment of sleep disorders. Evid Rep Technol Assess (Summ). 2004;108:1–7.
182. Leone H, Polsonetti BW. Amantadine for traumatic brain injury: does it improve cognition and reduce agitation? J Clin Pharm Ther. 2005;30(2):101–4.
183. Sawyer E, Mauro LS, Ohlinger MJ. Amantadine enhancement of arousal and cognition after traumatic brain injury. Ann Pharmacother. 2008;42(2):247–52.
184. Kraus MF, Smith GS, Butters M, et al. Effects of the dopaminergic agent and NMDA receptor antagonist amantadine on cognitive function, cerebral glucose metabolism and D2 receptor availability in chronic traumatic brain injury: a study using positron emission tomography (PET). Brain Inj. 2005;19(7):471–9.
185. Meythaler JM, Brunner RC, Johnson A, et al. Amantadine to improve neurorecovery in traumatic brain injury-associated diffuse axonal injury: a pilot double-blind randomized trial. J Head Trauma Rehabil. 2002;17(4):300–13.
186. Sedney CL, Orphanos J, Bailes JE. When to consider retiring an athlete after sports-related concussion. Clin Sports Med. 2011;30(1):189–200, xi.
187. Binder LM. Persisting symptoms after mild head injury: a review of the postconcussive syndrome. J Clin Exp Neuropsychol. 1986;8(4):323–46.
188. Binder LM, Rohling ML. Money matters: a meta-analytic review of the effects of financial incentives on recovery after closed-head injury. Am J Psychiatry. 1996;153(1):7–10.
189. Johnston KM, McCrory P, Mohtadi NG, et al. Evidence-based review of sport-related concussion: clinical science. Clin J Sport Med. 2001;11(3):150–9.
190. Silverberg ND, Iverson GL. Etiology of the post-concussion syndrome: physiogenesis and psychogenesis revisited. NeuroRehabilitation. 2011;29(4):317–29.
191. Al Sayegh A, Sandford D, Carson AJ. Psychological approaches to treatment of postconcussion syndrome: a systematic review. J Neurol Neurosurg Psychiatry. 2010;81(10):1128–34.
192. Leddy JJ, Sandhu H, Sodhi V, et al. Rehabilitation of concussion and post-concussion syndrome. Sports Health. 2012;4(2):147–54.
193. Guskiewicz KM, Marshall SW, Bailes J, et al. Recurrent concussion and risk of depression in retired professional football players. Med Sci Sports Exerc. 2007;39(6):903–9.
194. Ponsford J, Willmott C, Rothwell A, et al. Factors influencing outcome following mild traumatic brain injury in adults. J Int Neuropsychol Soc. 2000;6(5):568–79.

195. Preiss-Farzanegan SJ, Chapman B, Wong TM, et al. The relationship between gender and postconcussion symptoms after sport-related mild traumatic brain injury. PM R. 2009;1(3):245–53.
196. Chamelian L, Feinstein A. The effect of major depression on subjective and objective cognitive deficits in mild to moderate traumatic brain injury. J Neuropsychiatry Clin Neurosci. 2006;18(1):33–8.
197. Luis CA, Vanderploeg RD, Curtiss G. Predictors of postconcussion symptom complex in community dwelling male veterans. J Int Neuropsychol Soc. 2003;9(7):1001–15.
198. McCauley SR, Boake C, Levin HS, et al. Postconcussional disorder following mild to moderate traumatic brain injury: anxiety, depression, and social support as risk factors and comorbidities. J Clin Exp Neuropsychol. 2001;23(6):792–808.
199. Field M, Collins MW, Lovell MR, et al. Does age play a role in recovery from sports-related concussion? A comparison of high school and collegiate athletes. J Pediatr. 2003;142(5):546–53.
200. Grady MF. Concussion in the adolescent athlete. Curr Probl Pediatr Adolesc Health Care. 2010;40(7):154–69.
201. Pellman EJ, Lovell MR, Viano DC, et al. Concussion in professional football: recovery of NFL and high school athletes assessed by computerized neuropsychological testing—Part 12. Neurosurgery. 2006;58(2):263–74; discussion 263–274.
202. Pickles W. Acute general edema of the brain in children with head injuries. N Engl J Med. 1950;242(16):607–11.
203. Aldrich EF, Eisenberg HM, Saydjari C, et al. Diffuse brain swelling in severely head-injured children. A report from the NIH Traumatic Coma Data Bank. J Neurosurg. 1992;76(3):450–4.
204. Bruce DA, Alavi A, Bilaniuk L, et al. Diffuse cerebral swelling following head injuries in children: the syndrome of "malignant brain edema". J Neurosurg. 1981;54(2):170–8.
205. Bauer R, Fritz H. Pathophysiology of traumatic injury in the developing brain: an introduction and short update. Exp Toxicol Pathol. 2004;56(1–2):65–73.
206. McDonald JW, Johnston MV. Physiological and pathophysiological roles of excitatory amino acids during central nervous system development. Brain Res Brain Res Rev. 1990;15(1):41–70.
207. Mihalik JP, Blackburn JT, Greenwald RM, et al. Collision type and player anticipation affect head impact severity among youth ice hockey players. Pediatrics. 2010;125(6):e1394–401.
208. Ommaya AK, Goldsmith W, Thibault L. Biomechanics and neuropathology of adult and paediatric head injury. Br J Neurosurg. 2002;16(3):220–42.
209. Meares S, Shores EA, Taylor AJ, et al. Mild traumatic brain injury does not predict acute postconcussion syndrome. J Neurol Neurosurg Psychiatry. 2008;79(3):300–6.
210. Ruff RM, Camenzuli L, Mueller J. Miserable minority: emotional risk factors that influence the outcome of a mild traumatic brain injury. Brain Inj. 1996;10(8):551–65.
211. Bryant RA, Harvey AG. Postconcussive symptoms and posttraumatic stress disorder after mild traumatic brain injury. J Nerv Ment Dis. 1999;187(5):302–5.
212. Wetjen NM, Pichelmann MA, Atkinson JL. Second impact syndrome: concussion and second injury brain complications. J Am Coll Surg. 2010;211(4):553–7.
213. Giza CC, Hovda DA. The neurometabolic cascade of concussion. J Athl Train. 2001;36(3):228–35.
214. Cantu RC. Second-impact syndrome. Clin Sports Med. 1998;17(1):37–44.
215. McCrea HJ, Perrine K, Niogi S, et al. Concussion in sports. Sports Health. 2013;5(2):160–4.
216. Thomas M, Haas TS, Doerer JJ, et al. Epidemiology of sudden death in young, competitive athletes due to blunt trauma. Pediatrics. 2011;128(1):e1–8.
217. McCrory P, Davis G, Makdissi M. Second impact syndrome or cerebral swelling after sporting head injury. Curr Sports Med Rep. 2012;11(1):21–3.
218. Bailes JE, Dashnaw ML, Petraglia AL, et al. Cumulative effects of repetitive mild traumatic brain injury. Prog Neurol Surg. 2014;28:50–62.

219. Bailes JE, Petraglia AL, Omalu BI, et al. Talavage T. Role of subconcussion in repetitive mild traumatic brain injury. J Neurosurg. 2013;119(5):1235–45.
220. Omalu BI, DeKosky ST, Minster RL, et al. Chronic traumatic encephalopathy in a National Football League player. Neurosurgery. 2005;57(1):128–34; discussion 128–134.
221. Manley G, Gardner AJ, Schneider KJ, et al. A systematic review of potential long-term effects of sport-related concussion. Br J Sports Med. 2017;51:969–77.
222. McAllister T, McCrea M. Long-term cognitive and neuropsychiatric consequences of repetitive concussion and head-impact exposure. J Athl Train. 2017;52(3):309–17. https://doi.org/10.4085/1062-6050-52.1.14.
223. Noy S, Krawitz S, Del Bigio MR. Chronic traumatic encephalopathy-like abnormalities in a routine neuropathology service. J Neuropathol Exp Neurol. 2016;75(12):1145–54. https://doi.org/10.1093/jnen/nlw092.
224. Iverson GL, Luoto TM, Karhunen PJ, Castellani RJ. Mild chronic traumatic encephalopathy neuropathology in people with no known participation in contact sports or history of repetitive neurotrauma. J Neuropathol Exp Neurol. 2019;78(7):615–25. https://doi.org/10.1093/jnen/nlz045.
225. Dashnaw ML, Petraglia AL, Bailes JE. An overview of the basic science of concussion and subconcussion: where we are and where we are going. Neurosurg Focus. 2012;33(6):E5: 1–9.
226. Saulle M, Greenwald BD. Chronic traumatic encephalopathy: a review. Rehabil Res Pract. 2012;2012:816069.
227. Blaylock RL, Maroon J. Immunoexcitotoxicity as a central mechanism in chronic traumatic encephalopathy—a unifying hypothesis. Surg Neurol Int. 2011;2:107.
228. Turner RC, Lucke-Wold BP, Robson MJ, et al. Repetitive traumatic brain injury and development of chronic traumatic encephalopathy: a potential role for biomarkers in diagnosis, prognosis, and treatment? Front Neurol. 2012;3:186.
229. Small GW, Kepe V, Siddarth P, et al. PET scanning of brain tau in retired national football league players: preliminary findings. Am J Geriatr Psychiatry. 2013;21(2):138–44.

Chapter 11
Sport-Related Structural Brain Injury

Alan R. Tang, Aaron M. Yengo-Kahn, Christopher M. Bonfield, Allen K. Sills, and Scott L. Zuckerman

Introduction

Sport-related structural brain injury (SRSBI) is defined as intracranial trauma seen on neuroimaging incurred by an athlete during sport or other life activities. Though sport-related concussion (SRC) receives much of the attention when discussing the topic of head injuries in sports and are significantly more common, SRSBI has potential to cause permanent neurologic deficits and/or death and may require emergent brain or spine surgery. Distinguished from SRC by the presence of positive imaging findings of intracranial trauma, SRSBI includes subarachnoid hemorrhage (SAH), epidural hemorrhage (EDH), subdural hemorrhage (SDH), intraparenchymal hemorrhage (IPH), diffuse cerebral edema (DCE), and diffuse axonal injury (DAI) [50]. Cases of SRSBI are medical emergencies, require hospital admission, often warrant intensive care unit (ICU) monitoring, with or without surgery.

Since SRSBI represent a more severe form of SRC, a general understanding of the epidemiology of SRC is worthy of discussion. SRC comprises up to 9% of all athletic injuries in the United States (U.S.), with approximately 3.8 million emergency department (ED) visits documented between 2001 and 2018 for sports and recreation-related traumatic brain injuries (TBI) [23, 46]. Following more than a

A. R. Tang · A. M. Yengo-Kahn · C. M. Bonfield · A. K. Sills · S. L. Zuckerman (✉)
Vanderbilt Department of Neurosurgery, Vanderbilt University Medical Center, Nashville, TN, USA

M. E. Oppenlander (ed.), *Neurosurgical Care of Athletes*,
https://doi.org/10.1007/978-3-030-88227-3_11

decade of increasing rates of in-game SRC, rates have plateaued from 2014 to 2017, specifically a decrease in recurrent and practice SRC rates [27, 46]. Furthermore, in a study of 13,000 U.S. high school students, being male, white, in a higher grade, and participating in competitive sports were associated with a higher lifetime prevalence of reporting a diagnosed concussion, and participating in contact sports was associated with a higher odds of being diagnosed with more than one concussion [45]. Although much attention has been given to SRC stemming from collision sports such as American football (football), ice hockey, and lacrosse, lower contact sports, including international football (soccer), basketball, and cheerleading, have also been implicated [32, 34].

Given their low prevalence, a lack of information exists regarding pathophysiology, epidemiology, and outcomes following SRSBI [28]. Similarly, consensus regarding SRSBI management and return-to-play (RTP) is lacking, leaving neurosurgeons with little guidance to manage these complex situations. This chapter highlights the pathophysiology, epidemiology, treatment, and long-term outcomes in athletes suffering SRSBI.

Definition/Pathology

SRSBI is defined as intracranial trauma seen on neuroimaging incurred by an athlete during sport or other life activities. Athletes diagnosed with a concussion during play with subsequent neuroimaging findings positive for SDH, EDH, SAH, IPH, DAI, or DCE are considered to have suffered an SRSBI (Figs. 11.1, 11.2, and 11.3). Fractures alone without parenchymal damage are not typically considered SRSBI, as long as the brain is uninvolved [50]. The pathology of SRSBI is heterogeneous, and ranges from the well-described SDH to the relatively poorly understood and controversial Second Impact Syndrome (SIS) [1]. Common mechanisms of injury are similar to SRC, including head-to-head, head-to-opponent, and head-to-ground mechanisms [39, 49]. Though most SRSBI occur during sport, injuries that occur during other activities but involve an RTP decision are also grouped under SRSBI due to the ensuing discussion between neurosurgeon and athlete/family.

Subdural Hemorrhage

SDH is defined as intracranial bleeding between the dura and arachnoid layers of meninges. It is the most-reported form of SRSBI, as well as the most common cause of sport-related fatality [10]. The pathophysiology of subdural hemorrhage involves rupture of bridging veins traversing the subdural space, leading to intracranial hemorrhage not confined between suture lines, and potentially rapid increases in

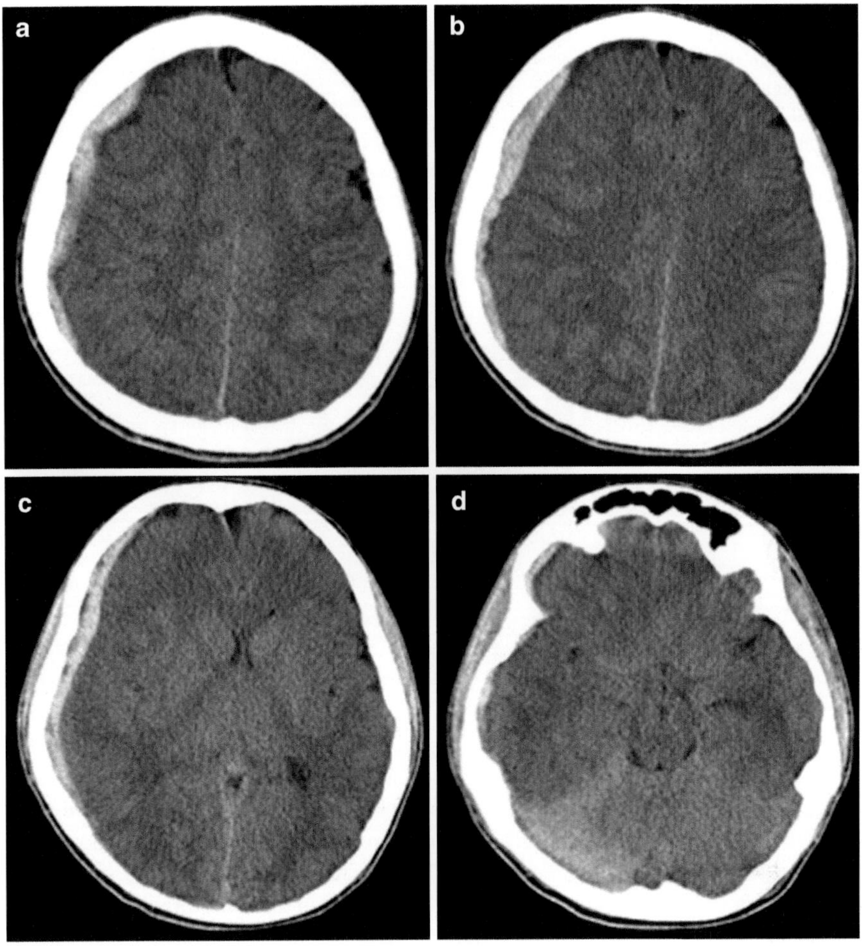

Fig. 11.1 Non-contrast CT of head for SDH SRSBI. (**a**, **b**) 9-mm acute right convexity subdural hemorrhage with associated effacement of ipsilateral sulci and midline shift; (**c**) 8-mm of midline shift related to hemorrhage with significant effacement of lateral ventricles; (**d**) extension of subdural towards floor of anterior and middle fossa with further layering along right tentorium, early right uncal herniation with effacement of crural cisterns. (With permissions from Yengo-Kahn et al. [49])

intracranial pressure leading to subsequent neurological deficit or death. SDH can be subcategorized by the period of time since bleeding as: minutes to hours being acute SDH (aSDH), or days to weeks being chronic SDH (cSDH). Radiographically, aSDH appears as an extra-axial crescent-shaped hyperdensity on non-contrast head computed tomography (CT), most common along the convexities, tentorium, or falx [44]. In contrast, cSDH typically presents as a hypodense extra-axial collection

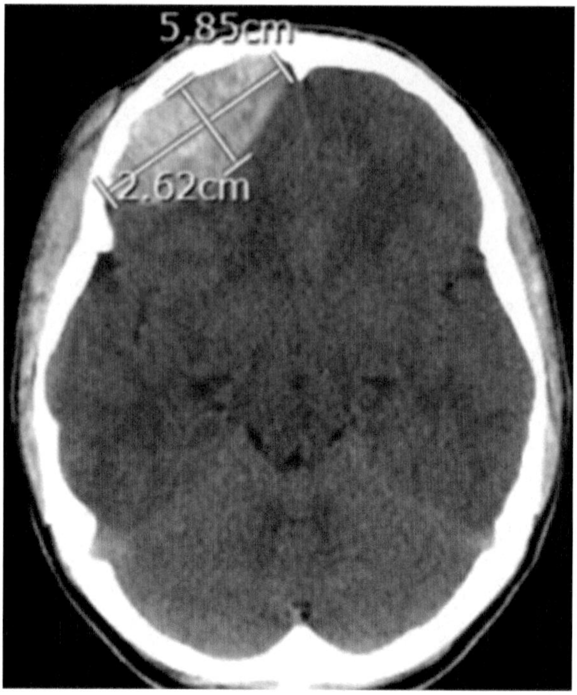

Fig. 11.2 Non-contrast CT of head for EDH SRSBI. Scan shows a 2.6-cm right, frontal epidural hematoma after heading resulting in a head-to-head collision in a soccer game. (With permissions from Mummareddy et al. [39])

along the cerebral convexity [47]. Both aSDH and cSDH presentations have been observed related to sports, ranging from collision-heavy sports such as football to low-impact sports such as race walking [10, 11]. Although the majority of SDH in SRSBI are aSDH, requiring immediate hospitalization and potential neurosurgical intervention, cSDH should not be ignored as a potential etiology as a cause of persistent and progressive symptoms in athletes following head trauma.

Of note, there is early evidence that cSDH potentially occurs more frequently in athletes with pre-existing arachnoid cysts, congenital cerebrospinal fluid collections enveloped in an arachnoid membrane [38, 51]. In athletes with existing arachnoid cyst who suffer acute or chronic SDH, evacuation of the hemorrhage is performed in conjunction with cyst fenestration [51]. Presently, there is no absolute contraindication for patients with an arachnoid cyst to participate in sports, given the unlikelihood of a hemorrhage occurring. Furthermore, no data exists to establish the true incidence and risk of SRSBI with an arachnoid cyst. Though reports of cSDH and arachnoid cysts exist, aSDH can certainly occur in the setting of arachnoid cysts, but is easily missed in the setting of an emergent craniotomy [51]. Furthermore, publication bias is likely at play, since a cSDH in a young athlete is more academically interesting than a traumatic aSDH. Overall, multi-institution studies are needed to establish prevalence of these rare injuries in the setting of arachnoid cysts.

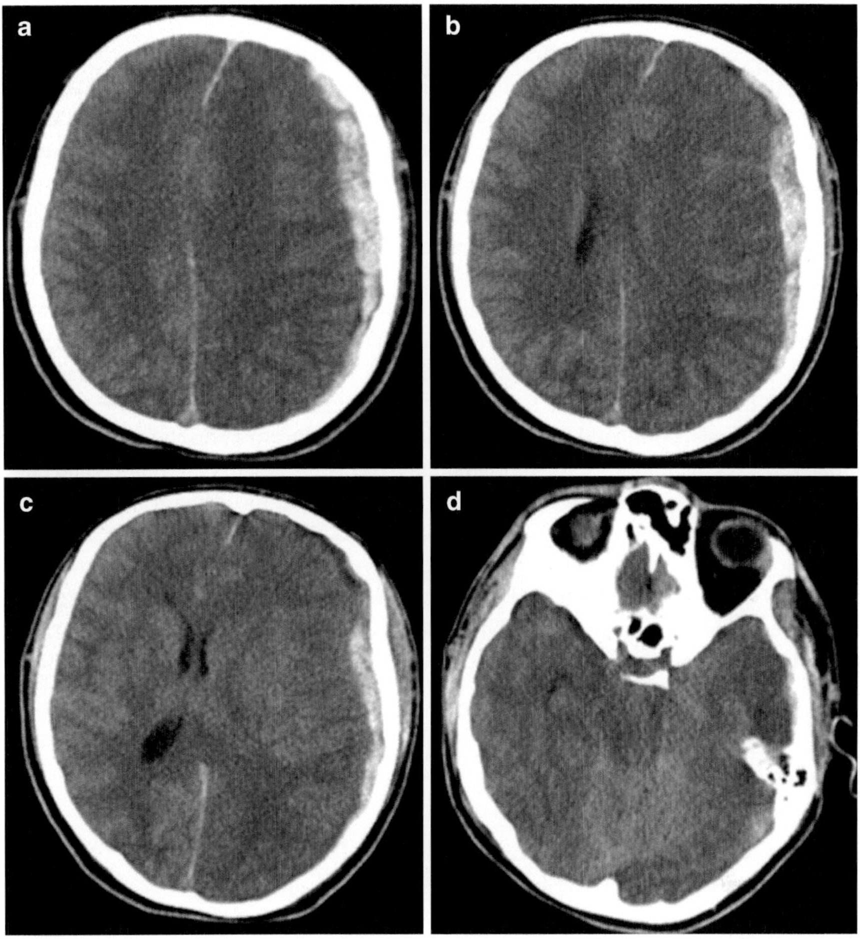

Fig. 11.3 Non-contrast CT of head for SDH SRSBI with DCE. (**a**) 12-mm acute left convexity subdural hemorrhage with effacement of bilateral sulci and clear midline shift; (**b**) acute hemorrhage again demonstrated with near total effacement of left lateral ventricle; (**c**) midline shift measured at 10-mm; (**d**) complete effacement of basal cisterns with uncal herniation. (With permissions from Yengo-Kahn et al. [49])

Subarachnoid Hemorrhage

SAH is defined as bleeding into the subarachnoid space between the arachnoid and pia layers enveloping the brain [50]. It can be further subcategorized by etiology and origin of bleeding. Traumatic SAH, as seen in SRSBI, is due to momentary brain oscillation secondary to rotational or linear acceleration of the head, and subsequent shearing of small cortical vessels [17]. CT imaging reveals isolated hyperdense foci along the cerebral sulci, and traumatic SAH can present concurrently with diffuse axonal injury, SDH, or other structural injuries [18]. Outside traumatic SAH, athletes rarely present with large-vessel damage or aneurysm rupture secondary to a traumatic event. Vertebral artery injury can be precipitated by trauma to the skull base or neck, caused by impact with a hockey puck, collision secondary to tackle in rugby, and direct blow impact from an opponent's foot in martial arts and kickboxing [12, 33, 37, 42]. These patients can present with symptoms such as headache, neck pain, or Horner's syndrome if the sympathetic plexus along the carotid artery is disrupted. Aneurysm rupture has been reported in a variety of sport settings, including soccer, hockey, and weightlifting, with several cases reporting fatalities [3, 24, 43]. In these cases, a pre-existing aneurysm and/or vascular malformation becomes disturbed by an external trauma or hemodynamic force, leading to aneurysmal SAH. Aneurysmal or AVM-related SAH are complex injuries and require primary treatment of the vascular abnormality by an open or endovascular approach. Like non-sport-related trauma, detection of an underlying aneurysm often portends a poor prognosis, compared to isolated traumatic SAH from a cortical vessel rupture alone [50]. As the literature for sport-related SAH is limited to case reports and case series, trends and outcomes must be extrapolated from the general neurosurgical literature rather than sport-specific data [26, 40, 42]. Overall, as long as no underlying lesion is found, acute management of sport-related, traumatic SAH is similar to non-sport SAH. However, the RTP discussion is more nuanced and requires resolution of any previous hemorrhage, along with an in-depth discussion of the risks/benefits of continued sport participation.

Epidural Hemorrhage

EDH is defined as bleeding between the skull and the dura mater. Most often, epidural hemorrhages occur due to high-impact trauma and are associated with skull fractures in the area of the middle meningeal arteries, although the venous sinuses may be implicated occasionally. EDH classically presents with acute loss of consciousness, followed by a lucid phase and subsequent rapid decompensation. EDH is classically identified as a biconvex, lens-shaped hyperdensity limited by cranial suture lines on head CT. It is considered a neurosurgical emergency. EDHs have been described in a variety of sport settings, including impact injuries in basketball and simultaneous head-to-head and ball-to-head contact during contested headers in soccer [14, 39]. Management is again similar to non-sport-related EDH, and often requires emergent craniotomy and evacuation.

Intraparenchymal Hemorrhage

IPH is defined as bleeding within the brain parenchyma. The spectrum of etiologies causing IPH is vast, ranging from trauma (brain contusions) to hypertension to tumors or vascular malformations. Within sport, IPHs have been documented most often when occurring concurrently with other forms of intracranial bleeding, such as traumatic SAH and SDH in soccer players, boxers, and ice hockey players, among other sports [16, 20–22]. Furthermore, traumatic IPH frequently occurs at bone-brain interfaces in the form of contusions. Small, deep-seated IPH or punctate IPH within the corpus callosum, hippocampi or the grey-white junction frequently reflects DAI rather than true contusions, and these injuries are rarely related to sports. Most important in any sport-related IPH is ruling out a primary vascular lesion through CTA and/or MRI.

Diffuse Cerebral Edema and Second-Impact Syndrome

Diffuse cerebral edema (DCE) is a commonly fatal condition that results from a failure of cerebral hemodynamic autoregulation [50]. DCE in the context of SRSBI can occur after any high-energy TBI. The proposed mechanism involves a rapid loss of cerebral autoregulation with a concurrent rise in catecholamines, effectively leading to an inability of the cerebral vasculature to accommodate the rapid rises in blood pressure [50]. However, some patients with DCE seem to fit a clinical entity known as Second Impact Syndrome (SIS). SIS occurs when an athlete who has suffered a recent SRC is returned to play prematurely, and sustains a second blow to the head or body. The second, inciting impact may be low energy and not head-related, including blows to the torso, and occurs while the athlete is still recovering from the first SRC. After the second impact, the brain loses its ability to autoregulate, DCE ensues, and the athlete loses consciousness quickly [50]. DCE can present in isolation as part of SIS, with no intracranial hemorrhages or mass effect observed, or concurrently with other structural brain injury, such as SDH, often worsening the first injury [41]. It must be noted that SIS is a controversial topic, with continued debate over its existence [1]. Some report its existence only in young, football athletes, while other researchers refute its existence at all [7, 35]. Regardless, it is critical for providers to both prophylactically caution against premature RTP and recognize the signs of an athlete presenting with DCE following an initial insult.

Epidemiology

With the little data that has been published, the overall incidence of SRSBI is low; the National Center for Catastrophic Sport Injury (NCCSI) noted that SRSBI was present in 14.7% (n = 11) of all reported sport-related catastrophic injuries [8]. Cantu and Mueller recorded 497 catastrophic brain injuries between 1945 and 1999; death was brain-related in 49% of these cases, with 16% related to cervical spine injuries, and 15% undefined [10].

Although the majority of attention in the discussion of SRSBI revolves around collision and high-impact sports, SRSBI is commonly observed in sports that are not considered high-impact. The NCCSI defines catastrophic injuries as fatalities, non-fatal (permanent severe-functional disability), and serious (no permanent functional disability but severe injury) [8]. Though the NCCSI data include more than just SRSBI, such as sudden cardiac death, the statistics are nonetheless relevant to a discussion of SRSBI. According to the NCCSI's report on high school sports, gymnastics had the highest rates of fatal (0.84) injuries per 100,000 participants, while cheerleading had the highest rate of both non-fatal (1.71 in males, 0.98 in females) and serious (1.71 in males, 1.80 in females) injuries per 100,000 participants. Of note, football remained a significant cause for fatal (0.38), non-fatal (1.14) and serious (1.12) catastrophic injuries in male high school athletes. At the collegiate level, skiing had the highest rate of direct fatal injuries per 100,000 participants in both males and females (4.62 and 5.59 per 100,000, respectively). Both gymnastics (5.37 in males, 3.72 in females) and hockey (3.56 in males) had a higher incidence of non-fatal injury than football (2.28) per 100,000 participants [9]. Again, though we cannot tease out which of these are specifically due to SRSBI, one can imagine that many are due to neurologic causes.

Collision sports such as football and rugby have also been implicated in a wide variety of SRSBI, ranging from intracranial bleeds to DCE. While football results in the most cases of SRSBI, several cases of SRSBI have also been reported in high-impact sports such as soccer and basketball. Specifically, headers in soccer have been implicated in SRSBI, typically resulting from head-to-head collision or head-to-elbow/body collisions, rather than the actual head-to-ball contact. Finally, individual combat sports such as martial arts and kickboxing have also reported cases of SRSBI [11, 12].

Diagnosis and Management

Many healthcare providers, including certified athletic trainers (ATs), primary care and emergency medicine providers, neuroradiologists, neuropsychologists, and neurosurgeons, are involved in the diagnosis and management of SRSBI. While SRC is a clinical diagnosis, involving somatic, cognitive, and behavioral symptoms, along with physical signs, sleep/wake disturbance, and balance impairment, the gold standard for SRSBI diagnosis remains head imaging. The challenge may be the decision of *when* to image. Though obvious, certain "red flag signs/symptoms" require emergent transfer to the ER and immediate imaging. These include somnolence, unequal pupils, progressive headache, unremitting nausea/vomiting, prolonged or delayed loss of consciousness, focal neurologic deficit (one-sided facial droop, weakness, numbness), significantly altered mental status, progressive alteration in behavior or mental status, and delayed seizure. Providers potentially caring for athletes with head injuries should be familiar with and be able to recognize these signs and symptoms. Specific additional education in this area may be necessary. Also, having a neurosurgeon accessible to covering certified athletic trainers (ATs) for urgent consultations can facilitate rapid triage and transport to a hospital setting with appropriate level of care. Furthermore, decision support tools such as validated prediction rules identifying clinically important TBI with imaging exist to support clinical decision-making [29].

Just as the case with SRC, once a diagnosis of SRSBI is suspected, an athlete must be immediately removed from play. Whereas an athlete with SRC can be monitored on the sideline, suspicion for an SRSBI requires immediate transfer to a hospital for head CT. If any of the "red flag signs/symptoms" are seen, calling emergency service dispatch (i.e., 9-1-1 in the USA) is most appropriate. Acute management hinges on prompt diagnosis, as the difference between fatal and positive outcomes may depend on early surgical intervention [49]. In evaluating an athlete for potential SRSBI in the emergent setting, it is critical to remain true to the tenets of acute trauma care: airway, breathing, and circulation. Positive neuroimaging of SRSBI should be further triaged as conservative management with close monitoring or immediate operative intervention, depending on the status of the patient.

Presently, there are no sport-specific guidelines or indications for surgical intervention in SRSBI, but we can rely on the general neurosurgical trauma literature regarding indications to operate. In general, indications for surgical intervention include size and volume criteria, as well as the presence of midline shift, appearance of cisterns, and other markers of mass effect [19]. Specifically, these criteria differ for the underlying etiology of TBI, with specific guidelines existing for aSDH, SAH, EDH, and IPH [4–6, 31]. Other indications for surgical intervention include rapid expansion of mass lesions within the first hours or days following admission, presenting as new or worsening neurologic deficit, and/or new or worsening radiographic findings [19]. In accordance with the Brain Trauma Foundation surgical management guidelines, an operation is indicated for all symptomatic patients with a space-occupying lesion [30]. The decision to operate involves many clinical factors, and operations may be performed immediately (e.g., for large EDH or aSDH) or only when intracranial pressures are refractory to medical and intensive care therapies (e.g., for DCE or IPH) [13].

Overall outcomes for surgical intervention are mixed. Little debate exists about evacuation of a space-occupying lesion; however, much more controversial is DCE to relieve refractory intracranial hypertension. The DECRA trial in 2011 found that, in general, trauma patients with severe diffuse traumatic brain injury and intracranial hypertension refractory to first-tier therapies, decompressive craniectomy decreased intracranial pressure, duration of mechanical ventilation, and time in the ICU when compared with standard care [13]. However, patients undergoing decompressive craniectomy were found to have significantly lower median Extended Glasgow Outcome Scale scores (i.e., worse functional outcomes) and an overall higher risk of an unfavorable outcome, despite a relatively low rate of complications [13]. The RESCUE-ICP trial in 2016 illustrated similar results; while decompressive craniectomy in patients with TBIs and refractory intracranial hypertension was associated with lower mortality rate when compared to standard therapy, higher rates of vegetative state and severe disability were seen [25]. In SRSBI, surgical intervention depends heavily on etiology of SRSBI and ranges from invasive monitoring to hemicraniectomy and is associated with a wide range of clinical outcomes [49].

Outcomes

The spectrum for SRSBI outcomes ranges from full recovery to death [39, 48, 49]. Outcomes vary depending on age and sport, with variability seen within each defined SRSBI pathology. Due to a lack of reliable incidence, prevalence, and outcomes data, meaningful evidence-based outcomes are not able to be provided. Some SRSBI patients are only mildly symptomatic upon presentation, and the most common presenting symptoms are headache and nausea in the setting of small SDH and/or SAH [50]. Temporary and potentially permanent neurologic deficits, along with death, are commonly seen in SRSBI.

Several published case studies highlight the broad spectrum of outcomes observed in SRSBI. Mummareddy et al. presented a case of a 16-year-old boy who suffered an EDH following a head-to-ball and head-to-head collision during a high school soccer game (Fig. 11.2) [39]. Although the patient denied loss of consciousness and complained only of a minor headache, he experienced blurred vision, along with worsening headache and nausea/vomiting. Radiographic imaging upon presentation revealed a 2.6-cm right frontal EDH, for which an emergent evacuation was performed. The patient's postoperative course was unremarkable, and at both 2-week and 3-month follow-up visits, he expressed no complaints or residual effects, eventually being cleared for return to full sporting activity.

Yengo-Kahn et al. highlighted the spectrum of SRSBI in a small case series of high school football players presenting with aSDH following in-game collisions [49]. Of note, two out of three patients had suffered a known previous SRC within 4 weeks of the catastrophic event. All three reported helmet-to-helmet trauma and subsequent loss of consciousness. Two of three patients required immediate surgical decompression, while the other patient was treated conservatively with an uncomplicated hospital course. The patient undergoing conservative management began home-schooling 5 months post-injury and continued to struggle with headaches and focal neurologic deficits at 6 months. Of the patients undergoing surgical intervention, one continued to have difficulty with exertional headaches, memory, and spatial navigation. Unfortunately, the final patient remained nonverbal and quadriplegic, with nutritional requirements met through a percutaneous endoscopic gastrostomy tube (Fig. 11.3). None of the patients in the case series returned to sport.

In their larger-scale case series, Boden et al. described 94 cases of SRSBI reported to the NCCSI, with the following distribution of outcomes: death (9%), permanent neurologic injury (51%), serious injury with full recovery (40%) [2]. Of note, SDH was the most common injury in the study, with 75 isolated SDH and 10 SDH with diffuse brain edema. Of note, 39% of athletes who experienced a catastrophic brain injury were playing with residual neurologic symptoms from a prior head injury. Most players received impact to the head via either tackling or being tackled.

Return to Play

While RTP in SRC patients is well-defined with the near universal use of a graduated activity paradigm, RTP decision-making is heterogeneous in the SRSBI population, with no official guidelines [36]. Often, neurosurgeons are left to make these challenging decisions, assuming significant liability. In general, RTP depends on a multitude of factors, including but not limited to age, symptomatology, initial injury etiology, treatment, and the type of sport the athlete is returning to. Prior studies have advised against RTP within the first year in athletes following craniotomy, so as to allow for complete bony fusion of the craniotomy site [15]. However, these studies are limited in scope and may not address adequately the additional nuances involving RTP with SRSBI. Returning to collision sports following craniotomy with resolution of the hemorrhage and symptoms is particularly controversial, with experts ranging in opinion from RTP at 3 months to no RTP advised. In our anecdotal experience, level of play is also a crucial factor to consider. In professional athletes with income-related factors and careers at stake, a more aggressive approach to RTP may be considered. Conversely, a younger athlete with little aspirations to play beyond high school, not returning to sport, or choosing a low-contact sport is more appropriate.

In a recent systematic review and expert opinion, several insights were offered on RTP considerations. In the acute setting and management of SRSBI in asymptomatic patients, operative indications are similar to non-athletes, including large hemorrhage size >10 mm, midline shift >5 mm, or increasing size on serial imaging. Anecdotally, factors that we discuss and consider important when deciding RTP are the following. There should be complete resolution of hemorrhage on standard imaging. All symptoms must resolve, with no neurologic deficit, as patients with persistent, severe motor deficits secondary to SRSBI should not be participating in high-level, contact sports. Furthermore, RTP is advised against in high-contact or collision sports following SRSBI with persistent hemorrhage on imaging; however, return to low-contact sport may be indicated. These patients are recommended to switch to a low-contact sport. Finally, RTP may be considered earlier for higher levels of sport, where expert medical personnel are available and on-call.

Conclusions

SRSBI is a rare and often underappreciated subcategory of sport-related head injury that requires additional attention, given the potentially devastating neurologic sequelae. Although difficult to ascertain the true incidence of SRSBI, it is important to remember that many sports are indicted in SRSBI, including both collision/high-impact and low-impact sports. Outcomes are heavily dependent on the initial presentation, as well as the availability and success of timely and appropriate treatment. Recognition and prompt diagnosis of SRSBI is critical. Finally, treatment and RTP guidelines are lacking for the SRSBI population; more investigation is warranted to understand and improve long-term outcomes in athletes suffering head trauma. Future investigations and research, as well as the establishment of treatment and RTP guidelines, serve as intriguing future directions.

References

1. Bailes JE, Patel V, Farhat H, et al. Football fatalities: the first-impact syndrome. J Neurosurg Pediatr. 2017;19(1):116–21.
2. Boden BP, Tacchetti RL, Cantu RC, et al. Catastrophic head injuries in high school and college football players. Am J Sports Med. 2007;35(7):1075–81.
3. Brunelle C, Hennecker JL, Scordidis V. Loss of consciousness after a minor trauma revealing an aneurysm rupture in a child. Arch Pediatr. 2012;19(8):815–8.
4. Bullock MR, Chesnut R, Ghajar J, et al. Surgical management of traumatic parenchymal lesions. Neurosurgery. 2006;58(3 Suppl):S25–46; discussion Si-iv.
5. Bullock MR, Chesnut R, Ghajar J, et al. Surgical management of acute epidural hematomas. Neurosurgery. 2006;58(3 Suppl):S7–15; discussion Si-iv.
6. Bullock MR, Chesnut R, Ghajar J, et al. Surgical management of acute subdural hematomas. Neurosurgery. 2006;58(3 Suppl):S16–24; discussion Si-iv.
7. Cantu RC. Second-impact syndrome. Clin Sports Med. 1998;17(1):37–44.
8. Cantu RC. Catastrophic sports injury research. Available at: https://nccsir.unc.edu/files/2019/10/2018-Catastrophic-Report-AS-36th-AY2017-2018-FINAL.pdf. 2018.
9. Cantu RC. Catastrophic sports injury research. Available at: https://nccsir.unc.edu/files/2019/10/2018-Catastrophic-Report-AS-36th-AY2017-2018-FINAL.pdf. 2019.
10. Cantu RC, Mueller FO. Brain injury-related fatalities in American football, 1945–1999. Neurosurgery. 2003;52(4):846–52; discussion 852–3.
11. Carmont MR, Mahattanakul W, Pigott T. Acquisition of a chronic subdural haematoma during training for competitive race walking? Br J Sports Med. 2002;36(4):306–7.
12. Cohen JE, Margolin E, Moscovici S, et al. Life-threatening massive subarachnoid hemorrhage after Taekwondo-associated head trauma. Isr Med Assoc J. 2010;12(8):509–10.
13. Cooper DJ, Rosenfeld JV, Murray L, et al. Decompressive craniectomy in diffuse traumatic brain injury. N Engl J Med. 2011;364(16):1493–502.
14. Datti R, Gentile SL, Pisani R. Acute intracranial epidural haematoma in a basketball player: a case report. Br J Sports Med. 1995;29(2):95–6.
15. Davis G, Marion DW, Le Roux P, et al. Clinics in neurology and neurosurgery–extradural and subdural haematoma. Br J Sports Med. 2010;44(16):1139–43.
16. Degen RM, Fink ME, Callahan L, et al. Brain contusion with aphasia following an ice hockey injury. Phys Sportsmed. 2016;44(3):324–6.
17. Demirçivi F, Ozkan N, Büyükkeçeci S, et al. Traumatic subarachnoid haemorrhage: analysis of 89 cases. Acta Neurochir. 1993;122(1–2):45–8.
18. Depreitere B, Van Lierde C, Maene S, et al. Bicycle-related head injury: a study of 86 cases. Accid Anal Prev. 2004;36(4):561–7.
19. Drake M, Bernard A, Hessel E. Brain death. Surg Clin North Am. 2017;97(6):1255–73.
20. Ellis MJ, Barnes J, Cordingley DM, et al. Management of an adolescent athlete with sports-related concussion and Intraparenchymal hemorrhage. Curr Sports Med Rep. 2018;17(1):7–9.

21. Ellis MJ, Leiter J, Hall T, et al. Neuroimaging findings in pediatric sports-related concussion. J Neurosurg Pediatr. 2015;16(3):241–7.
22. Ellis MJ, McDonald PJ, Cordingley D, et al. Retirement-from-sport considerations following pediatric sports-related concussion: case illustrations and institutional approach. Neurosurg Focus. 2016;40(4):E8.
23. Gessel LM, Fields SK, Collins CL, et al. Concussions among United States high school and collegiate athletes. J Athl Train. 2007;42(4):495–503.
24. Haykowsky MJ, Findlay JM, Ignaszewski AP. Aneurysmal subarachnoid hemorrhage associated with weight training: three case reports. Clin J Sport Med. 1996;6(1):52–5.
25. Hutchinson PJ, Kolias AG, Timofeev IS, et al. Trial of decompressive Craniectomy for traumatic intracranial hypertension. N Engl J Med. 2016;375(12):1119–30.
26. Kariyanna PT, Charles A, Ahmed MF, et al. Rare case of bilateral cerebellar hemorrhage in a male boxer. Am J Med Case Rep. 2019;7(10):236–9.
27. Kerr ZY, Chandran A, Nedimyer AK, et al. Concussion incidence and trends in 20 high school sports. Pediatrics. 2019;144(5)
28. Kucera KL, Yau RK, Register-Mihalik J, et al. Traumatic brain and spinal cord fatalities among high school and college football players – United States, 2005–2014. MMWR Morb Mortal Wkly Rep. 2017;65(52):1465–9.
29. Kuppermann N, Holmes JF, Dayan PS, et al. Identification of children at very low risk of clinically-important brain injuries after head trauma: a prospective cohort study. Lancet. 2009;374(9696):1160–70.
30. Lee JC, Rittenhouse K, Bupp K, et al. An analysis of Brain Trauma Foundation traumatic brain injury guideline compliance and patient outcome. Injury. 2015;46(5):854–8.
31. Long B, Koyfman A, Runyon MS. Subarachnoid hemorrhage: updates in diagnosis and management. Emerg Med Clin North Am. 2017;35(4):803–24.
32. Lovell MR, Solomon GS. Neurocognitive test performance and symptom reporting in cheerleaders with concussions. J Pediatr. 2013;163(4):1192–5.e1.
33. Malek AM, Halbach VV, Phatouros CC, et al. Endovascular treatment of a ruptured intracranial dissecting vertebral aneurysm in a kickboxer. J Trauma. 2000;48(1):143–5.
34. Marar M, McIlvain NM, Fields SK, et al. Epidemiology of concussions among United States high school athletes in 20 sports. Am J Sports Med. 2012;40(4):747–55.
35. McCrory P. Does second impact syndrome exist? Clin J Sport Med. 2001;11(3):144–9.
36. McCrory P, Meeuwisse W, Dvořák J, et al. Consensus statement on concussion in sport-the 5(th) international conference on concussion in sport held in Berlin, October 2016. Br J Sports Med. 2017;51(11):838–47.
37. McCrory PR, Berkovic SF, Cordner SM. Deaths due to brain injury among footballers in Victoria, 1968–1999. Med J Aust. 2000;172(5):217–9.
38. Miele VJ, Bailes JE, Martin NA. Participation in contact or collision sports in athletes with epilepsy, genetic risk factors, structural brain lesions, or history of craniotomy. Neurosurg Focus. 2006;21(4):E9.
39. Mummareddy N, Legarreta AD, Yengo-Kahn AM, et al. Sport-related structural brain injury in high school soccer: epidural hemorrhage after a "header". World Neurosurg. 2019;127:20–3.
40. Plog BA, Pierre CA, Srinivasan V, et al. Neurologic injury in snowmobiling. Surg Neurol Int. 2014;5:87.
41. Quintana LM. Second impact syndrome in sports. World Neurosurg. 2016;91:647–9.
42. Rughani AI, Lin CT, Ares WJ, et al. Helmet use and reduction in skull fractures in skiers and snowboarders admitted to the hospital. J Neurosurg Pediatr. 2011;7(3):268–71.
43. Sahjpaul RL, Abdulhak MM, Drake CG, et al. Fatal traumatic vertebral artery aneurysm rupture. Case report. J Neurosurg. 1998;89(5):822–4.
44. Vega RA, Valadka AB. Natural history of acute subdural hematoma. Neurosurg Clin N Am. 2017;28(2):247–55.
45. Veliz P, McCabe SE, Eckner JT, et al. Prevalence of concussion among US adolescents and correlated factors. JAMA. 2017;318(12):1180–2.

46. Waltzman D, Womack LS, Thomas KE, et al. Trends in emergency department visits for contact sports-related traumatic brain injuries among children – United States, 2001–2018. MMWR Morb Mortal Wkly Rep. 2020;69(27):870–4.
47. Yadav YR, Parihar V, Namdev H, et al. Chronic subdural hematoma. Asian J Neurosurg. 2016;11(4):330–42.
48. Yengo-Kahn A, Zuckerman SL. Letter: preventable deaths, video analysis, artificial intelligence, and the future of sport. Neurosurgery. 2020;86(3):E349–e350.
49. Yengo-Kahn AM, Gardner RM, Kuhn AW, et al. Sport-related structural brain injury: 3 cases of subdural hemorrhage in American High School Football. World Neurosurg. 2017;106:1055.e5–1055.e11.
50. Zuckerman SL, Kuhn A, Dewan MC, et al. Structural brain injury in sports-related concussion. Neurosurg Focus. 2012;33(6):E6: 1–12.
51. Zuckerman SL, Prather CT, Yengo-Kahn AM, et al. Sport-related structural brain injury associated with arachnoid cysts: a systematic review and quantitative analysis. Neurosurg Focus. 2016;40(4):E9.

Chapter 12
Neuroimaging and Blood Biomarkers of Sport Concussion

Ayobami L. Ward and Jacob R. Joseph

Introduction

Today, sports-related traumatic brain injury is more studied than ever before. Between 1.7 and 3 million concussions happen every year, of which around 300,000 are related to sports [25]. By nature of the injury, about 50% of concussions go unreported at time of presentation. Furthermore, without loss of consciousness, many athletes themselves are asked to self-report symptoms post-trauma, which may or may not happen [17]. Repeat concussions can have severe repercussions on the developing and developed brain, and scientific investigation has hoped to determine the best way of identifying traumatic brain injury when it takes place, both with imaging correlates and with blood biomarkers of injury that may distinguish injury in the hyperacute period. Concussion diagnostics are currently hampered by the lack of objective data. Research in sport-related concussion (SRC) is now moving towards more objectivity in both diagnosis and prognosis. In this chapter, we will discuss the current state of neuroimaging, fluid biomarkers, and their implications on where the field of sports-related concussion is moving.

A. L. Ward · J. R. Joseph (✉)
Department of Neurosurgery, University of Michigan, Ann Arbor, MI, USA
e-mail: ayward@med.umich.edu; jojacob@med.umich.edu

M. E. Oppenlander (ed.), *Neurosurgical Care of Athletes*,
https://doi.org/10.1007/978-3-030-88227-3_12

Neuroimaging in Sports-Related Concussion

Computed Tomography Imaging

For traumatic brain injury, the computed tomography (CT) scan is the first line imaging given its speed, cost, and ease of access. However, in relation to sports-related neurotrauma, the evidence clearly takes a divergent path. As SRC generally falls under the category of *mild uncomplicated TBI*, there are by definition no pathologic correlates seen on CT scan in concussion. It has been the consensus of multiple professional medical organizations that CT scan after acute sports-related concussion is not medically indicated. The American Academy of Neurology, for example, does not recommend the use of CT scan to *diagnose* a suspected sports-related concussion. However, mild *complicated* TBI is also possible with sports injury. These injuries, typically accompanied by "red-flag" symptoms, may require Emergency Department evaluation along with CT imaging. These symptoms may include loss of consciousness, post-traumatic amnesia, persistent Glasgow Coma Scale <15, focal neurologic deficit, evidence of skull fracture on examination, or signs of clinical deterioration [6]. It is important to note that while concussion and mild TBI are not indications for CT scans, neuroimaging in the aforementioned clinical context is to rule out moderate to severe traumatic brain injury, which may present with intracranial hemorrhage, cerebral contusions, or skull fractures depending on the mechanism and force of trauma applied to the skull. In consensus, the American Medical Society for Sports Medicine also states that CT scans should not be obtained unless the athlete in question demonstrates "worsening symptoms, pronounced amnesia, progressive balance dysfunction, or focal neurological deficits on examination," which may indicate signs of intracranial pathology, or "macrostructural" damage [8]. Similarly, the Centers for Disease Control present a variant of these guidelines, which are tailored to traumatic brain injury in the general population and take a more judicious approach to recommendations for CT scanning post TBI. These recommendations were adapted in part from early large multicenter cohort studies which attempted to determine clinical factors associated with the roughly 5–10% of patients with mild TBI who have positive imaging findings on CT [2, 16]. Furthermore, in relation to the pediatric population in which sports-related concussion is prevalent, there is evidence that CT scans in populations below 18 years of age was associated with an increased incidence of malignant and benign brain tumors [18, 19]. This further increases the need to limit arbitrary CT scans for straightforward presentations of SRC.

Magnetic Resonance Imaging

Athletes with concussion do not show structural lesions on CT and basic magnetic resonance (MR) imaging in the acute setting. However, Post-Concussive Syndrome is a well-studied and characterized phenomenon by which athletes may begin to demonstrate a wide array of clinical symptoms such as psychological distress, cognitive impairment, and neurologic symptoms. Furthermore, recurrent concussion is posited to lead to a stepwise decline in neuropsychological functioning in affected athletes. The current guidelines from the American Association of Neurology recommend return to play when "signs and symptoms of concussion have resolved, are off of all medications (i.e., related to headache) and have been cleared by a qualified healthcare professional trained in the management of concussion, such as a neurologist" [6]. Unfortunately, it can be difficult to objectively determine when or if the symptoms have completely resolved. Due to the pathophysiology of concussion taking place in the functional level rather than the macro-structural level of the parenchyma, structural neuroimaging such as CT and MR logically tend to be *normal* in many athletes [4].

Advanced MRI Techniques

There is a vested interest on the part of clinicians and regulators to determine exactly who among concussed athletes will develop more severe symptoms. Recent studies have shown that patients with multiple concussions have an increased rate of extremity injury, advanced neurologic pathology, and neuropsychologic disorders such as depression, which may not present until later in life [14, 28]. The pathophysiology of concussion involves, among other things, changes in ion physiology within the brain, as well as pathologic microstructural changes. This mechanism makes certain MR sequencing uniquely suited to evaluating traumatic brain injury. Newer, advanced multimodal MRI technologies (Diffusion Tensor Imaging, Functional MRI, Susceptibility Weighted Imaging, and Magnetic Resonance Spectroscopy) are currently being studied for their value in discovering microscopic changes in the CNS environment secondary to concussion in athletes and the general population.

The main player in advanced MR imaging for SRC is *diffusion tensor imaging*. This is a modality of magnetic resonance that focuses on two variables. The first is *fractional anisotropy (FA)*, which is essentially the directionality of water movement within axon fiber tracts. The second variable is *mean diffusivity (MD)*, which informs about the total water content of the fiber tracts, irrespective of direction of flow [21]. This allows researchers to not only view fiber tracts but, in the case of sports-related concussion, evaluate the integrity of the fiber tracts on a molecular scale. The basis of this investigation is simple—normal functional white matter tracts have high FA, that is—directional flow down the axon to its target. This creates a portion of the characteristic DTI image of millions of thin string like tracts moving together. Normal functioning white matter will also have a low MD value, which indicates the diffusion of water *outside* of the axon tracts. Typically, MD is higher in damaged tissues as a result of increased free diffusion across damaged myelin, which subsequently inhibits ion gradient stabilization leading to ion outflow and water movement. In contrast, FA decreases due to the loss of coherence in the main preferred diffusion direction, such that water is no longer flowing down the axon to the terminal, but haphazardly causing the weighted average movement in one direction to decrease. Damage to white matter tracts leads to alterations in this simple ratio. Studies into the areas of focal axonal disintegration have yielded evidence of decreases in FA and increases in MD in SRC patients acutely. These changes have been documented in the corpus callosum, corona radiata, temporal lobe, inferior longitudinal fasciculus, and internal capsule [1, 4, 27]. As a more practical example, decreased FA was seen in athletes who had a high frequency of heading (>855–1800 headings per year) in soccer. Strikingly, this finding was correlated with a lower cognitive function as tested by the CogState brief battery for mild TBI, suggesting that repeated "normal" head trauma had an effect on the integrity of axon tracts similar to that of concussion.

Fortunately, as DTI techniques have evolved and become more consistent, there has been a concerted effort to correlate the presence of DTI changes with changes in post concussive evaluation scales such as the Sports Concussion Assessment Tool. In one study in particular, investigators were able to show that SRC athletes' SCAT2 scores were able to predict the presence of DTI changes in the brain within 2 months of concussion [1]. Other studies have corroborated these findings, and correlated specific chronic SRC symptoms such as language, coordination, and visual deficits with anisotropic changes in the specific white matter tracts associated with those functions. Unfortunately, there is no consensus yet on the permanence of the microstructural changes seen in DTI imaging. There are data to suggest that microstructural changes may reverse between 2 days and 2 weeks post SRC, while others suggest a persistence of these changes as far out as 6 months to 3 years [9, 13, 15]. There is also evidence that recovery may be sex specific. One study demonstrated that the white matter changes seen on DTI were persistent for a longer period of time in female athletes who were part of a mixed gender study on SRC DTI changes [1].

In the last decade, functional MRI (fMRI) has emerged as a powerful tool for investigating changes in brain function with respect to SRC (Fig. 12.1). The underlying concept in fMRI is that resting neurons and active neurons differ in the amount of oxygen utilization, concomitant with their level of activity. As neurons increase activity, the level of deoxyhemoglobin present in the surrounding tissue should increase relative to non-active tissues. This activity results in an increase in paramagnetic deoxyhemoglobin, which can be quantified. This is known as blood oxygen level dependent imaging, or BOLD which is the lynchpin of fMRI sequencing [20]. The relative levels can then be compared between brain areas where functionally similar areas are said to have undergone "functional connectivity." Resting state (rs) fMRI studies over the last decade have demonstrated that athletes diagnosed with sports-related concussion show significantly altered functional connectivity within the first week post-injury [3, 30]. This is particularly significant, as this is the time during which most athletes are still symptomatic.

Further studies have demonstrated that this period of resting state functional impact persists well into the sub-acute phase to 1 month post-injury. This is particularly significant because this is generally when athletes are asymptomatic, demonstrating that functionally, neurons are still undergoing the process of repair [10, 29, 30].

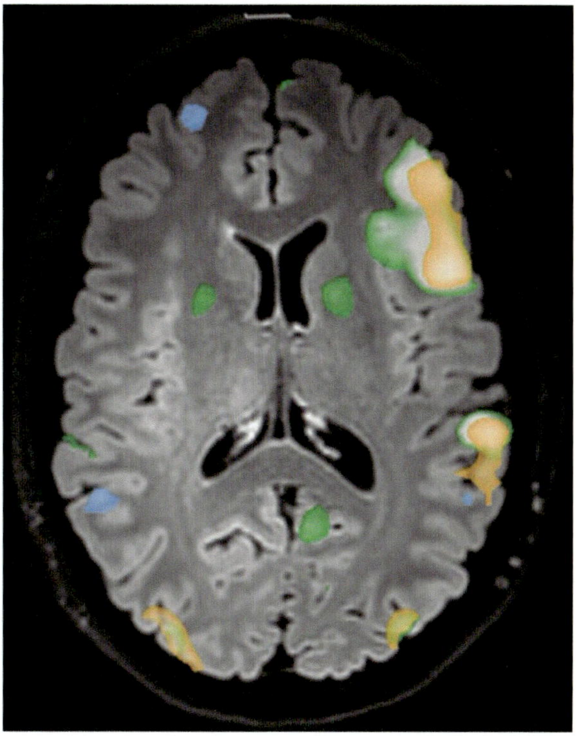

Fig. 12.1 Functional MRI study demonstrating left-sided language function

More recently, we have seen evidence of the underlying basis of many of the symptoms which typify concussion such as personality change [23], reaction time, as well as changes in the perception of pain. These have led to a particularly interesting finding. In 2014, Talavage et al. demonstrated in the study of SRC in population of high school athletes, fMRI had the ability to predict cognitive impairment in athletes that otherwise had no discernable symptoms of concussion. This deficit was linked to the dorsolateral prefrontal cortex [24], and markedly elevated in players who saw regular helmet-to-helmet contact such as lineman and defensive backs.

Other MR sequences have been investigated for potential use in SRC. Magnetic resonance spectroscopy (MRS), which has been used to evaluate intracranial tumors, has demonstrated changes in neuronal metabolism which may last weeks after initial injury, especially in the hippocampus and primary motor cortices [9, 26]. Studies have shown that there is a decrease in N-acetylasparate (NAA) in white matter after SRC. However, as neurometabolic changes can be dependent on many factors which are not always controlled, the value of these findings is not yet understood. High-resolution T1-weighted MR imaging is capable of providing highly detailed anatomical images of the brain and some studies have indicated that some athletes who have been cleared to play demonstrate evidence of parenchymal atrophy [7]. However, since the advent of DTI, the use of standard T1 imaging has not been as thoroughly investigated, as it does not reveal information about the likely microstructural changes taking place.

Blood Biomarkers for Sports-Related Concussion

Macro-structural imaging correlates, as described previously in this chapter, may not indicate the extent of the injury within the first few hours of trauma, which may lead to delayed care. Microstructural imaging such as DTI, fMRI, and MRS have not yet been approved for regular use in acute sports-related concussion. It is for this reason that the current research into blood biomarkers associated with trauma is expanding. One of the primary responses to acute traumatic brain injury is an acute inflammatory response mediated by cytokine release. In response to this injury, there is local breakdown of the blood brain barrier, which allows the normally isolated CNS milieu to interact with the serum. Thus, markers of damage may become present in the serum or plasma. The benefit of this pathophysiology is that diagnosis, risk stratification, and treatment of TBI could potentially be detected in a relatively simple fashion, as opposed to biomarkers in cerebrospinal fluid, or imaging techniques, which may be expensive and time consuming. However, given the individual variability in presentations, low quantity of TBI biomarkers in blood, variability in clearance rates of biomarkers, and several other reasons, there has not been a clinical role for blood biomarkers in clinical practice so far. Improvements in the reliability of biomarker assays have been instrumental in the recent advances in the field. There are several blood biomarkers currently under investigation in relation to SRC, which can grossly be categorized into biomarkers of neuronal, axonal, or astroglial injury (Fig. 12.2).

Neuronal Injury

Biomarkers for neuronal injury include ubiquitin C-terminal hydrolase-L1 (UCH-L1) and brain derived neurotrophic factor (BDNF), amongst others. UCH-L1, a protein found in neuronal cytoplasm, has been well studied in TBI. However, it is also present in peripheral nerves and other non-CNS organs. In severe TBI, increases in UCH-L1 have been shown consistently. In mild TBI, UCH-L1 has been shown to have the ability to predict the likelihood of a positive CT scan with a traumatic intracranial lesion. However, its utility in CT-negative mild TBI is less certain. Other neuronal markers such as BDNF and neuron-specific enolase (NSE) have demonstrated little success in the diagnosis or management of SRC.

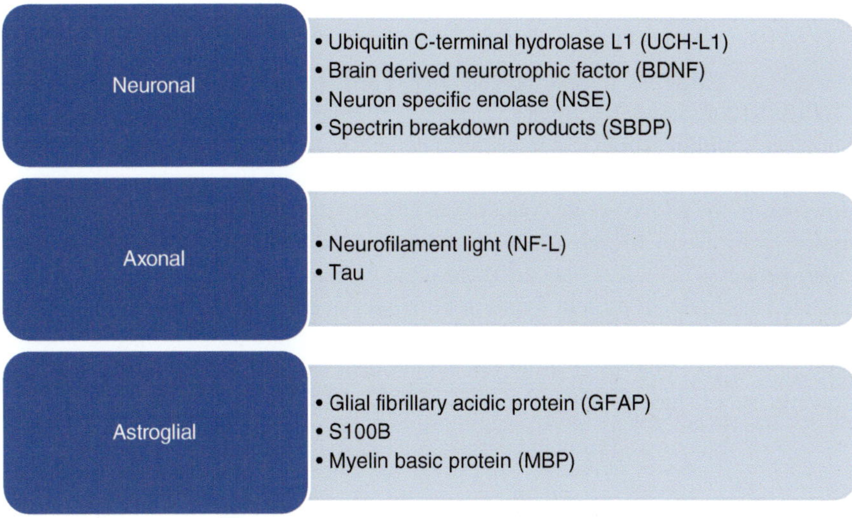

Fig. 12.2 Categories of blood biomarkers for sports related concussion

Axonal Injury

The most promising biomarkers for axonal injury include tau protein and neurofilament-light (NF-L). Tau is a microtubule-associated protein which is responsible for microtubule stabilization in the milieu of the cell. This protein is especially important within axons, in which it is utilized to transport neurotransmitter vesicles down the axon to the terminal. Aggregation of tau protein in the general population has been implicated as the inciting factor in the initiation of the neuropathology of Alzheimer's disease [11, 22]. Tau has been most notably implicated in the presence of chronic traumatic encephalopathy, the step-wise degeneration of cognitive function seen in repeated cranial trauma in boxing and other contact sports with high velocity head trauma [5]. Tau has also been investigated as a possible biomarker for TBI. Investigation of Olympic athletes after rounds of boxing in 2012 demonstrated that there were elevations in the levels of tau in these patients, although there were no symptoms of concussion. Serum tau has also been shown to rise in concussed hockey players, and was shown to predict time to return-to-play. Neurofilament-light is a significant component of the axonal skeleton. A study of collegiate football players found that concentrations of NF-L increased over the course of a season. Furthermore, elevations in serum NF-L were found starting at 1 hour post-injury, and its elevations were correlated to time to return-to-play. Further studies have shown that NF-L is able to accurately distinguish acute SRC from controls. Other less well-studied axonal proteins include breakdown products of alpha-2 spectrin.

Astroglial Injury

Markers of astroglial injury include glial fibrillary acidic protein (GFAP) and S100-B. S100ß protein's primary function is to bind and regulate intracellular calcium levels within astrocytes. It has been demonstrated by several groups that there are physiologic increases in the serum level of S100ß with simple physical exertion. However, in the case of acute concussion, elevations in its levels have been demonstrated to forewarn the presence of intracranial hemorrhage within closed head injury patients [12]. GFAP is one of the most well-studied proteins in TBI. It is an intermediate filament protein found in astrocytes and has been shown to be able to detect mild TBI, and may be more specific than other biomarkers. In SRC specifically, GFAP is able to distinguish symptomatic athletes with high accuracy. However, other studies have not replicated these results.

Future of Blood and Imaging Biomarkers in SRC

SRC is a difficult clinical diagnosis due to patient heterogeneity in presentation, reliance on self-reporting, lack of patient education, and variability in providers, amongst other reasons. A move toward more objective data is necessary in order to achieve large-scale improvements in clinical outcomes of SRC. Both blood and imaging biomarkers continue to be an area of intense interest in SRC due to their objectivity. However, research in biomarkers has continued to be hamstrung by a reliance on clinical diagnosis of SRC as a benchmark. Numerous studies have demonstrated that asymptomatic athletes without clinical diagnosis of SRC show biomarker evidence of brain injury [24]. The cause of this is unclear. In addition, many of the studies cited here demonstrate statistically significant changes in biomarkers, but the within-subject variability is extreme. This greatly limits the current practicality of biomarker tests for clinical use today. Nevertheless, it is anticipated that improvements in imaging techniques and fluid assays may help circumvent these issues in the future.

Conclusion

Advanced neuroimaging techniques and blood biomarkers hold great promise for the future of SRC diagnosis and management. It is anticipated that they will eventually become a part of standard clinical practice. Further research is needed prior to the realization of this goal.

Bibliography

1. Bazarian JJ, et al. Subject-specific changes in brain white matter on diffusion tensor imaging after sports-related concussion. Magn Reson Imaging. 2012;30(2):171–80.
2. Borg J, et al. Diagnostic procedures in mild traumatic brain injury: results of the WHO Collaborating Centre Task Force on Mild Traumatic Brain Injury. J Rehabil Med. 2004;36.0:61–75.
3. Churchill NW, et al. Neuroimaging of sport concussion: persistent alterations in brain structure and function at medical clearance. Sci Rep. 2017;7(1):1–9.
4. Gardner A, et al. A systematic review of diffusion tensor imaging findings in sports-related concussion. J Neurotrauma. 2012;29(16):2521–38.
5. Giza CC, Hovda DA. The new neurometabolic cascade of concussion. Neurosurgery. 2014;75. suppl_4:S24–33.
6. Giza CC, et al. Summary of evidence-based guideline update: evaluation and management of concussion in sports: report of the Guideline Development Subcommittee of the American Academy of Neurology. Neurology. 2013;80(24):2250–7.
7. Guenette JP, Shenton ME, Koerte IK. Imaging of concussion in young athletes. Neuroimag Clin. 2018;28(1):43–53.
8. Harmon KG, et al. American Medical Society for Sports Medicine position statement on concussion in sport. Br J Sports Med. 2019;53(4):213–25.
9. Henry LC, et al. Acute and chronic changes in diffusivity measures after sports concussion. J Neurotrauma. 2011;28(10):2049–59.
10. Johnson B, et al. Alteration of brain default network in subacute phase of injury in concussed individuals: resting-state fMRI study. NeuroImage. 2012;59(1):511–8.
11. Jucker M, Walker LC. Self-propagation of pathogenic protein aggregates in neurodegenerative diseases. Nature. 2013;501(7465):45–51.
12. Kiechle K, et al. Subject-specific increases in serum S-100B distinguish sports-related concussion from sports-related exertion. PLoS One. 2014;9(1):e84977.
13. Lipton ML, et al. Multifocal white matter ultrastructural abnormalities in mild traumatic brain injury with cognitive disability: a voxel-wise analysis of diffusion tensor imaging. J Neurotrauma. 2008;25(11):1335–42.
14. Manley G, et al. A systematic review of potential long-term effects of sport-related concussion. Br J Sports Med. 2017;51(12):969–77.
15. Mayer AR, Hanlon FM, Ling JM. Gray matter abnormalities in pediatric mild traumatic brain injury. J Neurotrauma. 2015;32(10):723–30.
16. McAllister TW, et al. Neuroimaging findings in mild traumatic brain injury. J Clin Exp Neuropsychol. 2001;23(6):775–91.
17. McCrea M, et al. Unreported concussion in high school football players: implications for prevention. Clin J Sport Med. 2004;14(1):13–7.
18. Meulepas JM, et al. Radiation exposure from pediatric CT scans and subsequent cancer risk in the Netherlands. JNCI J Natl Cancer Inst. 2019;111(3):256–63.
19. Miglioretti DL, et al. The use of computed tomography in pediatrics and the associated radiation exposure and estimated cancer risk. JAMA Pediatr. 2013;167(8):700–7.
20. Ogawa S, et al. Brain magnetic resonance imaging with contrast dependent on blood oxygenation. Proc Natl Acad Sci. 1990;87(24):9868–72.
21. Osborn AG, Hedlund GL, Salzman KL. Osborn's brain E-book. Elsevier Health Sciences; 2017.
22. Prusiner SB. A unifying role for prions in neurodegenerative diseases. Science. 2012;336(6088):1511–3.
23. Sours C, et al. Hyper-connectivity of the thalamus during early stages following mild traumatic brain injury. Brain Imaging Behav. 2015;9(3):550–63.
24. Talavage TM, et al. Functionally-detected cognitive impairment in high school football players without clinically-diagnosed concussion. J Neurotrauma. 2014;31(4):327–38.

25. Thunnan DJ, Branche CM, Sniezek JE. The epidemiology of sports-related traumatic brain injuries in the United States: recent developments. J Head Trauma Rehabil. 1998;13(2):1–8.
26. Vagnozzi R, et al. Assessment of metabolic brain damage and recovery following mild traumatic brain injury: a multicentre, proton magnetic resonance spectroscopic study in concussed patients. Brain. 2010;133(11):3232–42.
27. Virji-Babul N, et al. Diffusion tensor imaging of sports-related concussion in adolescents. Pediatr Neurol. 2013;48(1):24–9.
28. Waltzman D, et al. Concussion reporting, return to learn, and return to play experiences in a sample of private preparatory high school students. Brain Inj. 2020;34(9):1193–201.
29. Zhang K, et al. Are functional deficits in concussed individuals consistent with white matter structural alterations: combined FMRI & DTI study. Exp Brain Res. 2010;204(1):57–70.
30. Zhu DC, et al. A potential biomarker in sports-related concussion: brain functional connectivity alteration of the default-mode network measured with longitudinal resting-state fMRI over thirty days. J Neurotrauma. 2015;32(5):327–41.

Chapter 13
Active Rehabilitation and Return to Play After Concussion

Matthew T. Lorincz, Katharine Seagly, Andrea Almeida, and Bara Alsalaheen

Introduction

An estimated 1.6–3.8 million sports-related concussions (SRCs) occur each year in the United States. This number is difficult to estimate, as many individuals who meet criteria for concussion fail to seek medical care [1], but also because there is no way to know if all reported concussions are true concussions, given the diagnosis is based on self-report of non-specific symptoms which may or may not be related to brain injury [2, 3]. Concussion continues to be conceptualized broadly as functional impairment due to brain neurometabolic and neuropathological changes that occur after biomechanical trauma [4]. These functional changes can result in signs and symptoms that include somatic complaints, vestibular abnormalities, balance disturbance, cognitive change, psychosocial disruptions, sleep irregularities, and/or autonomic dysfunction [5]. The diagnosis remains a clinical one, and there is no one test, biomarker, or imaging study that can confirm a concussion [5]. Historically, concussion was characterized as a homogenous injury for which rest was considered the mainstay of treatment. We now have a better understanding of the complex, diverse nature of concussion, where the best treatment option is an individualized

M. T. Lorincz (✉)
University of Michigan, Michigan NeuroSport, Ann Arbor, MI, USA
e-mail: Lorincz@umich.edu

K. Seagly
University of Michigan, Traumatic Brain Injury Rehabilitation Program, Ann Arbor, MI, USA
e-mail: kseagly@umich.edu

A. Almeida · B. Alsalaheen
University of Michigan-Flint, Flint, MI, USA
e-mail: Almeidaa@umich.edu; Alsalahe@umich.edu

M. E. Oppenlander (ed.), *Neurosurgical Care of Athletes*,
https://doi.org/10.1007/978-3-030-88227-3_13

approach that entails active rehabilitation and a biopsychosocial approach [3, 6]. Due to the heterogeneous nature of the injuries and the people who sustain them, multidisciplinary teams consisting of physicians, neuropsychologists, physical therapists, athletic trainers, and psychotherapy providers are vital to the successful and active management of concussion.

Concussion incidence peaks between 9 and 22 years, when group athletics are most popular [7]. The age-adjusted rate of SRC increased 108% from 73.1 per 100,000 in 2001 to 152.0 per 100,000 in 2012. Increases occurred in all age groups and across sexes. Males had over twice the age-adjusted SRC rate compared to females, 205.1 to 97.1 per 100,000 [1]. While SRC is being diagnosed at higher rates, and public and provider concern appears to be at an all-time high, data suggest that the large majority of concussions result in a time-limited disruption of functional abilities [8, 9]. Normal recovery in adults is reported to be within 14 days and within 30 days in children [10]. Unfortunately, 10–30% of those who sustain a concussion have a prolonged recovery experience [5]. The etiology of prolonged recovery remains a point of disagreement among many researchers, wherein some believe it may be due to ongoing concussion-specific pathophysiology [11], while others cite research showing quick return to baseline for proposed concussion biomarkers [12], or simply question the validity of many biomarkers given the potential for confounds. While it is unlikely that brain injury is the primary driver of symptoms in concussed athletes beyond the first several weeks, for recovery to occur, these symptoms do need to be addressed, with acknowledgement of the complex biopsychosocial factors that contribute to symptom experience in those with more prolonged recovery. For a large portion of concussed athletes a contributing factor in prolonged symptom experience is lack of early education on concussion recovery and inadequate treatment of initial concussion symptoms and other downstream factors [6]. Appropriate education on a biopsychosocial recovery model and a brief course of active rehabilitation early on post-injury can prevent prolonged symptom experience.

The biopsychosocial model of concussion includes injury-related, or biological factors such as neuro-metabolic changes and medication effects, but also focuses on the person who sustained the injury, including their pre-morbid dispositions and their post-injury adjustment (Fig. 13.1) [7, 13]. The biopsychosocial model of concussion lends itself well to an active multidisciplinary approach for SRC care. It allows for a holistic conceptualization of all factors that may be driving symptom report, thus increasing the likelihood that non-injury factors maintaining symptoms will be addressed in addition to the brain injury itself. With a multidisciplinary team, each team member can not only address biological, psychological, and social factors that fall under their area of expertise, but importantly, the team as a whole can send a unified message that includes accurate education on concussion recovery, setting the expectation for return to prior meaningful activities, including return to sport in most cases, and increasing exposure to activities in a graded fashion that allows for successful recovery.

The most current guidelines suggest that after a short period of rest, the first 24–48 hours, a gradual symptom-limited return to school, work, and sport should be

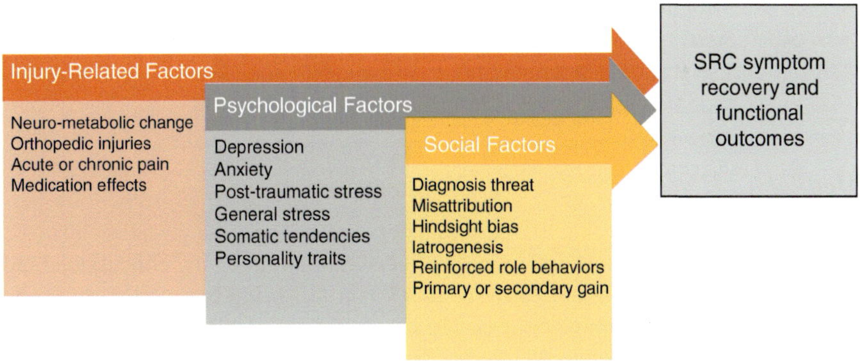

Fig. 13.1 The Biopsychosocial model as applied to Sports Related Concussion (SRC)

undertaken [5]. Since these recommendations, a growing body of evidence suggests that not only should the approach be gradual but that in the normal concussion recovery period, actively engaging in sub-symptom threshold exercise, as described in the Concussion Exercise Tolerance Testing section below, facilitates recovery [14, 15]. A major goal of an active rehabilitation strategy is safe return to sport. The current guidelines suggest a stepwise exercise progression whose aim is to safely test for symptom provocation in a graded progression of increasing risk. Although evidence supports that exercise facilitates recovery, a knowledge gap exists as to the optimal timing of initiation, type, duration, frequency, and intensity of exercise through recovery of concussion [5]. Studies have also demonstrated that active rehabilitation strategies, including time-limited psychotherapy focused on concussion education, increasing coping mechanisms and behavioral activation, as well as brief courses of cervical and vestibular therapy can lead to improvement of symptom experience and accelerated return to play [6, 16, 17].

Foundations of Active Rehabilitation of Concussion

Concussion History

Initiation of an active rehabilitation management plan for concussion recovery begins with a thorough assessment based on the clinical symptom experience and associated exam findings, contextualized within each individual's biopsychosocial history, including non-injury factors that may be contributing to symptom experience [18]. The clinical evaluation should focus first on gathering the acute neurologic indices of brain injury, including length of loss of consciousness and length of post-traumatic amnesia, to allow for a better understanding of the concussion severity. As recovery proceeds, the focus shifts to identifying current symptom presentations, their associated physical exam findings, and potential biopsychosocial underpinnings, which can then be used to guide individualized active rehabilitation [19]. Many of the symptoms experienced following concussion may have been occurring prior to the injury, therefore it is important to ask about pre-existing symptoms.

Headache History

Given headache is the most common reported symptom following concussion, and as symptom presentation and cause of head pain following concussion are quite variable, it is of the utmost importance to undertake a comprehensive history. Information should be gathered regarding the onset of headache, the precise character and location of the headache, and clinical course to identify specific triggers. The factors leading to head pain can also be multifaceted with spinal, musculoskeletal, and vestibular contributions. Clinicians should ask about red flag symptoms that may include focal neurologic symptoms with the headache, progressively worsening severity, intractable vomiting associated with headache, altered level of consciousness, or positional component to headache. If red flags are present, structural abnormalities should be considered and neuroimaging is warranted. Migraine-like features such as photophobia, phonophobia, nausea, and dizziness can be described with the headache, all being relatively constant in the first days following an injury, and gradually improving in duration and severity over the first 1–2 weeks. It is typical that cognitive and physical exertion can cause a transient increase in headache severity. As time since injury increases, the likelihood that headache is directly related to ongoing concussion pathophysiology decreases, and treatment approaches should evolve over time in accordance. The history, including specific triggers, and physical exam findings, should be used to guide active rehabilitation for headache that can include vestibular, or spine physical therapy (Fig. 13.2).

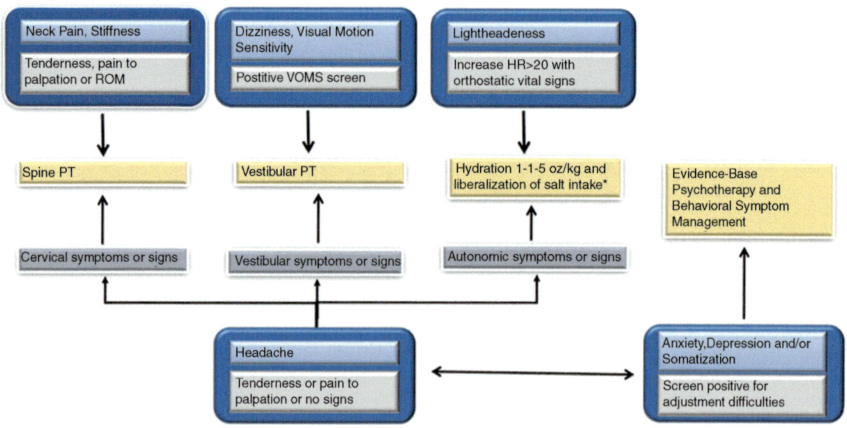

Fig. 13.2 Summary of active rehabilitation of concussion. Light blue boxes –symptoms. Gray boxes –signs or screen of issue. Yellow boxes – therapy. * Increased hydration and salt intake should only be undertaken when medically safe. ROM range of motion, HR heart rate

Neck Pain History

As neck injury is commonly associated with concussion, and can mimic or cause many symptoms similar to those attributed to concussion, it is critical to engage in a comprehensive approach to neck pain and develop an individualized active rehabilitation plan. Initial severe neck pain, especially with reported weakness and/or sensory changes, represents a medical emergency and requires immediate stabilization and urgent medical evaluation. Musculoskeletal symptoms vary in location and duration. Musculoskeletal pain is typically sub-occipital, in the cervical paraspinal region, and can also involve musculature into the anterior neck and shoulders. These types of musculoskeletal symptoms can be a major contributor or sole cause of head pain, with referred neck pain presenting as headache or head pain (i.e., cervicogenic headache). Musculoskeletal symptoms are not typically associated with photophobia or phonophobia but can be associated with dizziness and/or nausea. Common cervicogenic presentations are headaches that are frontal or occipital, worse in the morning, and improve as the day goes on. These headaches are often described as dull, pressure-like, or throbbing. Psychological stress can contribute to muscle tightness and related cervicogenic presentations. It is noteworthy that post-concussive cervicogenic changes can be the underlying source driving dizziness, headache, and imbalance even in the absence of neck pain [20]. The subset of patients whose presentation is largely cervicogenic usually does not fit other clinical trajectories in terms of vestibular impairment or neurocognitive deficits. These individuals should be evaluated by a physical therapist early on and provided with targeted interventions in order to optimize recovery.

History of Vestibular-Related Symptoms

Vestibular impairment is a common problem following concussion. If not identified or treated properly, can have negative psychological ramifications, delay return to usual activities for fear of provoking symptoms, and thus delayed recovery. It is widely appreciated that vestibular changes and subsequent avoidance of activity can contribute to many post-concussion symptoms. Previous investigations reported the prevalence of vestibular-related symptoms after concussion to range from 28% to 90%, though many studies are based solely on self-report of nonspecific symptoms, and thus the true prevalence of concussion-related vestibular and ocular motor symptom remains unknown [21–24]. Importantly, post-concussion vestibular and ocular motor symptom report, regardless of etiology, is associated with poorer recovery outcomes including longer symptom duration [21–23, 25–27], longer time to return to school [21, 27], and longer times to achieve medical clearance to return to sport [21, 27].

Clinicians should seek to determine factors contributing to dizziness, including peripheral or central vestibular dysfunction, migraine, cervicogenic and psychosocial causes, as these can lead to varying treatment approaches. A detailed history will help identify symptoms provoked by vestibular dysfunction, as well as provide context regarding pre-injury and post-concussion non-injury contributory factors. It is important to ask about difficulty with reading, diplopia, blurred vision, headache with oculomotor activities, eye strain, and difficulty with visual scanning, which can manifest as difficulty in school and related poor academic or work performance. Vestibular-related symptoms can be described in a variety of ways, including dizziness, balance problems, blurred vision, headache, nausea, sensitivity to light, sensitivity to sound, fogginess, and motion sensitivity. Patients may also describe a variety of associated symptoms, including headache, nausea, or eye fatigue that may present with dizziness triggered by activities such as reading, riding in a car, or walking in a busy environment. Commonly, patients have co-impairment of the ocular motor systems that causes difficulties associated with alignment, convergence, version, and accommodation, resulting in trouble reading, unstable vision, and trouble focusing [28]. Regardless of underlying cause, promoting adaptation or habituation in the vestibular system via vestibular therapy is the preferred initial approach. It is noteworthy to indicate that patients with persistent oculomotor symptoms that started or worsened after concussion may exhibit with oculomotor findings on exam. Despite being poorly understood and not well supported in primary concussion literature [29, 30], a specific therapeutic approach broadly referred to as vision therapy can be considered to address these findings. It is important to point out that vision therapy is a controversial topic in rehabilitation of concussion with only relatively low quality evidence [29, 30]. It is of the utmost importance to view these symptoms within the context of psychosocial factors, including anxiety, somatic response to stress, and diagnosis threat. Even in the case of vestibular symptom experience due to non-injury factors, promoting adaptation or habituation to symptom experience, as well as setting the expectation for improvement, can be very helpful for making functional gains.

Cognitive Symptoms

Following concussion, cognitive symptom experience is commonly reported. Many report difficulties with concentration, confusion, memory deficits, and feeling slowed down or mentally foggy. Objective neuropsychological data support cognitive change acutely following concussion, though with a small effect size overall and most significant effects in verbal and visual memory domains in the first week post-injury. By 3 months post-injury, effect sizes across cognitive domains were non-significant in numerous meta-analyses, indicating concussion has an initial small effect on neuropsychological functioning that dissipates quickly [9]. When perceived cognitive sequelae extend beyond this period, they are almost certainly unrelated to brain injury and more likely associated with pre-injury vulnerabilities and/or psychosocial factors. When treating cognitive symptom experience following concussion, it is important to educate patients that cognitive effects from concussion are mild and quickly improve. Treatment of prolonged symptom experience should focus on functional gains rather than TBI etiology. Validation of a patient's cognitive experience can be very helpful in moving them forward functionally, whereas reinforcing this experience as being due to brain injury generally is not [31].

Other Historical Considerations

Disturbances in sleep are commonly seen after concussion [32]. Individuals may describe poor sleep quality in addition to difficulty falling and/or staying asleep. Many report sleeping more than usual or the need for increased sleep, with ongoing daytime fatigue and drowsiness. It is vital to actively address sleep disturbances as they may contribute to and worsen other symptoms, as well as delay recovery. Provision of information on good sleep hygiene, as well as highlighting the connection between emotional adjustment and sleep quality are useful tools when sleep is disrupted.

Because concussion can result in non-specific symptoms that often overlap with preexisting conditions, it is important for the clinician to inquire about history of; headache or migraine, prior concussion, other neurologic co-morbidities, mood disorders, psychological health, prior coping mechanisms, behavioral patterns, personality traits, learning disabilities such as attention deficit disorder (ADD), all or nothing thinking, and history of trauma. It is then critical to differentiate post injury symptoms from those experienced prior to concussion or exacerbated by the psychological stress of the event. Additional information regarding, family history of migraine, other neurologic co-morbidities is also important.

The Concussion Physical Examination

The next step guiding active rehabilitation of concussion is the physical examination. The physical exam should begin with a brief measure of cognitive status, interpreted within the context of the patient's history. Many practitioners use the Standardized Assessment of Concussion (SAC), which is a validated sideline tool; however, this measure loses sensitivity and specificity after 72 hours post-injury [8]. Therefore, during any in-office exam, a well-validated brief measure of cognitive status can be used instead. These can include the Montreal Cognitive Assessment, Mini-Mental Status Examination, or Cognitive Log, with this latter measure being developed specifically for cognitive screening after TBI. It is important to note that these are merely screes of cognitive function, and should not be over-interpreted. None of these measures include embedded performance validity indicators, and thus do not guarantee optimal engagement in the screening, which may result in over-pathologizing. Given effect size on cognition is small, even in the acute phase post-concussion, severe impairment on brief measure of cognitive status is inconsistent with the known cognitive sequelae of concussion and should be seen as a red flag, warranting a referral to a neuropsychologist who specializes in concussion.

Orthostatic vitals should also be performed to identify signs of possible autonomic dysfunction [33], and a detailed head, eyes, ears, nose, and throat (HEENT) exam should be completed looking for abrasions, lacerations, bruising, and rhinorrhea or otorrhea, as well as observing for pain to palpation. A thorough cervicogenic musculoskeletal examination should include cervical range of motion (ROM), assessment of cervical musculature, flexibility and strength evaluation, and testing for cervical ligamentous instability. A more detailed cervicogenic examination also includes screening for ligamentous instability and vascular integrity, followed by a symptom-guided examination that includes examination of movement quality and generalized joint hypermobility (GJH), myofascial tension to palpation, joint mobility, muscle strength and endurance, proprioception, and special tests for upper extremity radicular symptoms [17, 34]. It is important to note that a cervical musculoskeletal examination may extend to examine the thoracic spine and/or the temporomandibular joint for potential sources of musculoskeletal dysfunction contributing to symptoms (i.e., headache) [17]. If point tenderness along the spinous processes or step-off is noted, urgent advanced imaging (either computerized tomography [CT] scan or magnetic resonance imaging [MRI]) should be obtained to rule out fracture or ligamentous injury.

The neurologic examination should also include cranial nerve evaluation and assessment of coordination, gait, dynamic balance testing, strength, reflexes, and sensation. Due to its utility in diagnosis and management, specialized testing of the vestibular system should be included as part of the physical exam [17, 35]. A vestibular ocular motor assessment based on the vestibular ocular motor screen (VOMS) assess for symptoms provoked during smooth pursuits, horizontal and vertical saccades, Horizontal and vertical VOR, VOR cancellation, and convergence [36]. In addition to evoked symptoms, a clinician may observe performance based abnormalities such as saccadic intrusions with smooth pursuit, hypometria/hypermetria with horizontal or vertical saccades, nystagmus, catch-up saccades during vestibulo-ocular reflex testing, or difficulty performing near point convergence and accommodation [37]. Any of these findings noted with reports of headache, dizziness, nausea, or motion sensitivity can not only aid in the diagnosis of concussion but also guide referral decisions to establish a formal vestibular evaluation and subsequent active rehabilitation with vestibular therapy. A vestibular physical therapist can conduct a thorough and symptom-guided assessment examining the following domains: gaze stability, postural stability, ocular motor control, and visual motion sensitivity testing (i.e., visual vertigo) and provide the individualized therapy plan.

Concussion Exercise Tolerance Testing

Properly dosed exercise is an important component of active recovery from concussion. With commonly available exercise and monitoring equipment, determining the type and intensity of exercise likely to be of benefit is relatively straightforward and can be incorporated into the outpatient concussion evaluation [15]. In general, this consists of determining the exercise intensity that provokes symptoms and using this as a basis for recommendation of exercise at an intensity less than that which provoked symptoms, known as sub-symptom exercise, that should be consistently performed during the acute phase of recovery. If symptoms do not remit as time since injury increases, engagement in exercise with some symptom provocation, with development of improved symptom coping, may be warranted. Abstaining from exercise and activity in general for long periods post-injury is contraindicated. A treadmill or stationary exercise bike can be used during the supervised exercise testing to determine the amount of exercise that provokes symptoms, or the symptom exercise threshold [38, 39]. As motion sensitivity and dizziness are frequent following concussion, a stationary bike that reduces head movement may be preferred as the initial exercise equipment used to determine the exercise symptom threshold and performance of exercise.

Once it has been determined that it is safe to undergo a supervised exercise session, the patient is fitted with a chest strap heart rate monitor and queried as to symptoms they are experiencing prior to beginning the supervised exercise session [40]. The supervised exercise session is initiated with a very low exercise intensity (10–40 Watts). Intensity is gradually increased and symptoms, heart rate, and relative exertion are monitored serially. If there is no significant symptom provocation during the supervised aerobic exercise, the exercise intensity is increased in order to reach ~90% of the patient's age-predicted maximum heart rate. Typically, an increase in any symptom by three or more points on a ten-point scale is considered clinically significant and is used to determine the maximum acceptable exercise symptom threshold.

Active Rehabilitation Approaches for Concussion

Cervical Physical Therapy

Based on the results of a thorough cervical musculoskeletal examination, a physical therapist will implement a targeted therapeutic program to address identified impairments (Fig. 13.2). The cervical physical therapy (CPT) program is usually completed in 3–6 visits [20, 41], and may include therapeutic exercises to target muscle strength, range of motion, posture, joint position, and/or sensorimotor function [17]. CPT may include manual therapy to the cervical and/or thoracic spines, as indicated [17]. Studies examining the effectiveness of cervical physical therapy after concussion have documented that CPT can independently and in combination with other therapies (e.g., vestibular interventions), lead to improvement in symptoms, and is associated with accelerated return to play [17, 42]. This evidence from clinical trials is augmented by findings of other studies reporting the beneficial effects of cervical musculoskeletal interventions to improve symptoms and function after concussion [41, 43]. It is important to consider that cervical musculoskeletal impairments can coexist with vestibular impairments [41], complicating initial clinical presentation.

Therefore, a physical therapist with advanced training in both areas will be able to thoroughly assess, prioritize, and successfully implement a comprehensive therapeutic program targeting overlapping cervical and vestibular impairments [44].

Vestibular Physical Therapy

Due to of the high prevalence and the prognostic utility of vestibular-related symptoms, accurate identification and targeted interventions are an essential component of active concussion rehabilitation to improve recovery outcomes. Based on the findings of the vestibular history and examination, a vestibular physical therapist will implement an individualized vestibular physical therapy program targeting identified impairments [35]. The vestibular therapy exercises are dosed to cause transient and mild increase in symptoms to facilitate habituation. Once an exercise is no longer causing a transient increase in symptoms, the exercise is progressed to the next level in order to derive a functional benefit. Vestibular therapy exercises are progressed by altering one or more of the following exercise modifiers: posture, surface, base of support, trunk position, arm position, direction and speed of head movement, direction and speed of body movement, visual input presence and complexity, or dual task [45].

Previous investigations documented the beneficial effects of vestibular rehabilitation to reduce dizziness and balance changes [46], and to expedite recovery times [42]. Moreover, preliminary evidence suggests the feasibility and the potential beneficial effects of early vestibular physical therapy initiated within 10 days from injury [47]. These benefits were documented when vestibular therapy exercises were delivered in isolation or in conjunction with other physical therapy interventions (i.e., cervical physical therapy) for a median of four visits [41, 46]. It is important to consider that changes in vestibular function can co-exist with cervical musculoskeletal changes, and also can be due to psychosomatic factors, complicating initial clinical presentation and course of recovery [17]. Therefore, a physical therapist with advanced training in these areas, and a thorough understanding of the biopsychosocial model of concussion, will be able to thoroughly assess, prioritize, and successfully implement a comprehensive therapeutic program targeting overlapping vestibular, cervical, and psychosocial factors [17, 44].

Psychological Assessment and Treatment Following Concussion

Psychological symptoms may be directly related to concussion, but can be influenced by downstream factors such as removal from school, work, or sport. Psychological factors are a known etiology for prolonged symptom experience post-SRC. Psychological risk factors for prolonged symptom experience include history of trauma, depression or anxiety, chronic pain or other medically unexplained physical or cognitive symptoms, and other life stressors [6]. While these factors play a greater role for some with SRC than others, everyone recovering from an acute injury goes through a period of psychological adjustment. This could be brief and uncomplicated, or may be extensive and complex, requiring specialized psychological care. In either case, early education about the role of psychological factors in concussion recovery is warranted and has been shown to improve post-injury outcomes [6, 48]. In particular, psychoeducation about physical and cognitive manifestations of stress, increasing participation in valued activities while managing symptom experience with pacing, limiting avoidance despite emotional discomfort, and learning present-centered coping such as meditation and mindfulness are suggested as treatment targets for anyone with SRC. Behavioral sleep hygiene techniques should also be implemented to optimize sleep after concussion, including a regular sleep schedule, relaxing routines as bedtime approaches, limiting non-sleep-related activities in the bedroom, and learning strategies for decreasing unhelpful, ruminative thoughts. Short term pharmacologic intervention, such as use of melatonin can be implemented. Quite commonly, sleep quantity and quality improves with the gradual initiation of sub-symptom physical activity and other values-based activities.

Psychotherapy specific to concussion recovery is often not needed, particularly if adequate psychoeducation is provided acutely to those who sustain concussion. However, for some with significant psychological risk pre-injury, post-concussion psychotherapy is indicated, and should focus specifically on better understanding of the biopsychosocial model of symptom maintenance and pre-injury risk factors that are at play, as well as improving psychological coping generally. This can include any evidence-based psychotherapy process, though methods that are transdiagnostic tend to be well suited given they are appropriate for any maladaptive psychological tendencies [49]. Normalization of uncomfortable emotions such as anxiety, anger, and sadness, setting SMART (Specific, Measurable, Achievable, Relevant, and Time-limited) goals to improve behavioral activation, using strategies to redirect focus away from symptoms and towards present-centered values-guided action, and using strategies for decreasing unhelpful thought patterns are all recommended, with the overarching goal being that the patient can get back to his or her life despite perceived residual symptom experience. A unified message from all treatment providers, including physicians, psychologists, therapists, and trainers, regarding the contribution of psychosocial factors in symptom experience is essential to ensure buy-in and optimize functional outcomes.

Exercise as Active Rehabilitation During Concussion Recovery

An initial step toward returning to sport is returning to activities of daily living as well as to light to moderate cognitive and physical activity, with an emphasis on meaningful activities. Examples of light to moderate cognitive activity include conversations with friends and loved ones, pleasure reading, listening to music and short periods of schoolwork. Examples of light physical activity include light activities around home and short walks. Pacing for symptom management early post-injury, and gradually increasing the intensity and duration of sub-symptom threshold activities and exercise aids recovery [14, 15]. Early during recovery, care partners should encourage a return to sub-symptom activity and exercise. Studies looking at the role of exercise in recovery of concussion have determined that both too little and too much exercise may prolong recovery [50]. Evidence suggests that after a short period of rest, returning to activity and exercise that does not significantly worsen symptoms, sub-symptom threshold exercise, facilitates recovery [14, 15]. The correct intensity can be determined by concussion exercise tolerance testing, as above. A heart rate or watts target that is ~80% of the symptom exercise threshold can be given as the exercise goal for exercises done on their own. The at home sub-symptom exercise generally consists of a five-minute warm up, gradually building the heart rate or watts to the sub-symptom exercise goal, then maintaining the exercise intensity at approximately the sub-symptom exercise goal for the duration of the exercise session. This is then followed by a five-minute cool down. The initial recommended exercise duration is 15 minutes and this can be lengthened to 30–45 minutes per day, as tolerated. As recovery proceeds, the duration, intensity, and type of exercises that are tolerated increase and at subsequent office visits a new sub-symptom threshold for exercise can be determined and new parameters for at home sub-symptom exercise recommended. As recovery ensues, dynamic and sport-specific exercise can be added. Most commonly, a medicine ball-based exercise is used as the first dynamic exercise initially with visual fixation followed by visual tracking [51]. Patients who tolerate medicine ball exercises without significant symptom provocation, or are further in their recovery, may advance to agility drills. Similar to the medicine ball exercises, these drills are designed to stress the vestibular system, but also add multiple planes of movement, including changes of speed and direction, rotations, twists, inversions, increasing visual motion integration and sport specific drills, along with continued cardiovascular exertion. The dynamic exercises are individualized with gradually increasing difficulty as tolerated. At their highest intensity, all of the sport-specific exercises should approximate game speed.

Exercise During the Return to Play Progression and as a Biomarker of Recovery of Sport-Related Concussion

A major goal of active rehabilitation of concussion is safe return to sport. Return to play decisions can be complex; therefore, it is essential to understand the sport in question and its risks [52]. The progression should be overseen by a health care provider trained in the evaluation and management of concussion. The return to play process is begun with sub-symptom threshold exercise and then gradually proceeds through a stepwise progression, increasing exercise intensity, duration, and complexity (Table 13.1) [5]. Exercise performed while symptomatic from concussion should not be considered the return to play progression, but is part of active

Table 13.1 Graduated Return-to-Sports progression

Stage of activity	Activity	Stage objective
Relative rest	Symptom-limited activities of daily living; light walking	Gradual reintroduction of activities involved with daily living and school/work.
Cardiovascular activity	Light to moderate aerobic exercise without resistance training on stationary bike or walking	Increase cerebral blood flow and heart rate.
Sport-specific non-contact exercise	Progressive aerobic exercise with sports-specific activity (drills) without head impact. May start progressive resistance training.	Interval training by adding fluctuations in heart rate and adding cognitive activity while increasing movement.
Non-contact training practice	Complex training drills, conditioning drills [can add limited controlled contact drills (e.g., pushing or hitting sleds or dummies)].	Increase cognitive demand and assess processing speed and coordination. Assess for recurrence of symptoms after adding limited controlled magnitude of force.
Unrestricted training	Participation in training activity only after medical clearance.	Assess for recurrence of symptoms. Assess functional skills by coaching staff. Ensure self-confidence and readiness to play.
Full return to play	Participation in full activity without restrictions	Full game day participation.

rehabilitation of concussion. Once a patient is at their preinjury state at rest and progressing with sub-symptoms threshold exercise without symptoms, the level of exercise that has been tolerated during the recovery phase can be used as a guide as to where to begin the return to play progression. As an example, if jogging has not precipitated symptoms during the recovery phase, more intense running, such as sprints can be initiated as the next stage in the progression, in conjunction with non-contact training practice. The goal of the return to play process is to safely test for symptom provocation in a stepwise progression of increasing risk. If symptoms develop during or after the activity at an individual stage, the following day the same stage can be attempted again. When asymptomatic at a given stage, the following stage may be undertaken the following day. A slower progression may be used for children or as clinically warranted [53–56]. The ability to perform exercise achieving a near maximum predicted heart rate and incorporating sport specific agility without symptoms can be used to determine readiness for return to full practice and full contact practice [57].

Returning to Academics and Work

Another major goal of an active rehabilitation approach to concussion recovery is successful return to learn and/or work. Although cognitive sequelae of concussion are mild and resolve quickly, cognitive inefficacy, disruption of usual routines, headache, dizziness, and other psychological factors can impact returning to learn, school, and work. Academic accommodations can be part of the active rehabilitation plan and may optimize recovery, particularly a step-wise return to activities that accommodates the known recovery trajectory for concussion, but is not too drawn out as this can serve to delay return to school or work, and increase maladaptive avoidance. Guidelines have been developed that can be used as a framework to facilitate a return to academics, but recommendations must be individualized [58]. It is not expected that students will be symptom free during the return to learn process. The gradual transition to preinjury performance can begin with completing school work at home in short 10–15 minute intervals. Once a student has manageable symptom levels during school work, typically not more than a few days to weeks post-injury, a gradual transition to the school environment can be undertaken. The return to learn plans should be developed in collaboration with school personnel, physicians, and associated treatment team. The return to the school environment can be eased by at first returning part-time with the use of breaks to alleviate symptoms. Students should not be expected to make up all missed work and stay current during the recovery process. A plan for completing the minimal requirements for missed work while performing essential work should be developed. Examinations should not be taken while concussion symptoms are at unmanageable levels. The goal of these accommodations is to maintain the pace in the classroom activities and provide a smooth transition to full academic activities. The return to work process should also be step-wise. Injured employees should work with their employers to arrange reasonable work accommodations allowing them to work part time, with breaks and with restriction of duties that provoke unmanageable symptoms, though it is expected that full return to work is possible within a few days to weeks post-injury. Inability to maintain academic progress and lost wages are common sources of psychological stress, and development of return to learn and work plans are critical to avoid this complication and prolonging symptom burden. Successful return to school must occur prior to full return to sport.

The care team should take an active approach in working with the school athletic trainers, school counselors and/or employers to facilitate reasonable accommodations for a smooth return to school and/or work. As focus on pain and other uncomfortable symptom experiences can impact one's ability to attend and process information, which in turn can result in reduced recall, it is important to determine the often somatic and psychosocial underpinnings of cognitive complaints. Cognitive screening can be completed during the clinic visit to assess for these complaints, but formal neuropsychological evaluation may be warranted to determine all factors contributing to prolonged report of cognitive deficits. Without academic accommodations, the student athlete may become overwhelmed and fall behind, which can then lead to increased depression and/or anxiety due to altered academic trajectory. It is important to realize that in the adolescent population, school and sport are activities that are key to developing self-identity. When these are removed or restricted, it can have negative ramifications, including new or worsening anxiety or depression. It is vital to identify and address these concerns; otherwise psychological issues can become more severe as recovery becomes prolonged, and can become the sole symptom generator over time. Actively identifying these issues early on, providing accurate education about the expectation of a quick cognitive recovery, and developing a treatment plan such as individualized evidence-based psychotherapy with a trained school counselor, psychologist, or social worker can help optimize recovery from concussion.

Conclusion

Although concussions are a recoverable injury, a significant minority of patients will develop prolonged symptoms. Due to insufficient understanding of prognostic factors that may identify patients who are likely to develop prolonged symptoms, and given the sometimes debilitating multidimensional effects of concussion, a biopsychosocial, active rehabilitation approach to concussion is warranted. This approach is found through proper identification of impairments via a detailed history and a comprehensive, multifaceted biopsychosocial assessment. Patients should then receive targeted rehabilitation approaches matching previously identified impairments. The targeted rehabilitation approach will vary in individual patients based on identified biopsychosocial vulnerabilities and post-concussion changes. Underpinning these interventions are: timely return to valued activities; sub-symptom threshold exercises; step-wise return to school, sport, and work commitments; and development of coping mechanisms for managing the psychological stress that often accompanies concussion-associated life disruptions.

Bibliography

1. Pierpoint LA, Collins C. Epidemiology of sport-related concussion. Clin Sports Med. 2021;40(1):1–18.
2. Iverson GL, Lange RT. Examination of "postconcussion-like" symptoms in a healthy sample. Appl Neuropsychol. 2003;10(3):137–44.
3. Waljas M, Iverson GL, Lange RT, Hakulinen U, Dastidar P, Huhtala H, et al. A prospective biopsychosocial study of the persistent post-concussion symptoms following mild traumatic brain injury. J Neurotrauma. 2015;32(8):534–47.
4. Barkhoudarian G, Hovda DA, Giza CC. The molecular pathophysiology of concussive brain injury. Clin Sports Med. 2011;30(1):33–48, vii-iii.
5. McCrory P, Meeuwisse W, Dvorak J, Aubry M, Bailes J, Broglio S, et al. Consensus statement on concussion in sport-the 5(th) international conference on concussion in sport held in Berlin, October 2016. Br J Sports Med. 2017;51(11):838–47.
6. Mittenberg W, Tremont G, Zielinski RE, Fichera S, Rayls KR. Cognitive-behavioral prevention of postconcussion syndrome. Arch Clin Neuropsychol. 1996;11(2):139–45.
7. Zemek RL, Farion KJ, Sampson M, McGahern C. Prognosticators of persistent symptoms following pediatric concussion: a systematic review. JAMA Pediatr. 2013;167(3):259–65.
8. McCrea M, Guskiewicz KM, Marshall SW, Barr W, Randolph C, Cantu RC, et al. Acute effects and recovery time following concussion in collegiate football players: the NCAA Concussion Study. JAMA. 2003;290(19):2556–63.

9. Rohling ML, Binder LM, Demakis GJ, Larrabee GJ, Ploetz DM, Langhinrichsen-Rohling J. A meta-analysis of neuropsychological outcome after mild traumatic brain injury: re-analyses and reconsiderations of Binder et al. (1997), Frencham et al. (2005), and Pertab et al. (2009). Clin Neuropsychol. 2011;25(4):608–23.
10. Davis GA, Anderson V, Babl FE, Gioia GA, Giza CC, Meehan W, et al. What is the difference in concussion management in children as compared with adults? A systematic review. Br J Sports Med. 2017;51(12):949–57.
11. Kamins J, Bigler E, Covassin T, Henry L, Kemp S, Leddy JJ, et al. What is the physiological time to recovery after concussion? A systematic review. Br J Sports Med. 2017;51(12):935–40.
12. Smoliga JM. Interpreting biomarker data after concussion and repeated subconcussive head impacts: challenges in evaluating brain protection. JAMA Neurol. 2020.
13. Iverson GL, Lange RT, Brooks BL, Rennison VL. "Good old days" bias following mild traumatic brain injury. Clin Neuropsychol. 2010;24(1):17–37.
14. Leddy JJ, Haider MN, Ellis MJ, Mannix R, Darling SR, Freitas MS, et al. Early subthreshold aerobic exercise for sport-related concussion: a randomized clinical trial. JAMA Pediatr. 2019;173(4):319–25.
15. Popovich M, Almeida A, Freeman J, Eckner JT, Alsalaheen B, Lorincz M, et al. Use of supervised exercise during recovery following sports-related concussion. Clin J Sport Med. 2019.
16. McCarty CA, Zatzick D, Stein E, Wang J, Hilt R, Rivara FP, et al. Collaborative care for adolescents with persistent postconcussive symptoms: a randomized trial. Pediatrics. 2016;138(4).
17. Quatman-Yates CC, Hunter-Giordano A, Shimamura KK, Landel R, Alsalaheen BA, Hanke TA, et al. Physical therapy evaluation and treatment after concussion/mild traumatic brain injury. J Orthop Sports Phys Ther. 2020;50(4):CPG1–CPG73.
18. Collins MW, Kontos AP, Okonkwo DO, Almquist J, Bailes J, Barisa M, et al. Statements of agreement from the targeted evaluation and active management (TEAM) approaches to treating concussion meeting held in Pittsburgh, October 15–16, 2015. Neurosurgery. 2016;79(6):912–29.
19. Charek DB, Collins M, Kontos A. Office-based concussion evaluation, diagnosis, and management: adult. 158. Netherlands: Elsevier Health Sciences; 2018. p. 91–105.
20. Kennedy E, Quinn D, Chapple C, Tumilty S. Can the neck contribute to persistent symptoms post concussion? A prospective descriptive case series. J Orthop Sports Phys Ther. 2019;49(11):845–54.
21. Corwin DJ, Wiebe DJ, Zonfrillo MR, Grady MF, Robinson RL, Goodman AM, et al. Vestibular deficits following youth concussion. J Pediatr. 2015.
22. Ellis MJ, Cordingley D, Vis S, Reimer K, Leiter J, Russell K. Vestibulo-ocular dysfunction in pediatric sports-related concussion. J Neurosurg Pediatr. 2015;16(3):248–55.
23. Pearce KL, Sufrinko A, Lau BC, Henry L, Collins MW, Kontos AP. Near point of convergence after a sport-related concussion: measurement reliability and relationship to neurocognitive impairment and symptoms. Am J Sports Med. 2015;43(12):3055–61.
24. Gallaway M, Scheiman M, Mitchell GL. Vision therapy for post-concussion vision disorders. Optom Vis Sci. 2017;94(1):68–73.
25. Lau BC, Kontos AP, Collins MW, Mucha A, Lovell MR. Which on-field signs/symptoms predict protracted recovery from sport-related concussion among high school football players? Am J Sports Med. 2011;39(11):2311–8.
26. Anzalone AJ, Blueitt D, Case T, McGuffin T, Pollard K, Garrison JC, et al. A positive vestibular/ocular motor screening (VOMS) is associated with increased recovery time after sports-related concussion in youth and adolescent athletes. Am J Sports Med. 2017;45(2):474–9.
27. Corwin DJ, Zonfrillo MR, Master CL, Arbogast KB, Grady MF, Robinson RL, et al. Characteristics of prolonged concussion recovery in a pediatric subspecialty referral population. J Pediatr. 2014;165(6):1207–15.
28. Akhand O, Balcer LJ, Galetta SL. Assessment of vision in concussion. Curr Opin Neurol. 2019;32(1):68–74.
29. Ciuffreda KJ, Rutner D, Kapoor N, Suchoff IB, Craig S, Han ME. Vision therapy for oculomotor dysfunctions in acquired brain injury: a retrospective analysis. Optometry. 2008;79(1):18–22.

30. Scheiman M, Mitchell GL, Cotter S, Cooper J, Kulp M, Rouse M, et al. A randomized clinical trial of treatments for convergence insufficiency in children. Arch Ophthalmol. 2005;123(1):14–24.
31. Delis DC, Wetter SR. Cogniform disorder and cogniform condition: proposed diagnoses for excessive cognitive symptoms. Arch Clin Neuropsychol. 2007;22(5):589–604.
32. Hoffman NL, Weber ML, Broglio SP, McCrea M, McAllister TW, Schmidt JD, et al. Influence of postconcussion sleep duration on concussion recovery in collegiate athletes. Clin J Sport Med. 2020;30 Suppl 1:S29–35.
33. Purkayastha S, Stokes M, Bell KR. Autonomic nervous system dysfunction in mild traumatic brain injury: a review of related pathophysiology and symptoms. Brain Inj. 2019;33(9):1129–36.
34. Tiwari D, Goldberg A, Yorke A, Marchetti GF, Alsalaheen B. Characterization of cervical spine impairments in children and adolescents post-concussion. Int J Sports Phys Ther. 2019;14(2):282–95.
35. Alsalaheen B, Carender W, Grzesiak M, Munday C, Almeida A, Lorincz M, et al. Changes in vestibular/ocular-motor screen scores in adolescents treated with vestibular therapy after concussion. Pediatr Phys Ther. 2020;32(4):331–7.
36. Mucha A, Collins MW, Elbin RJ, Furman JM, Troutman-Enseki C, DeWolf RM, et al. A brief vestibular/ocular motor screening (VOMS) assessment to evaluate concussions: preliminary findings. Am J Sports Med. 2014;42(10):2479–86.
37. Ventura RE, Balcer LJ, Galetta SL. The neuro-ophthalmology of head trauma. Lancet Neurol. 2014;13(10):1006–16.
38. Haider MN, Johnson SL, Mannix R, Macfarlane AJ, Constantino D, Johnson BD, et al. The buffalo concussion bike test for concussion assessment in adolescents. Sports Health. 2019;11(6):492–7.
39. Leddy JJ, Baker JG, Kozlowski K, Bisson L, Willer B. Reliability of a graded exercise test for assessing recovery from concussion. Clin J Sport Med. 2011;21(2):89–94.
40. Leddy JJ, Willer B. Use of graded exercise testing in concussion and return-to-activity management. Curr Sports Med Rep. 2013;12(6):370–6.
41. Grabowski P, Wilson J, Walker A, Enz D, Wang S. Multimodal impairment-based physical therapy for the treatment of patients with post-concussion syndrome: a retrospective analysis on safety and feasibility. Phys Ther Sport. 2016;23:22–30.
42. Schneider KJ, Meeuwisse WH, Nettel-Aguirre A, Barlow K, Boyd L, Kang J, et al. Cervicovestibular rehabilitation in sport-related concussion: a randomised controlled trial. Br J Sports Med. 2014;48(17):1294–8.
43. Kennedy E, Quinn D, Tumilty S, Chapple CM. Clinical characteristics and outcomes of treatment of the cervical spine in patients with persistent post-concussion symptoms: a retrospective analysis. Musculoskelet Sci Pract. 2017;29:91–8.
44. Alsalaheen B, Landel R, Hunter-Giordano A, Shimamura KK, Quatman-Yates C, Hanke T, et al. A treatment-based profiling model for physical therapy management of patients following a concussive event. J Orthop Sports Phys Ther. 2019;49(11):829–41.
45. Alsalaheen B, Whitney SL, Mucha A, Morris LO, Furman JM, Sparto PJ. Exercise prescription patterns in patients treated with vestibular rehabilitation after concussion. Physiother Res Int. 2013;18(2):100–8.
46. Alsalaheen B, Mucha A, Morris LO, Whitney SL, Furman JM, Camiolo-Reddy CE, et al. Vestibular rehabilitation for dizziness and balance disorders after concussion. J Neurol Phys Ther. 2010;34(2):87–93.
47. Reneker JC, Hassen A, Phillips RS, Moughiman MC, Donaldson M, Moughiman J. Feasibility of early physical therapy for dizziness after a sports-related concussion: a randomized clinical trial. Scand J Med Sci Sports. 2017;27(12):2009–18.
48. Hanks RA, Rapport LJ, Seagly K, Millis SR, Scott C, Pearson C. Outcomes after concussion recovery education: effects of litigation and disability status on maintenance of symptoms. J Neurotrauma. 2019;36(4):554–8.
49. Barlow DH, Farchione TJ, Bullis JR, Gallagher MW, Murray-Latin H, Sauer-Zavala S, et al. The unified protocol for transdiagnostic treatment of emotional disorders compared with

diagnosis-specific protocols for anxiety disorders: a randomized clinical trial. JAMA Psychiat. 2017;74(9):875–84.
50. Grool AM, Aglipay M, Momoli F, Meehan WP 3rd, Freedman SB, Yeates KO, et al. Association between early participation in physical activity following acute concussion and persistent post-concussive symptoms in children and adolescents. JAMA. 2016;316(23):2504–14.
51. Popovich M, Sas A, Almeida AA, Freeman J, Alsalaheen B, Lorincz M, Eckner JT. Symptom provocation during aerobic and dynamic supervised exercise challenges in adolescents with sport-related concussion. J Athl Train. 2021. In press.
52. Almeida A, Kutcher J. Sports and performance concussion. In: Daroff RB, et al., editors. Neurology in clinical practice. 7th ed. Phildelphia, PA: Elsevier; 2014.
53. Giza CC, Kutcher JS, Ashwal S, Barth J, Getchius TSD, Gioia GA, et al. Summary of evidence-based guideline update: evaluation and management of concussion in sports: report of the Guideline Development Subcommittee of the American Academy of Neurology. Neurology. 2013;80(24):2250.
54. Guay JL, Lebretore BM, Main JM, DeFrangesco KE, Taylor JL, Amedoro SM. The era of sport concussion: evolution of knowledge, practice, and the role of psychology. Am Psychol. 2016;71(9):875.
55. Guskiewicz KM, Bruce SL, Cantu RC, Ferrara MS, Kelly JP, McCrea M, et al. Recommendations on management of sport-related concussion: summary of the national athletic trainers' association position statement. Neurosurgery. 2004;55(4):891.
56. Harmon KG, Drezner J, Gammons M, Guskiewicz K, Halstead M, Herring S, et al. American Medical Society for Sports Medicine Position Statement: Concussion in Sport. Clin J Sport Med. 2013;23(1):1.
57. Marshall CM, Chan N, Tran P, DeMatteo C. The use of an intensive physical exertion test as a final return to play measure in concussed athletes: a prospective cohort. Phys Sportsmed. 2019;47(2):158–66.
58. O'Neill JA, Cox MK, Clay OJ, Johnston JM, Novack TA, Schwebel DC, et al. A review of the literature on pediatric concussions and return-to-learn (RTL): implications for RTL policy, research, and practice. Rehabil Psychol. 2017;62(3):300–23.

Chapter 14
Sports Concussions: Is There a Role for Alternative Treatments?

Khaled J. Zaza, Hussam Abou-Al-Shaar, Vincent J. Miele, and Joseph C. Maroon

Introduction

Around 3.8 million sports-related concussions occur in the United States each year; and up to 50% of those go unreported [1]. Sports-related concussions are commonly referred to as mild traumatic brain injuries (TBI) that affect a wide range of recreational and professional sports athletes. Mild TBIs typically result from biomechanical forces that induce complex cellular metabolic cascades. This impairs neuronal membrane and transmitter function and causes ionic shifts that increase intracellular glutamate and calcium [2]. The resulting transient clinical symptoms often reflect a functional injury from disruption of brain networks, which cannot be depicted grossly with neuroimaging. Despite the complex pathophysiological constellation of neurologic and musculoskeletal symptoms, the majority (80–90%) of sports-related concussive episodes resolve spontaneously in 7–10 days [3].

Traditional treatment has hence involved complete physical and mental rest with low light and low sound stimulating environments until symptom resolution. However, complete rest is better substituted with controlled submaximal activity after 72 hours of injury to hasten recovery [4]. Despite that, the overall

K. J. Zaza
Department of Anesthesiology and Perioperative Medicine, University of Pittsburgh Medical Center, Pittsburgh, PA, USA

H. Abou-Al-Shaar · V. J. Miele · J. C. Maroon (✉)
Department of Neurological Surgery, University of Pittsburgh Medical Center, Pittsburgh, PA, USA
e-mail: maroonjc@upmc.edu

M. E. Oppenlander (ed.), *Neurosurgical Care of Athletes*,
https://doi.org/10.1007/978-3-030-88227-3_14

management paradigms of mild TBIs remains controversial with varying success rates of different therapies. This might be attributed to the lack of general consensus and concrete evidence as well as the absence of Food and Drug Administration (FDA)-approved pharmacological interventions. Thus, physicians often target such symptoms with corticosteroids and anti-inflammatory drugs that inhibit arachidonic acid or modify monoamine function, glutamate receptor antagonists, calcium channel blockers, or thyrotrophin-releasing hormones [5]. Many nonpharmaceutical alternatives such as dietary supplements, vitamins, and minerals have already been utilized in the management of neurodegenerative conditions. These agents have also shown promising results in the management of a wide array of neurologic sequelae resulting from repetitive concussive head injury such as post-concussion syndrome (PCS), prolonged PCS, and post-traumatic stress disorder (PTSD) (Fig. 14.1) [2, 6].

Proper assessment and evaluation remain an integral part in managing concussed patients for optimal delivery of effective care. This includes both onsite tools of assessment and further comprehensive neuropsychological testing. The following chapter discusses the scientific basis of proposed supplements and their potential implications in the treatment of sports concussion and prevention of its short- and long-term sequelae such as PCS.

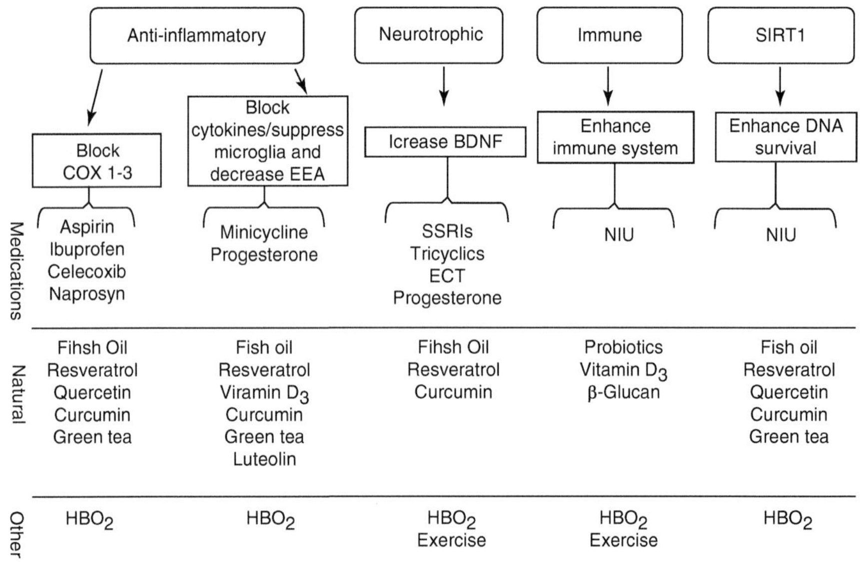

Fig. 14.1 Both pharmacological agents and nonpharmaceutical alternatives target similar pathways responsible for immunoexcitotoxicity post brain injury. Natural alternatives may be as effective without the undesirable side effects associated with their pharmacological counterparts. (Courtesy of Maroon et al. [5])
Abbreviations: BDNF brain-derived neurotrophic factor, COX cyclooxygenase, ECT electroconvulsive therapy, EAA excitatory amino acids, HBO2 hyperbaric oxygen, NIU no pharmacological agents in use, SIRT1 sirtuin 1, SSRI selective serotonin reuptake inhibitor

Supplements

Omega-3-Fatty Acids

Omega-3-Fatty Acids (O3FAs) have been found to have significant health benefits in neurological disease prevention and treatment [7]. O3FAs are among the most popular supplements for the management of concussions partly due to their promising neuroprotective effects in animal experiments [8], and their role as a natural anti-inflammatory [9]. The growing evidence behind their medicinal properties and health benefits have made fish oil capsules and oils, which contain O3FAs, the most common dietary supplement in the United States [10].

Fatty acids comprise the bilipid membrane of every cell in the human body. They are involved in many vital structural roles that enhance neuronal cell fluidity, stability, and neurotransmitter functions [11]. The brain especially comprises mostly fatty acids, of which 40% of those are docosahexaenoic acid (DHA) [12, 13]. DHA, eicosapentaenoic acid (EPA), and α-Linolenic acid are the most important O3FAs with potential benefits in concussion and traumatic brain injury. They are referred to as omega-3 essential fatty acids (EFAs) because of the inability of the human body to endogenously synthesize them and therefore must be obtained from dietary nutrition sources, such as fish, walnuts, flaxseeds, and certain other vegetables. Deficiency in omega-3 EFAs can induce various forms of brain dysfunction and disrupt the normal composition and chemical properties of neuronal cell membranes, neurons, oligodendrocytes, and astrocytes leading to neurosensory and behavioral abnormalities [7, 13].

Animal studies have demonstrated that supplementation of O3FA in rats before sustaining a concussion can preserve learning and protect against reduced neuronal plasticity by normalizing protein levels associated with neuronal circuit function, cognitive processing, synaptic facilitation, neuronal excitability, and locomotor control [14]. When administered 30 days before TBI, they have shown to reduce the response to injury, evident by reduction in markers of cellular injury and apoptosis, axonal counts, and memory as assessed by water-maze testing [15].

Whereas supplementation of O3FAs prior to concussion seems beneficial, studies have also reported that supplementation in animals following TBI helps maintain genomic stability and cellular hemostasis [16], as well as decrease the amount of injury the brain sustains [17]. DHA supplementation significantly reduces the number of swollen, disconnected, and injured axons [11, 18]. The administration of EPA has also shown to attenuate neuronal cell death in rats suffering from an interruption in blood flow following injury [14]. Other studies have described that long-term treatment with EPA improved age-related reduction in blood flow in the brain and increased glucose metabolism [19]. Fish oil has also demonstrated the ability to attenuate TBI-induced deficits and dopamine release in the striatum, which could potentially benefit behavioral impairments [20].

Perhaps the main benefit of omega-3 EFAs lies within their ant-inflammatory properties that can potentially counter brain trauma-related inflammation [14, 18].

They are able to stabilize cell membranes and inhibit the release of pro-inflammatory prostaglandins such as arachidonic acid, a major mediator of the inflammatory response [11, 14, 21]. At the cellular level, cyclooxygenase (COX) enzyme maintains an equilibrium between the conversion of arachidonic acid (AA) from omega-6 EFA into proinflammatory prostaglandin E2 (PGE2) and anti-inflammatory prostaglandin E3 (PGE3) from EPA [10, 22]. As the percentage of EPA increases compared to the amount of AA within the phospholipid membrane of a cell, PGE2 production is downregulated through competitive inhibition and COX favors the anti-inflammatory PGE3 production (Fig. 14.2). Consequently, the inflammatory cascade is blunted, and the synthesis of inflammatory cytokines interleukin (IL)-1, tumor necrosis factor (TNF)-α, IL-6, and IL-8 is decreased [12, 23]. Downstream mediators of nuclear factor (NF)-κB pathway are also inhibited, which restricts chronic microglia activation [24]. While EPA is a precursor for resolvins [25], DHA is a precursor of both resolvins, and protectins synthesis; both of which halt inflammation [26] and possibly limit the damage from concussion.

Researchers have found that O3FAs increase neuronal survival following injury by activating cellular N-methyl-D-aspartate (NMDA) receptors [27], and

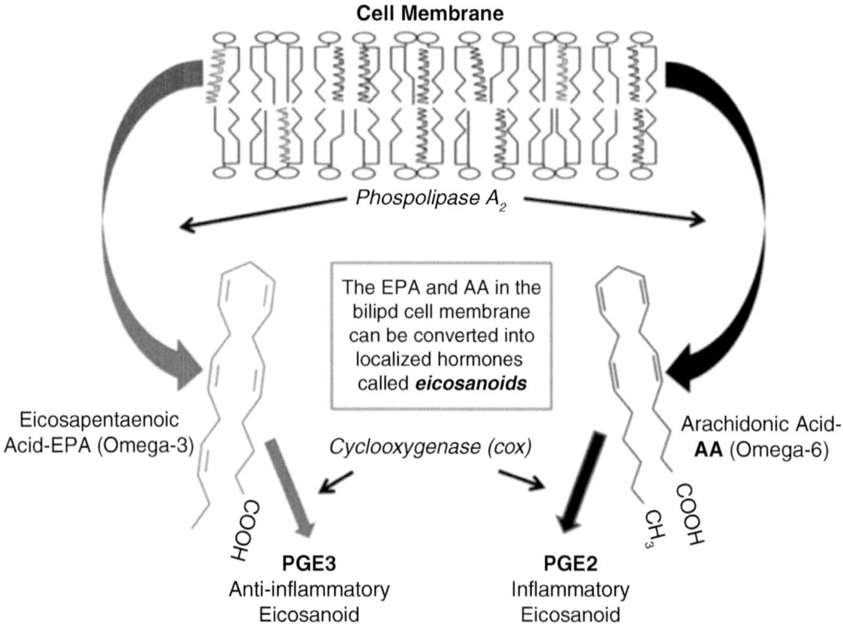

Fig. 14.2 The cell membrane contains various concentrations of both omega-3 EFA and omega-6 EFA. Following trauma or injury, COX enzyme maintains an equilibrium between the conversion of AA from omega-6 EFA into proinflammatory PGE2, and anti-inflammatory PGE3 from EPA. (Courtesy of Maroon et al. [5])

Abbreviations: EFA essential fatty acids, COX cyclooxygenase, AA arachidonic acid, PGE prostaglandin E, EPA eicosapentaenoic acid suppressing the toxic effects of the excitatory neurotransmitter glutamate, which activates amino-3-hydroxy-5-methylisoxazole-4-propionic acid (AMPA) receptors [28], following TBI. DHA helps attenuate the inhibition of antioxidant enzymes, downregulate nitrous oxide (NO) production, and inhibit intracellular Ca^{2+} influx and subsequent neuronal death following brain injury [11, 14, 19]. This also promotes neurogenesis through neuronal neurotrophic stimulated replication and growth [29]. Additionally, DHA undergoes oxidation following cerebral injury to produce neuroprotectin D1, a counter-proinflammatory messenger. This ultimately downregulates neutrophil infiltration and the expression of inflammatory TNF-α, IL-6, and COX-2 in microglial cells [30]. One study in American football players who received DHA supplementation observed a decrease in neurofilament light (NFL) levels across the football season [31]. NFL levels are known to increase to up to 400% after repetitive head trauma [32].

Adequate supplementation of omega-3 EFA has indeed shown to improve a wide range of brain-related conditions with a common underlying inflammatory cascade; which include PCS and chronic traumatic encephalopathy (CTE). They can supply the brain with the needed fatty acids for healing and reduce neurologic inflammation and its undesired complications.

The suggested dosing is a total of 1.5–5.0 g of approximately equal parts of EPA and DHA fish oil per day for the improvement of concussion symptoms [5, 31]. Omega-3 fish oils are readily available, highly safe, and well tolerated but should be used with caution in those on prescription anticoagulants because of their potential to increase bleeding [13]. Dosing requirements for those on other prescription medications or with underlying diseases should also be adjusted. Common side effects include belching, heartburn, bad breath, nausea, and loose stools.

Resveratrol

Resveratrol is a naturally occurring polyphenol found in many different plant sources. Polyphenols protect plants from microbial infections and excessive ultraviolet radiation [33]; and provide much of the nutritional benefits behind the consumption of fruits and vegetables. This entails significant anticancer, anti-inflammatory, antioxidant, and DNA-protective actions [34]. Resveratrol was discovered in 1940, and has since gained popularity due the aforementioned properties, and its ability to increase insulin sensitivity in both animals and humans [35]. Its consumption has also cleared β-amyloid and reduced the risk of Alzheimer's disease in population studies [36]. More importantly, resveratrol crosses the blood brain barrier (BBB) and possesses much of the neuroprotective effects and anti-inflammatory properties seen with O3FA supplementation. This includes the suppression of proinflammatory PGE2 synthesis, downregulation of TNF-α- and IL-1β-induced NF-κB and microglial activation [33, 37].

Following neurologic injury, free radicals induce lipid peroxidation of arachidonic acid in neuronal cell membranes [38]. This then leads to the formation of neurotoxic aldehydes that inhibit cellular protein function. Resveratrol contains multiple phenolic hydroxyl groups [38], which allow it to donate electrons and neutralize the superoxide and lipid peroxyl radicals produced following injury [39]. In animals, resveratrol is also able to attenuate glutamate release and ecotoxicity [40], reduce neutrophil infiltration, and improve Na^+/K^+-ATPase activity following TBI [21].

Researchers at the University of Pittsburgh found that administrating 100 mg/kg of resveratrol to rats after controlled brain injury, provided neuroprotective effects in the form of motor performance and visuospatial memory [21]. Other animal studies demonstrated reduced oxidative stress, neuronal loss, and lesion volume as well as improved behavioral measures of locomotion, anxiety, and memory [41]. Furthermore, resveratrol supplementation has been found to increase cerebral blood flow [42] and at higher doses extend animal life span [43], slow the development of chronic neurodegenerative disease, and improve patient outcomes following stroke, global cerebral ischemia, spinal cord injury, and TBI [44, 45].

Resveratrol is found in multiple natural dietary sources, including peanuts and chocolate, but is most concentrated in the plant *Polygonum cuspidatum* (Japanese knotweed) and the skins of red wine grapes [34, 37]. It is also commercially available in its bioactive trans- form as a dietary supplement [33]. The typical suggested supplement dose is between 50 to 500 mg/day. It is generally safe with no significant reported side effects; however, patients taking antiplatelet- or coagulation-altering products should be cautioned about the observed antiplatelet effects of resveratrol [33].

Vitamin D3

Vitamin D is one of the fat-soluble vitamins known for physiologic calcium homeostasis and bone health. Its active form, vitamin D3, is produced in the skin by ultraviolet B radiation from the sun and is involved in a number of cellular and tissue functions. It impacts immunity, inflammation, cardiovascular health as well as neuronal regulation [46, 47].

Vitamin D's cholesterol backbone allows it to easily traverse neural cell membranes in the brain where it is commonly referred to as vitamin D hormone (VDH). VDH functions as a neurosteroid and binds to nuclear vitamin D receptors to modulate neuronal gene transcription. Vitamin D deficiency increases inflammatory damage and behavioral impairment following experimental head injury [18]. When supplemented following TBI, VDH has been shown to reduce inflammation, necrosis, apoptosis, and cerebral edema [48], especially when administered with progesterone [49]. Patients supplemented with both Vitamin D3 and progesterone experienced better recovery rates following severe TBI [48]; the combination is thought to induce reductions in astrocyte activation and NF-kB phosphorylation [50].

In general, VDH is known to inhibit the upregulation of the proinflammatory cytokines IL-6, IL-17, TNF-α, and IFN-γ by inhibiting NF-κB [51] and increasing IL-10 levels; the anti-inflammatory cytokine known to be lower in the brains of patients with Alzheimer's disease [52]. However, its neuroprotective effects specifically are thought to be due to decreased glutamate-induced neuronal cell death [49] and downregulation of L-type calcium channels expression in neurons following TBI [53]. This is primarily via increasing phosphorylation, and subsequent activation, of mitogen activated protein kinase (MAPK) [49]. The upregulation of MAPK then induces the expression of antiapoptotic genes such as *Bcl-2*, which protects neurons from toxic injury.

The importance of Vitamin D intake and supplementation extends beyond concussive head injury. Vitamin D deficiency is seasonal and geographical, whereby risk is higher in winter and in southern parts of the United States [54]. It is a significant public health risk in the United States due to the use of sunblock, dark-colored skin, and decreased activity levels [55]. High-risk populations include institutionalized and hospitalized elderly patients as well as up to 30% of athletes [56].

Dietary sources of vitamin D include fatty fish, fish liver oils, fortified milk, cheese, beef, and egg yolks [55]. The current recommended dietary allowance is between 800 and 1000 IU/day, but the replacement dose in deficient athletes appears to lie between 35,000 and 50,000 IU/wk. [57]. Vitamin D supplementation is generally safe and should be tailored to blood levels. Excessive amounts may increase calcium in the blood and risk the development of kidney stones and arterial hardening.

Curcumin

Curcumin is a flavonoid compound found in the Indian spice turmeric; a flowering plant of the ginger family that provides the yellow pigment seen in many curries [58]. Flavonoids have been historically used to treat digestive disorders and promote wound healing [12, 22]. They have gained more popularity recently largely due to their potent anti-inflammatory, antioxidant, and antineoplastic effects [58]. The anti-inflammatory actions of curcumin arise from its ability to suppress messenger RNA (mRNA) production for proinflammatory mediators, activation of Nrf2, and inhibition of NF-κB, COX-1, and COX-2 [59]. This had made it comparable to nonsteroidal anti-inflammatory drugs (NSAIDs) in effect but with a safer side effect profile [5].

Curcumin is neuroprotectant after TBI in animals [38, 60]. It suppresses neuroinflammation, protects the brain from neurotoxins [39], and potentially promotes memory and cognitive function [61]. The polyphenolic derivatives of curcumin prevent post-traumatic perineuronal microgliosis and reactive astrogliosis [62], and promote neuronal survival and synaptic plasticity. They decrease oxidative stress [38, 60] and the edema following TBI and ischemic neurodegeneration by counteracting post-traumatic upregulation of astrocyte water channel aquaporin-4 [62, 63]. The antiapoptotic function of curcumin is similar to that of vitamin D, and that is by upregulating the expression of *Bcl-2* gene. The administration of curcumin both pre- and post-injury seems beneficial [61]. Yet, the therapeutic window for significant neuroprotection after injury seems to be less than 1 hour and far greater effects were observed when it was supplemented before injury [60].

Curcumin is safe and available for supplementation at nano-sized units for better gastrointestinal absorption. The suggested dosage of supplementation is 400–600 mg taken three times per day [5]. Extended use may cause stomach disturbance and ulcers in rare cases.

Magnesium and Vitamin B2 (Riboflavin)

Magnesium is an essential intracellular cation involved in the stability of polyphosphate compounds cells and a multitude of vital human processes, including protein synthesis, smooth muscle tone, energy metabolism, immune system regulation, and the maintenance of calcium and ionic transmembrane gradients [5]. It has been commonly prescribed as a laxative, antacid, or to correct abnormal nerve excitation or blood vessel spasm owing to its role in mitochondrial membrane stability and coupling of oxidative phosphorylation. More importantly, magnesium decline is thought to play a major role in the neuronal pathogenesis following TBI. Magnesium levels seem to be significantly lower after TBI in both animals and humans; this increases the likelihood of apoptosis by interrupting sufficient energy production during recovery [64]. Its administration attenuates immunoexcitotoxicity, especially in individuals with hypomagnesaemia.

Magnesium regulates the influx of Ca^{2+} in neurons by decreasing glutamate release, and acts as a noncompetitive inhibitor of NMDA receptors [65]. Following a concussion, the decrease in intracellular Mg levels and altered cellular membrane potentials result in transient neurologic dysfunction [64] and neural destruction seen in severe cases. Humans and animals with low cerebrospinal fluid (CSF) or serum magnesium levels experience worse neurological outcomes following ischemia and TBI [66]. The supplementation of magnesium post-injury improves both Glasgow outcome scale and Glasgow coma scale scores, but seems to have no mortality benefit in patients with severe TBI [67].

Magnesium similarly decreases edema and lesion size in animals by downregulating the transcription of aquaporin-4 channels [68]. The administration of magnesium has similarly improved functional outcomes in stroke patients and reduced the risk of cerebral palsy in preterm births [69]. Low cytosolic levels of magnesium have also been linked to the pathogenesis of migraine and cluster headaches as well as to the precipitation of seizures [70]. It may therefore have implications in post-concussion recovery period and post-traumatic seizures.

Vitamin B2 (Riboflavin) is a co-factor in oxidative metabolism and seems to also have therapeutic potential in the treatment of human TBI. Riboflavin administration following traumatic frontal cortex contusion in animals reduced lesion volume, edema formation, and expression of glial fibrillary acidic protein (GFAP), as well as significantly improved behavioral outcomes [71]. The combination of Mg chloride and riboflavin seems to have a synergistic effect therapeutically as their administration together in one animal study improved functional recovery to a greater extent when administered shortly after frontal cortical contusion injury [72]. Their combination may also reduce the frequency and severity of post-traumatic migraine headaches [73]. A randomized clinical trial of Mg, riboflavin, and Q10 supplementation demonstrated significantly reduced symptom severity migraine attacks [74].

More than 60% of Americans aged >20 years as well as the majority of athletes receive inadequate amounts of magnesium [75]. Magnesium is found naturally in nuts, whole grains, legumes, and vegetables, as well as in over-the-counter supplements with the recommended dosage being between 80 and 420 mg/day, depending on age and sex of the patient [76]. Apart from minor gastrointestinal side effects, patients on calcium channel blockers for high blood pressure, for example, should exercise caution due to the possibility of excessively low blood pressure drop when combined with magnesium [76].

N-Acetyl Cysteine

N-acetyl cysteine (NAC) is an acetyl derivative of the amino acid cysteine and is among the few supplements to have shown promising data in clinical trials. It is commonly used as an antidote for acetaminophen overdose and toxicity and has also shown to reduce recovery times in military blast mild TBI, when supplemented within 24 hours of injury [77]. In animal studies, its supplementation after TBI showed significant behavioral recovery when administered alone and in combination with minocycline or selenium [77]. NAC is safe, well-tolerated, and widely available over the counter, but physicians and patients should take note of its interaction with nitroglycerin causing vasodilation [78]. Mild side effects include nausea, vomiting, and gastrointestinal upset [78]. No recommended dose has been suggested and further studies are needed to elucidate its antioxidant properties in sports concussions.

Vitamins E and C

The supplementation of vitamins E and C have been studied in both animals and humans following concussive injuries. Ascorbic acid (vitamin C) is a water-soluble free radical scavenger that helps transform vitamin E to its active form; a lipid-soluble lipid peroxidation inhibitor present in high concentrations in the brain [61]. The inhibition of lipid peroxidation has been linked to neuroprotective effects following TBIs [38]. While the supplementation of vitamin E in rats post-concussion minimized functional neurologic deficits and microscopic brain damage, as well as reduced amyloid accumulation [63] and oxidative stress; the combination of both vitamins C and E has proved superior than supplementation with either alone [79]. This is evident by the reduced brain injury due to oxidative stress following their supplementation.

Patients supplemented with vitamin E after severe TBI experienced decreased mortality and increased Glasgow outcome scores, and had decreased edema and lesion size when treated with vitamin C. Treatment with both, however, was better than each treatment alone. Both vitamins are readily available, but vitamin E can cause hemorrhage at high dosages. Further studies are needed to evaluate their efficacy in sports concussions and recommend an appropriate supplementation dose for therapy.

Nicotinamide Ribose

Nicotinamide, or vitamin B3, is a precursor of neuronal nicotinamide adenine dinucleotide (NAD+). Its involvement in the many cellular metabolic and immune responses to pathophysiologic stress mechanisms makes it a subject of interest. Additionally, studies reported its enhanced ability to attenuate mediators of axonal degeneration when supplemented in rodents recovering from brain injury [80]. Elevated NAD concentrations reduced the damage caused by Sterile alpha and TIR motif-containing 1 (SARM1) protein, an essential mediator of axonal death during injury and disease [81]. An ongoing human clinical trial is currently being conducted to observe its effect in American football athletes (NCT02721537). No dosage recommendations have been proposed, but sources of nicotinamide ribose include dairy milk, yeast, and beer [80].

Melatonin

Melatonin is a hormone secreted by the pineal gland in the brain and is primarily responsible for regulating the sleep-wake cycle. It is commonly used to alleviate jet lag symptoms and adjust nocturnal rhythms in travelers. Its antioxidative, anti-apoptotic, neuroprotective, and anti-inflammatory properties [82] make it worth exploring as an alternative treatment in concussive head injuries, especially since sleep-wake disturbances are common following TBI [83]. Sleep disturbances have been shown to prolong healing and recovery times after concussions and affect the severity of post-concussive symptoms in athletes and nonathletes alike [84].

Brain injury seems to disrupt the synthesis and production of melatonin. Patients who experienced mild-severe TBIs have shown decreased sleep efficiency, increased wake after sleep onset, delayed melatonin secretion, and significantly lower levels of evening melatonin production associated with less rapid eye movement (REM) sleep when compared to controls [83]. Melatonin has showed neuroprotective properties in animals following TBI [82]. Additionally, a systematic review in children with TBIs concluded that melatonin appears to be promising for the management of sleep impairment [85] and another similar clinical trial by the University of Calgary is currently underway (NCT01874847). Melatonin may also be effective in treating and decreasing the frequency of primary headache disorders such as migraines and cluster headaches which represent another common complaint throughout the delayed phase of concussive symptoms [86].

Melatonin is a widely available safe supplement that holds promise in the management of sports concussions sleep symptoms. A dose of 0.5–5 mg, followed by a maintenance dose after realignment, has been suggested. Further studies are warranted to validate its use and effectiveness in sports concussions.

Caffeine

Caffeine, the most commonly used psychoactive agent in the world, is a central nervous system stimulant of the methylxanthine class. It also affects the cardiovascular system and is extremely popular worldwide, especially among athletes. It is known to enhance memory, alertness, and physical performance. It is of concern to the concussive sports patient because of its alternating effects in the short- versus long-term. Caffeine inhibits the adenosine 1 (A1) and A2A receptors [87] responsible for suppressing glutamate release and excessive inflammatory cytokine production [88]. It therefore interferes with the neuroprotective actions of adenosine in ischemic-hypoxic conditions. The adverse outcomes as a result of caffeine supplementation in mild TBI [88] are possibly due to the increased intracellular calcium concentration and activation of adenylyl cyclase, as a result of IP-3 receptor stimulation [87].

Conversely, the chronic ingestion of caffeine has shown to be beneficial in animal and humans experiencing severe TBI [88, 89]. The difference in effectiveness of caffeine between mild and severe TBIs could be explained by the differences in cAMP concentrations in CSF. The elevated CSF caffeine levels following severe TBI in humans showed outcome benefits [89]. This could be due to the increased A1 receptor expression following chronic caffeine ingestion, which helps suppress inflammation and glutamate release.

Caffeine is widely available as a supplement, and is found in tea, chocolate, soft drinks, and energy drinks. No dosage recommendations have been suggested, but further studies are needed to determine its efficacy, safety, and adverse effect profiles following TBI. Physicians involved in neurocognitive testing and return of play following concussion should take note of altered reaction times following caffeine ingestion close to assessment.

Green Tea

Green tea is produced from the leaves of the plant species *Camellia sinensis* (L.) Kuntze [89]. It is among the most popular consumed beverages and has shown to possess pharmacologically active polyphenols that are of benefit to a variety of diseases, including cancer, obesity, diabetes, cardiovascular disease, and neurodegenerative diseases. Its antioxidant and anti-inflammatory properties make it a subject of interest in the management of concussive head injuries.

Tea polyphenols directly scavenge reactive oxygen and nitrogen species, inhibit the activity of nitric oxide synthase, xanthine oxidase, cyclooxygenases, lipoxygenases, NF-κB, and activator protein-1. Epigallocatechin-3 galate (EGCG) is the most abundant polyphenol or catechin in green tea and is behind many of those anti-inflammatory and neuroprotective benefits. Studies have shown that EGCG inhibits TNF-α activation of IL-8 gene expression through the inhibition of NF-κB [89]. The inhibition of NF-κB is achieved by inhibiting the degradation of IL-1 receptor-associated kinase (IRAK), an enzyme responsible for the activation of NF-κB, or by interfering with the cell receptor binding of IL-1β [90]. EGCG may also have post-transcriptional anti-inflammatory effects by destabilizing proinflammatory mRNA [90]. The neuroprotective benefits of EGCG have been mainly observed in neurodegenerative diseases. This is through the inhibition of *N*-methyl-D-aspartate-induced cellular damage in neurons and the production of antioxidant enzymes such as glutathione S-transferases and superoxide dismutase. EGCG was also found to suppress the neurotoxicity induced by Aβ, as it activates glycogen synthase kinase-3β (GSK-3β) and inhibits the cytoplasmic nonreceptor tyrosine kinase Abl/FE65, which is primarily involved in neuronal development and nuclear translocation [91].

Green tea and its extracts are safe and widely available for use. The usual recommendation is around 300–400 mg/day or around four cups, but further studies are needed to validate its efficacy in mild TBIs.

Branched Chain Amino Acids

Branched-chain amino acids (BCAAs) have an aliphatic side chain and a branch. They are abundant in humans and comprise almost one-third of all amino acids present in our bodies. The three known proteinogenic BCAAs, valine, leucine, and isoleucine, play a vital role in muscle protein synthesis and have been popularized among athletes and bodybuilders as muscle building supplements. They also cross the BBB and contribute to the synthesis of neurotransmitters glutamate and gamma aminobutyric acid. Neurometabolic cascades associated with concussive brain injuries have been shown to decrease levels of BCAAs [92] and their supplementation following severe TBI allowed patients to exhibit cognitive benefits per disability rating scale scores [91]. BCAAs are the building blocks of protein and are found in meats, dairy, nuts, beans, and are also available in pill or powder form. Further research is required to examine their effect in mild TBI and supplementation in sports concussions.

Creatine

Creatine is an amino acid naturally synthesized in gastrointestinal tract from the amino acids glycine, arginine, and methionine [90]. It is phosphorylated by creatine kinase to phosphocreatine [90] to supply metabolically active areas of the body, such as skeletal muscles, heart, and brain with energy. It is among the most studied supplements in sports science and is popular among athletes that seek to increase their strength performance and muscle building activities [90]. Studies have shown neuroprotective effects in animals subjected to a creatine rich diet following brain injury [93]. This is of particular importance because creatine and phosphocreatine levels are decreased after mild TBI.

Neuroprotection is believed to be related to the maintenance of mitochondrial bioenergetics. This is achieved by the replenishment of cellular ATP levels, resulting in the reduction of mitochondrial permeability, free oxygen radicals, and calcium levels. In pediatric patients, creatine supplementation following severe TBI improved short- and long-term outcomes. This included less time being intubated, less time in the intensive care unit, and improved amnesia acutely; and communication, behavior, and cognitive benefits long-term [94]. Creatine is widely available as a supplement and can also be obtained from protein rich foods such as poultry, meat, and fish. It is often dosed at 5 g/day, but further studies are needed to validate its use in mild TBIs and sports concussions.

Key Learning Points

- The majority of sports-related concussive episodes (80–90%) resolve spontaneously in 7–10 days.
- Nonpharmaceutical therapies include O3FAs, resveratrol, vitamin D, curcumin, magnesium, vitamins B3, E, C, melatonin, green tea, creatine, BCAAs, and caffeine, among others.
- FDA has not approved the use of any dietary supplement or alternative therapies for the prevention of concussions or the reduction of post-concussion symptoms.

Conclusions

We have described the use and scientific basis of several anti-inflammatory supplements or alternative remedies that have shown to attenuate brain injury, excitotoxic cell signaling, and microglial activation. More recently, additional alternative therapies have been explored in the management of concussive head injuries and headaches with varying effects, including cranial nerve blocks, botulinum toxin injections, acupuncture, transcranial direct stimulation, physiotherapy, electroconvulsive therapy, and hyperbaric oxygen [5, 95, 96].

In general, little has been investigated regarding the management of sports concussions with supplements and medications. As of now, the FDA has not approved the use of any dietary supplement for the prevention of concussions or the reduction of post-concussion symptoms. Long-term clinical trials are still required to document their efficacy in humans, particularly in regard to mild TBIs. Compared to other forms of concussions (assault or collision), sports-related concussions seem less likely to result in PCS [1]. Though, PCS can be devastating to athletes and their careers, and require further medical attention along with the appropriate social support. Prevention is certainly the most important step in management, followed by the initial recognition of a concussive episode and prompt management.

References

1. Harmon KG, Drezner JA, Gammons M, et al. American Medical Society for Sports Medicine position statement: concussion in sport. Br J Sports Med. 2013;47(1):15–26.
2. Dashnaw ML, Petraglia AL, Bailes JE. An overview of the basic science of concussion and subconcussion: where we are and where we are going. Neurosurg Focus. 2012;33(6):1–9.
3. McCrory P, Meeuwisse WH, Aubry M, et al. Consensus statement on concussion in sport: the 4th International Conference on Concussion in Sport held in Zurich, November 2012. Br J Sports Med. 2013;47(5):250–8.
4. Jackson WT, Starling AJ. Concussion evaluation and management. Med Clin North Am. 2019;103(2):251–61.
5. Maroon JC, Lepere DB, Blaylock RL, Bost JW. Postconcussion syndrome: a review of pathophysiology and potential nonpharmacological approaches to treatment. Phys Sportsmed. 2012;40(4):73–87.
6. Petraglia AL, Maroon JC, Bailes JE. From the field of play to the field of combat: a review of the pharmacological management of concussion. Neurosurgery. 2012;70(6):1520–33.
7. Gómez-Pinilla F. Brain foods: the effects of nutrients on brain function. Nat Rev Neurosci. 2008;9(7):568–78.
8. Lewis M, Ghassemi P, Hibbeln J. Therapeutic use of omega-3 fatty acids in severe head trauma. Am J Emerg Med. 2013;31(1):273.e5–273.e2.73E8.
9. Curtis CL, Hughes CE, Flannery CR, Little CB, Harwood JL, Caterson B. n-3 fatty acids specifically modulate catabolic factors involved in articular cartilage degradation. J Biol Chem. 2000;275(2):721–4.
10. Calder PC. n-3 polyunsaturated fatty acids, inflammation, and inflammatory diseases. Am J Clin Nutr. 2006;83(6 Suppl):1505S–19S.
11. Mills JD, Bailes JE, Sedney CL, Hutchins H, Sears B. Omega-3 fatty acid supplementation and reduction of traumatic axonal injury in a rodent head injury model. J Neurosurg. 2011;114(1):77–84.
12. Maroon JC, Bost JW, Borden MK, Lorenz KM, Ross NA. Natural antiinflammatory agents for pain relief in athletes. Neurosurg Focus. 2006;21(4):E11.
13. Maroon JC, B. J. Fish oil: the natural anti-inflammatory. Laguna Beach, CA: Basic Health Publications, Inc.; 2006.
14. Wu A, Ying Z, Gomez-Pinilla F. Dietary omega-3 fatty acids normalize BDNF levels, reduce oxidative damage, and counteract learning disability after traumatic brain injury in rats. J Neurotrauma. 2004;21(10):1457–67.
15. Mills JD, Hadley K, Bailes JE. Dietary supplementation with the omega-3 fatty acid docosahexaenoic acid in traumatic brain injury. Neurosurgery. 2011;68(2):474–81.
16. Wu A, Ying Z, Gomez-Pinilla F. Omega-3 fatty acids supplementation restores mechanisms that maintain brain homeostasis in traumatic brain injury. J Neurotrauma. 2007;24(10):1587–95.
17. Bailes JE, Mills JD. Docosahexaenoic acid reduces traumatic axonal injury in a rodent head injury model. J Neurotrauma. 2010;27(9):1617–24.

18. Yates A, Norwig J, Maroon JC, et al. Evaluation of lipid profiles and the use of omega-3 essential Fatty Acid in professional football players. Sports Health. 2009;1(1):21–30.
19. Bazan NG. Omega-3 fatty acids, pro-inflammatory signaling and neuroprotection. Curr Opin Clin Nutr Metab Care. 2007;10(2):136–41.
20. Shin SS, Dixon CE. Oral fish oil restores striatal dopamine release after traumatic brain injury. Neurosci Lett. 2011;496(3):168–71.
21. Singleton RH, Yan HQ, Fellows-Mayle W, Dixon CE. Resveratrol attenuates behavioral impairments and reduces cortical and hippocampal loss in a rat controlled cortical impact model of traumatic brain injury. J Neurotrauma. 2010;27(6):1091–9.
22. Maroon JC, Bost JW. Omega-3 fatty acids (fish oil) as an anti-inflammatory: an alternative to nonsteroidal anti-inflammatory drugs for discogenic pain. Surg Neurol. 2006;65(4):326–31.
23. Mayer K, Meyer S, Reinholz-Muhly M, et al. Short-time infusion of fish oil-based lipid emulsions, approved for parenteral nutrition, reduces monocyte proinflammatory cytokine generation and adhesive interaction with endothelium in humans. J Immunol. 2003;171(9):4837–43.
24. Lonergan PE, Martin DS, Horrobin DF, Lynch MA. Neuroprotective actions of eicosapentaenoic acid on lipopolysaccharide-induced dysfunction in rat hippocampus. J Neurochem. 2004;91(1):20–9.
25. Barrett EC, McBurney MI, Ciappio ED. ω-3 fatty acid supplementation as a potential therapeutic aid for the recovery from mild traumatic brain injury/concussion. Adv Nutr. 2014;5(3):268–77.
26. Kohli P, Levy BD. Resolvins and protectins: mediating solutions to inflammation. Br J Pharmacol. 2009;158(4):960–71.
27. Högyes E, Nyakas C, Kiliaan A, Farkas T, Penke B, Luiten PG. Neuroprotective effect of developmental docosahexaenoic acid supplement against excitotoxic brain damage in infant rats. Neuroscience. 2003;119(4):999–1012.
28. Strokin M, Chechneva O, Reymann KG, Reiser G. Neuroprotection of rat hippocampal slices exposed to oxygen-glucose deprivation by enrichment with docosahexaenoic acid and by inhibition of hydrolysis of docosahexaenoic acid-containing phospholipids by calcium independent phospholipase A2. Neuroscience. 2006;140(2):547–53.
29. Robson LG, Dyall S, Sidloff D, Michael-Titus AT. Omega-3 polyunsaturated fatty acids increase the neurite outgrowth of rat sensory neurones throughout development and in aged animals. Neurobiol Aging. 2010;31(4):678–87.
30. Lu DY, Tsao YY, Leung YM, Su KP. Docosahexaenoic acid suppresses neuroinflammatory responses and induces heme oxygenase-1 expression in BV-2 microglia: implications of antidepressant effects for ω-3 fatty acids. Neuropsychopharmacology. 2010;35(11):2238–48.
31. Oliver JM, Jones MT, Kirk KM, et al. Effect of docosahexaenoic acid on a biomarker of head trauma in American football. Med Sci Sports Exerc. 2016;48(6):974–82.
32. Papa L, Ramia MM, Edwards D, Johnson BD, Slobounov SM. Systematic review of clinical studies examining biomarkers of brain injury in athletes after sports-related concussion. J Neurotrauma. 2015;32(10):661–73.
33. Maroon JC, Bost JW, Maroon A. Natural anti-inflammatory agents for pain relief. Surg Neurol Int. 2010;1:80.
34. Maroon JC. The longevity factor: how resveratrol and red wine activate genes for a longer and healthier life. New York: Atria; 2009.
35. Maroon JC, Bost J. Concussion management at the NFL, college, high school, and youth sports levels. Clin Neurosurg. 2011;58:51–6.
36. Marambaud P, Zhao H, Davies P. Resveratrol promotes clearance of Alzheimer's disease amyloid-beta peptides. J Biol Chem. 2005;280(45):37377–82.
37. Lopez MS, Dempsey RJ, Vemuganti R. Resveratrol neuroprotection in stroke and traumatic CNS injury. Neurochem Int. 2015;89:75–82.
38. Hall ED, Vaishnav RA, Mustafa AG. Antioxidant therapies for traumatic brain injury. Neurotherapeutics. 2010;7(1):51–61.
39. Mendes Arent A, de Souza LF, Walz R, Dafre AL. Perspectives on molecular biomarkers of oxidative stress and antioxidant strategies in traumatic brain injury. Biomed Res Int. 2014;2014:723060.

40. Li C, Yan Z, Yang J, et al. Neuroprotective effects of resveratrol on ischemic injury mediated by modulating the release of neurotransmitter and neuromodulator in rats. Neurochem Int. 2010;56(3):495–500.
41. Sönmez U, Sönmez A, Erbil G, Tekmen I, Baykara B. Neuroprotective effects of resveratrol against traumatic brain injury in immature rats. Neurosci Lett. 2007;420(2):133–7.
42. Wightman EL, Reay JL, Haskell CF, Williamson G, Dew TP, Kennedy DO. Effects of resveratrol alone or in combination with piperine on cerebral blood flow parameters and cognitive performance in human subjects: a randomised, double-blind, placebo-controlled, cross-over investigation. Br J Nutr. 2014;112(2):203–13.
43. Baur JA, Pearson KJ, Price NL, et al. Resveratrol improves health and survival of mice on a high-calorie diet. Nature. 2006;444(7117):337–42.
44. Karuppagounder SS, Pinto JT, Xu H, Chen HL, Beal MF, Gibson GE. Dietary supplementation with resveratrol reduces plaque pathology in a transgenic model of Alzheimer's disease. Neurochem Int. 2009;54(2):111–8.
45. Richard T, Pawlus AD, Iglésias ML, et al. Neuroprotective properties of resveratrol and derivatives. Ann N Y Acad Sci. 2011;1215:103–8.
46. Abou Al-Shaar H, Bohlega SA. Vitamin D deficiency in muscle. In: Angelini C, editor. Acquired neuromuscular disorders – pathogenesis, diagnosis and treatment. Switzerland: Springer; 2016. p. 155–62.
47. Bacchetta J, Ranchin B, Dubourg L, Cochat P. Vitamine D : un acteur majeur en santé ? [Vitamin D revisited: a cornerstone of health?]. Arch Pediatr. 2010;17(12):1687–95.
48. Lawrence DW, Sharma B. A review of the neuroprotective role of vitamin D in traumatic brain injury with implications for supplementation post-concussion. Brain Inj. 2016;30(8):960–8.
49. Atif F, Sayeed I, Ishrat T, Stein DG. Progesterone with vitamin D affords better neuroprotection against excitotoxicity in cultured cortical neurons than progesterone alone. Mol Med. 2009;15(9–10):328–36.
50. Tang H, Hua F, Wang J, et al. Progesterone and vitamin D combination therapy modulates inflammatory response after traumatic brain injury. Brain Inj. 2015;29(10):1165–74.
51. Chen Y, Kong J, Sun T, et al. 1,25-Dihydroxyvitamin D_3 suppresses inflammation-induced expression of plasminogen activator inhibitor-1 by blocking nuclear factor-κB activation. Arch Biochem Biophys. 2011;507(2):241–7.
52. Lio D, Licastro F, Scola L, et al. Interleukin-10 promoter polymorphism in sporadic Alzheimer's disease. Genes Immun. 2003;4(3):234–8.
53. Brewer LD, Thibault V, Chen KC, Langub MC, Landfield PW, Porter NM. Vitamin D hormone confers neuroprotection in parallel with downregulation of L-type calcium channel expression in hippocampal neurons. J Neurosci. 2001;21(1):98–108.
54. Maruyama-Nagao A, Sakuraba K, Suzuki Y. Seasonal variations in vitamin D status in indoor and outdoor female athletes. Biomed Rep. 2016;5(1):113–7.
55. Hall LM, Kimlin MG, Aronov PA, et al. Vitamin D intake needed to maintain target serum 25-hydroxyvitamin D concentrations in participants with low sun exposure and dark skin pigmentation is substantially higher than current recommendations. J Nutr. 2010;140(3):542–50.
56. Backx E, van der Avoort C, Tieland M, et al. Seasonal variation in vitamin D status in elite athletes: a longitudinal study. Int J Sport Nutr Exerc Metab. 2017;27(1):6–10.
57. Owens DJ, Tang JC, Bradley WJ, et al. Efficacy of high-dose vitamin D supplements for elite athletes. Med Sci Sports Exerc. 2017;49(2):349–56.
58. Araújo CC, Leon LL. Biological activities of Curcuma longa L. Mem Inst Oswaldo Cruz. 2001;96(5):723–8.
59. Jiang H, Tian X, Guo Y, Duan W, Bu H, Li C. Activation of nuclear factor erythroid 2-related factor 2 cytoprotective signaling by curcumin protect primary spinal cord astrocytes against oxidative toxicity. Biol Pharm Bull. 2011;34(8):1194–7.
60. Samini F, Samarghandian S, Borji A, Mohammadi G, Bakaian M. Curcumin pretreatment attenuates brain lesion size and improves neurological function following traumatic brain injury in the rat. Pharmacol Biochem Behav. 2013;110:238–44.

61. Petraglia AL, Winkler EA, Bailes JE. Stuck at the bench: potential natural neuroprotective compounds for concussion. Surg Neurol Int. 2011;2:146.
62. Laird MD, Sukumari-Ramesh S, Swift AE, Meiler SE, Vender JR, Dhandapani KM. Curcumin attenuates cerebral edema following traumatic brain injury in mice: a possible role for aquaporin-4? J Neurochem. 2010;113(3):637–48.
63. Ashbaugh A, McGrew C. The role of nutritional supplements in sports concussion treatment. Curr Sports Med Rep. 2016;15(1):16–9.
64. Barkhoudarian G, Hovda DA, Giza CC. The molecular pathophysiology of concussive brain injury – an update. Phys Med Rehabil Clin N Am. 2016;27(2):373–93.
65. Mcintosh TK, Saatman KE, Raghupathi R. Review: calcium and the pathogenesis of traumatic CNS injury: cellular and molecular mechanisms. Neuroscientist. 1997;3(3):169–75.
66. McIntosh TK, Faden AI, Yamakami I, Vink R. Magnesium deficiency exacerbates and pretreatment improves outcome following traumatic brain injury in rats: 31P magnetic resonance spectroscopy and behavioral studies. J Neurotrauma. 1988;5(1):17–31.
67. Li W, Bai YA, Li YJ, et al. Magnesium sulfate for acute traumatic brain injury. J Craniofac Surg. 2015;26(2):393–8.
68. Ghabriel MN, Thomas A, Vink R. Magnesium restores altered aquaporin-4 immunoreactivity following traumatic brain injury to a pre-injury state. In: Hoff JT, Keep RF, Xi G, Hua Y, editors. Brain Edema XIII. Acta Neurochirurgica Supplementum, vol. 96. Vienna: Springer; 2006.
69. Reeves SA, Gibbs RS, Clark SL. Magnesium for fetal neuroprotection. Am J Obstet Gynecol. 2011;204(3):202.e1–202.e2024.
70. Lodi R, Montagna P, Soriani S, et al. Deficit of brain and skeletal muscle bioenergetics and low brain magnesium in juvenile migraine: an in vivo 31P magnetic resonance spectroscopy interictal study. Pediatr Res. 1997;42(6):866–71.
71. Slutsky I, Sadeghpour S, Li B, Liu G. Enhancement of synaptic plasticity through chronically reduced Ca2+ flux during uncorrelated activity. Neuron. 2004;44(5):835–49.
72. Barbre AB, Hoane MR. Magnesium and riboflavin combination therapy following cortical contusion injury in the rat. Brain Res Bull. 2006;69(6):639–46.
73. Teigen L, Boes CJ. An evidence-based review of oral magnesium supplementation in the preventive treatment of migraine. Cephalalgia. 2015;35(10):912–22.
74. Gaul C, Diener HC, Danesch U, Migravent® Study Group. Improvement of migraine symptoms with a proprietary supplement containing riboflavin, magnesium and Q10: a randomized, placebo-controlled, double-blind, multicenter trial. J Headache Pain. 2015;16:516.
75. Lukaski HC. Magnesium, zinc, and chromium nutriture and physical activity. Am J Clin Nutr. 2000;72(2 Suppl):585S–93S.
76. Sen AP, Gulati A. Use of magnesium in traumatic brain injury. Neurotherapeutics. 2010;7(1):91–9.
77. Hoffer ME, Balaban C, Slade MD, Tsao JW, Hoffer B. Amelioration of acute sequelae of blast induced mild traumatic brain injury by N-acetyl cysteine: a double-blind, placebo controlled study. PLoS One. 2013;8(1):e54163.
78. Bavarsad Shahripour R, Harrigan MR, Alexandrov AV. N-acetylcysteine (NAC) in neurological disorders: mechanisms of action and therapeutic opportunities. Brain Behav. 2014;4(2):108–22.
79. Ishaq GM, Saidu Y, Bilbis LS, Muhammad SA, Jinjir N, Shehu BB. Effects of α-tocopherol and ascorbic acid in the severity and management of traumatic brain injury in albino rats. J Neurosci Rural Pract. 2013;4(3):292–7.
80. Chi Y, Sauve AA. Nicotinamide riboside, a trace nutrient in foods, is a vitamin B3 with effects on energy metabolism and neuroprotection. Curr Opin Clin Nutr Metab Care. 2013;16(6):657–61.
81. Gerdts J, Summers DW, Milbrandt J, DiAntonio A. Axon self-destruction: new links among SARM1, MAPKs, and NAD+ metabolism. Neuron. 2016;89(3):449–60.
82. Naseem M, Parvez S. Role of melatonin in traumatic brain injury and spinal cord injury. ScientificWorldJournal. 2014;2014:586270.

83. Ponsford JL, Ziino C, Parcell DL, et al. Fatigue and sleep disturbance following traumatic brain injury–their nature, causes, and potential treatments. J Head Trauma Rehabil. 2012;27(3):224–33.
84. Hinds A, Jungquist CR, Leddy JJ, Seemant F, Baker JG, Willer B. Sleep disturbance in patients with chronic concussive effects. Concussion. 2016;1(3):CNC15.
85. Keegan LJ, Reed-Berendt R, Neilly E, Morrall MC, Murdoch-Eaton D. Effectiveness of melatonin for sleep impairment post paediatric acquired brain injury: evidence from a systematic review. Dev Neurorehabil. 2014;17(5):355–62.
86. Gelfand AA, Goadsby PJ. The role of melatonin in the treatment of primary headache disorders. Headache. 2016;56(8):1257–66.
87. Lusardi TA. Adenosine neuromodulation and traumatic brain injury. Curr Neuropharmacol. 2009;7(3):228–37.
88. Li W, Dai S, An J, et al. Chronic but not acute treatment with caffeine attenuates traumatic brain injury in the mouse cortical impact model. Neuroscience. 2008;151(4):1198–207.
89. Sachse KT, Jackson EK, Wisniewski SR, et al. Increases in cerebrospinal fluid caffeine concentration are associated with favorable outcome after severe traumatic brain injury in humans. J Cereb Blood Flow Metab. 2008;28(2):395–401.
90. Hall M, Trojian TH. Creatine supplementation. Curr Sports Med Rep. 2013;12(4):240–4.
91. Aquilani R, Boselli M, Boschi F, et al. Branched-chain amino acids may improve recovery from a vegetative or minimally conscious state in patients with traumatic brain injury: a pilot study. Arch Phys Med Rehabil. 2008;89(9):1642–7.
92. Jeter CB, Hergenroeder GW, Ward NH 3rd, Moore AN, Dash PK. Human mild traumatic brain injury decreases circulating branched-chain amino acids and their metabolite levels. J Neurotrauma. 2013;30(8):671–9.
93. Scheff SW, Dhillon HS. Creatine-enhanced diet alters levels of lactate and free fatty acids after experimental brain injury. Neurochem Res. 2004;29(2):469–79.
94. Sakellaris G, Kotsiou M, Tamiolaki M, et al. Prevention of complications related to traumatic brain injury in children and adolescents with creatine administration: an open label randomized pilot study. J Trauma. 2006;61(2):322–9.
95. Dobney DM, Miller MB, Tufts E. Non-pharmacological rehabilitation interventions for concussion in children: a scoping review. Disabil Rehabil. 2019;41(6):727–39.
96. Wright JK, Zant E, Groom K, Schlegel RE, Gilliland K. Case report: treatment of mild traumatic brain injury with hyperbaric oxygen. Undersea Hyperb Med. 2009;36(6):391–9.

Chapter 15
Chronic Traumatic Encephalopathy: Past, Present, and Future

Aneek Patel, Hussam Abou-Al-Shaar, Mansour Mathkour, and Joseph C. Maroon

Historical Context

Dementia Pugilista

In the early twentieth century, Dr. Harrison Martland observed a series of similar clinical findings in former boxers that appeared somewhat overlapping but clinically distinct from any existing neurological or psychiatric diagnosis. He noted "parkinsonian" motor issues affecting gait and speech along with substantial cognitive decline. In 1928, he published a series of 23 such cases and coined the term *punch drunk syndrome* to describe these changes [1].

Several others observed similar clinical findings in individuals subjected to chronic head trauma. In 1937, with additional cases, Dr. Millspaugh used the more elegant term, *dementia pugilista* [2]. On gross pathology, the brains of former boxers were found to have cerebral atrophy, ventriculomegaly, callosal thinning, scarred cerebellar tonsils, and substantia nigral pallor. Clinicians began to shift more attention to neurobehavioral changes that anecdotally seemed to occur in higher numbers among boxers [3]. However, the condition remained poorly described or understood, largely limited to correlations between nonspecific clinical findings with an

A. Patel
Department of Neurosurgery, New York University School of Medicine, New York, NY, USA

H. Abou-Al-Shaar · J. C. Maroon (✉)
Department of Neurological Surgery, University of Pittsburgh Medical Center, Pittsburgh, PA, USA
e-mail: maroonjc@upmc.edu

M. Mathkour
Department of Neurosurgery, Tulane Medical Center, New Orleans, LA, USA

M. E. Oppenlander (ed.), *Neurosurgical Care of Athletes*,
https://doi.org/10.1007/978-3-030-88227-3_15

array of gross pathological changes. Although the condition was largely considered rare for former boxers, the term chronic traumatic encephalopathy (CTE) was first used in 1940 by Bowman and Blau, acknowledging the pattern of recurrent head trauma that seemed to be associated with the described clinical and gross pathological changes [4–6].

Corsellis et al. were the first to note neuropathological changes in the brains of former boxers in 1973; they appreciated ventricular dilation and cavum septum pellucidum on gross pathology, but importantly also noted neurofibrillary tangles [7]. Although the discovery did not cause widespread concern—largely because the condition seemed particularly confined to boxers—the study eventually prompted a re-analysis of Corsellis' case along with additional autopsies in 1990. This second neuropathological study notably found a high prevalence of amyloid plaques, which had not previously been described in association with CTE [4].

Stepping Out of the Ring

CTE first garnered national attention in 2005, when Omalu et al. published the autopsy of former Steelers center Michael Webster—the first autopsy reporting CTE outside of boxing—after he unexpectedly died due to coronary atherosclerotic disease complications 12 years after retiring from the National Football League (NFL). On gross pathology, his brain had no cerebral atrophy or cerebellar scarring and mild pallor of the substantia nigra. Neuropathologically, however, his brain was found to have sparse tau neurofibrillary tangles and diffuse amyloid plaques, as well as mild gliosis and neural loss in the frontal, parietal, and temporal cortices. Importantly, his pathological findings were correlated with neurobehavioral changes prior to his death, including parkinsonism, major depressive disorder, and cognitive impairment in the absence of any family history of Alzheimer's disease [8]. In the following year, the group published the autopsy findings of a second former NFL player, Terry Long, who in this case had committed suicide and had also been previously diagnosed with major depressive disorder. Grossly, his brain showed mild substantia nigral pallor, a cavum septum pellucidum, and no cerebral atrophy. Neuropathologically, tau neurofibrillary tangles were found diffusely. However, amyloid plaques and Lewy bodies were absent [9].

Defining CTE

With rising national discussions about a poorly understood connection between head trauma and neuropsychiatric changes with potential neuropathological underpinnings—and its implications on a major athletic industry that extended into youth activities—there was a priority to understand and to clearly delineate the nature of CTE from a pathological and behavioral standpoint.

Neuropathological Criteria

In 2013, McKee et al. published the largest case series on CTE at the time, autopsying the brains of 85 individuals with a history of repeated head trauma (a combination of contact athletes and military veterans) and comparing them with 18 age-matched controls. In their study, they found that 80% of the brain donors who had experienced chronic head trauma had neuropathological findings consistent with what they understood to be CTE [10]. At its core, these findings comprised tau-positive neurofibrillary and astrocytic tangles that were perivascularly concentrated. To better stratify the extent of disease progression, they proposed the first pathological classification system for CTE, embracing its definition as a progressive tauopathy with perivascular patterns that are distinct enough from other tau processes to warrant a unique diagnosis. This 4-level staging system quantified the number of perivascular tau aggregations seen on autopsy, with spread to temporal lobe structures and then eventually diffuse cerebral lesions in later stages. Notably, amyloid plaques were inconsistently found within the brains studied; moreover, amyloid was not used when constructing a staging model [10, 11].

In 2016, a consensus panel was held between the National Institute of Neurological Disorders and Stroke (NINDS) and National Institute of Biomedical Imaging and Bioengineering (NIBIB) to develop a unified neuropathological diagnostic model for CTE. To do so, they used ten cases from the 2015 McKee case series that had been stratified as stage III or IV to find pathological commonalities. The result was a tentative diagnostic criteria for CTE: p-tau and astroglial tangles distributed perivascularly and deep within cortical sulci [12]. The validity of those criteria was then tested by that body of pathologists on 25 brains of varying tauopathies. Of note, all of the cases studied were defined as late stage (Stages III or IV) disease. Consensus analysis showed that, although a promising start to teasing apart CTE from other tauopathies, the criteria could not be considered pathognomonic; 33% (Cohen's kappa) of pathologists disagreed when blindly reviewing the cases [12]. This can be compared to a kappa value of 90% for the diagnostic criteria for Alzheimer's disease [13].

Indeed, CTE remains difficult to distinguish from other tauopathies, and the overlap in pathological and behavioral findings across tauopathies makes it difficult to distinguish and diagnose CTE. Of the 68 patients with pathological findings for CTE by McKee et al. in 2015, 37% were found to have another diagnosed tauopathy [10]. Moreover, the NINDS/NIBIB had to account for this significant overlap between CTE and other tauopathies, determining that the presence of another tauopathy excluded an individual from being diagnosed with CTE [12].

To better understand the difficulty in basing a distinct diagnosis on abnormal tau proteins, it is helpful to understand the natural progression of abnormal tau proteins in healthy individuals and/or individuals that are *not* exposed to chronic head trauma. Tauopathy is a common condition—often affecting healthy individuals who show no signs of neurobehavioral deficits—that has been shown to increase naturally with age [14]. A random study of 2332 brains across all age groups found tau depositions in 89% of individuals in their fourth decade of life, with the prevalence and number of lesions per individual increasing consistently with each age group [15]. A large proportion of individuals found to have had abnormal tau aggregates postmortem, moreover, had no neuropsychiatric symptoms during life [16]. Therefore, the clinical significance of abnormal tau remains uncertain.

In 2017, Mez et al. reviewed the cases of 202 football players to study the prevalence and severity of CTE among the population. Of the 202 players, 111 had played in the NFL. The study, which employed the 2015 NINDS/NIBIB diagnostic criteria, found that 110 of the 111 NFL players and 87% of the players overall had some level of CTE. They found that 95 of the 111 players had severe CTE (stage III or IV, based on the 2015 NINDS/NIBIB tau lesion criteria), whereas 15 had mild CTE. Importantly, the median age of those patients with severe CTE was 71, whereas the median age of players with mild CTE was 44. Therefore, the natural progression of abnormal tau in healthy individuals should also be considered to account for this prevalence of severe CTE in older patients [17]. Nevertheless, the study demonstrated the prominence of symptomatic tauopathy in individuals exposed to repeated head trauma.

Clinicopathological Correlation

Interestingly, the 2017 Mez et al. study demonstrated an age-based heterogeneity in the prominent clinical features of CTE. Among the 111 NFL players studied, the younger cohort of mild CTE patients tended to have more behavioral or mood changes and a higher prevalence of substance use disorder. The older cohort of severe CTE patients presented primarily with cognitive symptoms, dementia, and motor deficits [17].

At present, CTE is a pathological diagnosis that can only be diagnosed postmortem. However, attempts have been made to reconcile pathological findings with the largely nonspecific clinical findings in CTE patients. Montenigro et al. proposed a set of criteria that can be used to clinically diagnose CTE by dividing the disease into a set of clinical subtypes that address the heterogeneity found among patients suspected of having CTE (Table 15.1). To be diagnosed, a patient must have a history of repeated head trauma, no overlapping neuropsychiatric disease, a core change in cognition, behavior, or mood, and at least two of the following: impulsivity, anxiety, apathy, paranoia, suicidality, headache, motor deficits, documented decline, or delayed onset of symptoms [18]. While useful in tying a largely pathological disease to clinical manifestations, the clinical findings are largely nonspecific and have not widely been implemented or validated.

Attempts to correlate the neuropathological underpinnings of CTE to clinical manifestations are further complicated by findings that, among patients who had experienced repeated head trauma, clinical findings have not seemed to differ between patients found to have and not to have CTE pathology [19]. Willer et al., when comparing 22 professional football and hockey players to age-matched

Table 15.1 Clinical diagnostic criteria for CTE proposed by Montenigro et al. [18]

Diagnostic criteria
1. History of multiple head impacts
2. No overlapping neuropsychiatric disorder
3. Clinical features present for ≥12 months
4. ≥1 core clinical feature (below)
5. ≥2 supporting features (below)
Core clinical features
Cognitive changes, behavioral changes, mood changes
Supporting features
Impulsivity, anxiety, apathy, paranoia, suicidality, headache, motor deficits, progressive decline, delayed onset

athletes in non-contact sports, found no cognitive or behavioral differences between the two groups, further suggesting that pathological findings do not necessarily manifest clinically [20]. Additionally, specific clinical findings for individual patients, which are most often reported retrospectively by interviewing those close to the patient, tend not to correlate with pathological underpinnings. In the 2017 study by Mez et al., for instance, the presence of reported behavioral changes such as memory deficits, attention, impulsivity, and explosivity did not ostensibly correlate with pathology of the hippocampus, entorhinal cortex, or amygdala, as would be highly expected [17]. Ultimately, while distinguishing CTE even pathologically is challenging, doing so clinically remains substantially more difficult; further research into clinical changes highly specific to CTE is warranted in order to better detect and diagnose CTE in living individuals.

Implications on Athletic Safety

The correlation between repeated head trauma and the potential development of CTE has raised concerns about the safety of athletes, spanning from professionals in the NFL to youths in recreational leagues. Stamm et al. found an increased incidence of adult-onset cognitive impairment in NFL players who started playing tackle football before the age of 12 compared to those that started playing after 12 [21]. The study quickly gained publicity, prompting widespread calls for further research into the risks of youth football and, often, calls for its abolishment. However, the study notably only sampled individuals who went on to play in the NFL rather than most youths, who only play recreationally. To the contrary, a similar study of 45 former NFL players that compared adult neurological complications between players that played before high school to those that did not was unable to replicate the findings of Stamm et al. [22]

Several other studies followed youths participating in tackle football and other contact sports longitudinally to better study its long-term neurological impact. A study by Savica et al. compared adults who played football in high school (from the years 1946 to 1956) to adults who went to high school during the same decade, but did not play football. They assessed both cohorts for the prevalence of dementia and neurodegenerative disease in later adulthood, including Parkinson's disease and amyotrophic lateral sclerosis, and found no significant difference between the groups [23]. It should be noted, additionally, that football in this decade was played with lower safety standards for protective equipment and concussion avoidance, and yet had no significant long-term cognitive implications.

Nevertheless, a link does persist between repeated head traumas in youth and CTE. While the age of exposure itself does not seem to correlate with the severity of CTE, early exposure has been mildly linked to an earlier onset of neurobehavioral symptoms [24]. For this reason, calls to enforce safety measures across all contact sports are certainly warranted and have been implemented nationally. To best guide the development of these safety measures, we must better understand what in particular within contact sports predisposes players to even mild risks of neurological sequelae. Concussions, independently, have not directly been correlated with the later development of CTE [25, 26]. In animal models, however, repeated head impacts have indeed been associated with neuropathological changes reflective of CTE. Much of our inability to fully understand the cause of CTE stems from the fact that it is difficult to comprehensively document the nature and extent of head trauma over time in large studies, as well as our inability to completely distinguish CTE from overlapping neurological disorders that present with similar clinical and histopathologic pictures [27]. Therefore, while concussions and repeated head impacts are not definitively connected to CTE, it is important to enforce strong safety measures, such as continually improving helmet designs at all athletic levels and close adherence to concussion protocols.

The NFL, too, has proactively worked to enforce strict safety measures that minimize the severity and frequency of head trauma. The NFL Engineering Committee has been reviewing footage of each reported concussion to find trends in impact distribution to better optimize rules and protocols. Deliberate blows using the crown of the head, for instance, were banned after it was found that this angle was highly prone to subsequent concussion. Such findings are also distributed nationally to be implemented in youth football programs through initiatives such as USA Football's Heads Up program, which trains coaches and players at all levels on best practices and proper training to minimize the incidence of concussions and the severity of head injury.

Future Directions

The high publicity of CTE and its implications have prompted much needed research. As contact sports are fundamental to American culture, the safety of their participants is essential. It is reasonable, then, that proactive measures be taken to minimize head injury in ways that are scientific and data-driven, since there is little downside to implementing and enforcing a higher standard of safety. However, much work needs to be done in the coming decade to elucidate a more precise etiology and pathophysiology of CTE in order to better develop safety measures preemptively and to more confidently diagnose and manage those who have developed it.

Two important steps are needed in order to better define CTE and, moreover, lend utility to its existence as a unique disease process. The first is to more concretely distinguish CTE from overlapping neurological and neurodegenerative disease processes. At present, the 2015 NINDS/NIBIB criteria—the current standard of diagnosis for CTE—do not exclude a diagnosis of CTE in the presence of neuropsychiatric comorbidities. In doing so, however, it becomes difficult to study the disease process independently and to make clinical decisions. The other necessary step is to better define and validate a clinicopathological diagnostic staging system for CTE. Currently, the diagnosis of CTE is purely pathological, meaning it can only be made postmortem. Although other neurological diseases such as Alzheimer's disease can only be diagnosed pathologically, they also have very specific clinical findings and patterns that can lead to working diagnoses in living patients that can actively guide management. CTE similarly needs a concrete, widely validated, clinicopathological model in order for it to be distinctly diagnosed, broadly studied, and precisely managed. Such studies are currently underway and should soon allow for a better clinicopathological understanding of the disease; in 2016, the NINDS funded a 5-year, multi-center study of approximately 1500 postmortem brains with longitudinal patient data led by the Dr. Douglas Smith from the University of Pennsylvania to correlate clinical behavior with neuropathological findings [28].

Also, research into biomarkers and detection on neuroimaging is needed to identify and stage CTE in vivo. Although there are no known biomarkers that can currently be used in the detection and diagnosis of CTE, there are several promising avenues of research. A disproportionate elevation in p-tau levels when compared to normal amyloid levels in the cerebrospinal fluid (CSF) of CTE patients has been hypothesized [18]. Recent investigations into the involvement of activated microglia in CTE tauopathy could also potentially be leveraged to search for microglial activation biomarkers, such as sTREM2, in the CSF [29]. Further research into the detection of specific anatomical changes on magnetic resonance imaging (MRI) or patterns specific for perivascular tau aggregations on positron emission tomography (PET) scan is also necessary to explore noninvasive and readily available methods for CTE screening.

In addition to better characterizing and detecting CTE, high-powered, longitudinal, controlled trials are needed to eliminate the high level of social and physiological confounders that currently make it difficult to study CTE in isolation. In order to do so, better record-keeping of the nature and severity of head injury over long periods of time is needed to isolate more precise risk factors for CTE to guide specific safety protocols, develop even more effective equipment, and ultimately determine the extent to which CTE is an independent disease process rather than an aggregate of mixed neuropsychiatric conditions and psychosocial factors.

The attention that CTE has brought to safety in contact sports is important; contact sports certainly predispose players at all levels to certain short- and long-term risks that can be mitigated with data-driven engineering and the implementation of specific safety protocols. However, the extent to which this disease process remains poorly defined and pathophysiologically understood should be factored in when making such decisions. As research into the condition grows to include more cases with more accurate data collection over longer periods of time, we will grow to better understand the clinical and pathological nature of CTE to ensure the continued safety of athletes at every level of their sport.

Conclusion

Chronic traumatic encephalopathy has been at the forefront of discussions concerning the safety and the implications for all contact sports. Ongoing collaborative efforts are essential to better define the problem.

References

1. Martland HS. Punch drunk. J Am Med Assoc. 1928;91(15):1103–7.
2. Millspaugh JA. Dementia pugilistica. US Naval Med Bull. 1937;35:297–303.
3. Roberts AH. Brain damage in boxers: a study of the prevalence of traumatic encephalopathy among ex-professional boxers. London: Pitman Medical & Scientific Pub. Co.; 1969.
4. Smith D, Johnson V, Trojanowski J, Stewart W. Chronic traumatic encephalopathy — confusion and controversies. Nat Rev Neurol. 2019;15.
5. Mez J, Stern RA, McKee AC. Chronic traumatic encephalopathy: where are we and where are we going? Curr Neurol Neurosci Rep. 2013;13(12):407.
6. Bowman KM, Blau A. Psychotic states following head and brain injury in adults and children. In: Injuries of the skull, brain and spinal cord: neuro-psychiatric, surgical, and medico-legal aspects. Baltimore, MD: Williams & Wilkins Co; 1940. p. 309–60.
7. Corsellis JA, Bruton CJ, Freeman-Browne D. The aftermath of boxing. Psychol Med. 1973;3(3):270–303.
8. Omalu BI, DeKosky ST, Minster RL, Kamboh MI, Hamilton RL, Wecht CH. Chronic traumatic encephalopathy in a National Football League player. Neurosurgery. 2005;57(1):128–34; discussion 128–134.
9. Omalu BI, DeKosky ST, Hamilton RL, et al. Chronic traumatic encephalopathy in a national football league player: part II. Neurosurgery. 2006;59(5):1086–92; discussion 1092–1083.
10. McKee AC, Stern RA, Nowinski CJ, et al. The spectrum of disease in chronic traumatic encephalopathy. Brain. 2013;136(Pt 1):43–64.
11. McKee AC, Stein TD, Kiernan PT, Alvarez VE. The neuropathology of chronic traumatic encephalopathy. Brain Pathol. 2015;25(3):350–64.
12. McKee AC, Cairns NJ, Dickson DW, et al. The first NINDS/NIBIB consensus meeting to define neuropathological criteria for the diagnosis of chronic traumatic encephalopathy. Acta Neuropathol. 2016;131(1):75–86.
13. Nagy Z, Vatter-Bittner B, Braak H, et al. Staging of Alzheimer-type pathology: an interrater-intrarater study. Dement Geriatr Cogn Disord. 1997;8(4):248–51.
14. Kovacs GG, Ferrer I, Grinberg LT, et al. Aging-related tau astrogliopathy (ARTAG): harmonized evaluation strategy. Acta Neuropathol. 2016;131(1):87–102.

15. Braak H, Thal DR, Ghebremedhin E, Del Tredici K. Stages of the pathologic process in Alzheimer disease: age categories from 1 to 100 years. J Neuropathol Exp Neurol. 2011;70(11):960–9.
16. Karantzoulis S, Randolph C. Modern chronic traumatic encephalopathy in retired athletes: what is the evidence? Neuropsychol Rev. 2013;23(4):350–60.
17. Mez J, Daneshvar DH, Kiernan PT, et al. Clinicopathological evaluation of chronic traumatic encephalopathy in players of American football. JAMA. 2017;318(4):360–70.
18. Montenigro PH, Baugh CM, Daneshvar DH, et al. Clinical subtypes of chronic traumatic encephalopathy: literature review and proposed research diagnostic criteria for traumatic encephalopathy syndrome. Alzheimers Res Ther. 2014;6(5):68.
19. Bieniek KF, Ross OA, Cormier KA, et al. Chronic traumatic encephalopathy pathology in a neurodegenerative disorders brain bank. Acta Neuropathol. 2015;130(6):877–89.
20. Willer BS, Zivadinov R, Haider MN, Miecznikowski JC, Leddy JJ. A preliminary study of early-onset dementia of former professional football and hockey players. J Head Trauma Rehabil. 2018;33(5):E1–8.
21. Stamm JM, Bourlas AP, Baugh CM, et al. Age of first exposure to football and later-life cognitive impairment in former NFL players. Neurology. 2015;84(11):1114–20.
22. Solomon GS, Kuhn AW, Zuckerman SL, et al. Participation in pre-high school football and neurological, neuroradiological, and neuropsychological findings in later life: a study of 45 retired National Football League Players. Am J Sports Med. 2016;44(5):1106–15.
23. Savica R, Parisi JE, Wold LE, Josephs KA, Ahlskog JE. High school football and risk of neurodegeneration: a community-based study. Mayo Clin Proc. 2012;87(4):335–40.
24. Alosco ML, Mez J, Tripodis Y, et al. Age of first exposure to tackle football and chronic traumatic encephalopathy. Ann Neurol. 2018;83(5):886–901.
25. Mainwaring L, Ferdinand Pennock KM, Mylabathula S, Alavie BZ. Subconcussive head impacts in sport: a systematic review of the evidence. Int J Psychophysiol. 2018;132(Pt A):39–54.
26. Tagge CA, Fisher AM, Minaeva OV, et al. Concussion, microvascular injury, and early tauopathy in young athletes after impact head injury and an impact concussion mouse model. Brain. 2018;141(2):422–58.
27. Maroon JC, Winkelman R, Bost J, Amos A, Mathyssek C, Miele V. Chronic traumatic encephalopathy in contact sports: a systematic review of all reported pathological cases. PLoS One. 2015;10(2):e0117338.
28. Penn Medicine Wins NIH Award to Study Progressive Brain Damage from Concussions and More Severe Traumatic Brain Injuries [press release]. Penn Medicine News: Penn Medicine, March 17 2016.
29. Zetterberg H, Blennow K. Chronic traumatic encephalopathy: fluid biomarkers. Handb Clin Neurol. 2018;158:323–33.

Index

M. E. Oppenlander (ed.), *Neurosurgical Care of Athletes*,
https://doi.org/10.1007/978-3-030-88227-3

D

Printed by Printforce, the Netherlands